PEDIATRIC ONCOLOGY

Carlos Rodriguez-Galindo
Matthew W. Wilson
(Editors)

Retinoblastoma

With 52 Figures and 19 Tables

Springer

Editors
Carlos Rodriguez-Galindo, M.D
Associate Professor of Pediatrics
Dana-Farber Cancer Institute and Children's Hospital
Harvard Medical School
Boston, MA
Carlos_Rodriguez-Galindo@dfci.harvard.edu

Matthew W. Wilson, M.D., FACS
Professor of Ophthalmology, Hamilton Eye Institute
University of Tennessee Health Science Center
Departments of Surgery and Pathology
St. Jude Children's Research Hospital
Memphis, TN
mwilson5@utmem.edu

ISBN 978-1-4899-7753-3 ISBN 978-0-387-89072-2 (eBook)
DOI 10.1007/978-0-387-89072-2
Springer New York Dordrecht Heidelberg London

Printed on acid-free paper

Springer is part of Springer Science+Business Media (www.springer.com)

Foreword

Although rare, retinoblastoma has been at the forefront of cancer research and treatment for the last three decades. The two-hit hypothesis of oncogenesis proposed by Alfred Knudson provided the conceptual framework for tumor suppressor gene research and led to the discovery of the retinoblastoma pathway as a key element in cancer development. More recently, the treatment of children with retinoblastoma has also provided a model for modern approach to the cancer patient; state of the art retinoblastoma treatment can only be conceived in the context of the multidisciplinary approach needed to address the oncologic, ophthalmologic, and developmental dimensions of these unfortunate children.

Treatment of retinoblastoma has evolved at a significant speed over the last two decades; ocular salvage approaches are now at the core of modern treatments, and assessment of visual and functional outcomes have become priority. New discoveries in retinoblastoma biology are leading the way to the development of targeted therapies that could revolutionize our current approaches to the treatment of this malignancy. But as we continue to make progress in this challenging field, we must not forget those less fortunate; while in the developed world eye preservation has become a priority, developing countries continue to face delays in diagnosis, poor access to care, and suboptimal treatment – the problem in the less developed world is cure.

In this book, we have invited a team of experts to address all those important aspects of retinoblastoma research and therapy - from biology to epidemiology to treatment. We hope that in subsequent editions we will be able to continue to provide updates on such exciting subjects.

As we finalize this work, we cannot forget those who preceded and mentored us, especially John L. Hungerford, FRCS, FRCOphth, Hans E. Grossniklaus, MD, Barrett G. Haik, MD, FACS, Anna T. Meadows, MD, and very especially the late Charles B. Pratt, MD. We also cannot forget our families and our patients, who have provided the inspiration to guide our careers. To all of them this work is dedicated.

Carlos Rodriguez-Galindo, MD
Boston,M A
Matthew W. Wilson, MD
Memphis,T N

Contributors

Guillermo L. Chantada, MD
PrincipalP hysician
Department of Hematology and Oncology
Hospital JP Garrahan
Buenos Aires
Argentina
gchantada@yahoo.com

Patricia Chévez-Barrios, MD
Associate Professor of Pathology and Laboratory Medicine
Department of Pathology
The Methodist Hospital
Weill College of Medicine of Cornell University
Houston, TX
USA
pchevez-barrios@tmhs.org

Helen Dimaras, MD
Ontario Cancer Institute
Princess Margaret Hospital
Toronto, ON
Canada

Ira J. Dunkel, MD
Department of Pediatrics
Memorial Sloan-Kettering Cancer Center
New York, NY
USA
dunkeli@mskcc.org

Michael Dyer, MD
Department of Developmental Neurobiology
St. Jude Children's Research Hospital
Memphis, TN
USA
michael.dyer@stjude.org

Anna Furmanchuk, MD
Ophthalmologist
Department of Oncology
Belarusian Scientific Research Centre For Pediatric Oncology and Hematology
Minsk
Belarus
furmanch@tut.by

Brenda L. Gallie, MD
Princess Margaret Hospital
Ontario Cancer Institute
Toronto, ON
Canada
gallie@attglobal.net

Dan S. Gombos, MD
Associate Professor of Ophthalmology
Department of Head and Neck Surgery
Section of Ophthalmology
The University of Texas MD.
Anderson Cancer Center
Houston, TX
USA
dgombos@mdanderson.org

Mary Ellen Hoehn, MD
AssistantP rofessor
Department of Ophthalmology
The Hamilton Eye Institute
University of Tennessee Health Science Center
Memphis, TN
USA
mehoehn@mac.com

Sandra Luna-Fineman, MD
California Pacific Medical Center
San Francisco, CA
USA
sluna123@comcast.net

Thomas E. Merchant, DO, PhD
Chief, Division of Radiation Oncology
St. Jude Children's Research Hospital
Memphis, TN
USA
thomas.merchant@stjude.org

Manuela Orjuela, MD
Assistant Professor of Clinical Public
Health and Clinical Pediatrics
Columbia University
New York, NY
USA
mao5@columbia.edu

Ibrahim Qaddoumi, MD, MS
Department of Oncology
St. Jude Children's Research Hospital
Memphis, TN
USA
ibrahim.qaddoumi@stjude.org

Carlos Rodriguez-Galindo, MD
Associate Professor of Pediatrics
Dana-Farber Cancer Institute and Children's
Hospital
Harvard Medical School
Boston, MA
USA
Carlos_Rodriguez-Galindo@dfci.harvard.edu

Judith Wilimas, MD
Department of Oncology
St. Jude Children's Research Hospital
Memphis, TN
USA
judy.wilimas@stjude.org

Matthew W. Wilson, MD
Professor of Ophthalmology
Department of Ophthalmology
The Hamilton Eye Institute
University of Tennessee Health Science Center
Memphis, TN
USA
Departments of Surgery and Pathology
St. Jude Children's Research Hospital Memphis, TN
USA
mwilson5@utmem.edu

Contents

1 Biology of Retinoblastoma
M.A. Dyer

1.1 Landmark Discoveries in Cancer Genetics 1
1.2 The Retinoblastoma Paradox 2
1.3 Secondary Genetic Lesions in Retinoblastoma 3
1.4 Preclinical Models of Retinoblastoma 5
1.5 Improving Retinoblastoma Treatment with Preclinical Studies 7
1.6 Cell of Origin for Retinoblastoma 7
1.7 Conclusions 8
References 8

2 Epidemiology
M. Orjuela

2.1 Introduction 11
2.2 Incidence 12
2.2.1 Population Differences in Incidence 12
2.2.2 Variation Within Countries: Subpopulations with Higher Incidence 14
2.2.3 Gender Differences 15
2.2.4 Biologic Underpinnings of Epidemiologic Studies on Retinoblastoma 15
2.3 Potential Hypotheses 16
2.3.1 Parental Occupations 16
2.3.2 Parental Age 16
2.3.3 In Vitro Fertilization (IVF) 17
2.3.4 UV Exposure 17
2.3.5 Nonoccupational Parental Exposures 18
2.3.6 Diet 18
2.3.7 Viral Agents 19
2.3.8 Diagnostic Interval 19
2.3.9 Screening and Media Campaigns 20
2.4 Summary 20
References 21

3 Clinical Features, Diagnosis, Pathology
P. Chévez-Barrios · D.S. Gombos

3.1 Introduction 25
3.2 Initial Presentation 25
3.3 Clinical History 26
3.4 Initial Examination 27
3.5 Differential Diagnosis 27
3.6 Examination Under Anesthesia 28
3.7 Fine Needle Aspiration Biopsy 30
3.8 Grouping and Staging of Retinoblastoma 30
3.9 Pathology 30
3.10 Histologic Features 32
3.11 Extraocular Extension, Metastasis, and Prognostic Factors 33
3.12 Metastasis 36
3.13 Prognostic Factors for Metastasis 37
3.14 Trilateral Retinoblastoma and Other Tumors 37
3.15 Processing of Eyes with Retinoblastoma for Histopathologic Examination 38
References 39

4 Genetics of Retinoblastoma and Genetic Counseling

H. Dimaras · B.L. Gallie

4.1 **Introduction** 41
4.2 **Molecular Genetic Progression of Retinoblastoma** 41
4.2.1 The *RB1* Gene, Protein, and Function 42
4.2.2 Cell of Origin 42
4.2.3 Transient Arrest: Senescence Halts Retinoma 43
4.2.4 Post-*RB1* Progressive Events 43
4.2.4.1 Genomic Gain of 1q: *KIF14* 43
4.2.4.2 Genomic Gain of 6p: *DEK* and *E2F3* 44
4.2.4.3 Genomic Gain of 2p: *NMYC* 44
4.2.4.4 Genomic Loss of 16q: *CDH11* 44
4.2.4.5 Deregulation of Apoptosis: Loss of Expression of $p75^{NTR}$ 45
4.2.5 Murine Models of Retinoblastoma 45
4.2.5.1 *RB1* Knockout Mouse Models 45
4.2.5.2 Viral Oncoprotein-induced Murine Retinoblastoma 45
4.2.5.3 Conditional *RB1* Knockout Murine Retinoblastoma Models 46
4.2.5.4 Limitations of Mouse Models 46
4.2.6 Summary: A Model of Retinoblastoma Development 46
4.3 **Genetic Counseling** 46
4.3.1 Heritability of Retinoblastoma 46
4.3.2 Role of Environmental Factors 48
4.3.3 Molecular Genetic Testing 48
4.3.4 *RB1* Test Strategies 48
4.3.4.1 Sporadic Bilateral or Familial Retinoblastoma 48
4.3.4.2 Sporadic Unilateral Retinoblastoma 49
4.3.4.3 Prenatal Testing 49
4.3.4.4 *RB1* Mutation Identification 49
4.3.4.5 Missense Mutations 49
4.3.4.6 Frameshift and Nonsense Mutations 50
4.3.4.7 Aberrant Splicing 50
4.3.4.8 Epigenetic Mutations 50
4.3.4.9 Translocations and Gross Deletions 50
4.3.4.10 Penetrance of Retinoblastoma 51
4.3.4.11 Mosaicism 51
4.3.4.12 Parent of Origin Effect 51
4.4 **Conclusions and Significance** 51
4.5 **Glossary** 52
References 52

5 Radiation Therapy in the Management of Retinoblastoma

T. E. Merchant

5.1 **Introduction** 55
5.2 **Treatment Methods** 56
5.3 **Extraocular and High-Risk Retinoblastoma** 60
5.4 **Secondary Malignant Tumors** 61
5.5 **Nonmalignant Side Effects from Radiation Therapy** 63
5.6 **Controversies in the Management of Retinoblastoma** 63
5.7 **Recommendations** 64
References 64

6 Chemotherapy in the Management of Retinoblastoma

C. Rodriguez-Galindo

6.1 **Introduction** 67
6.2 **Ocular Pharmacokinetics** 68
6.2.1 Ocular Drug Transporters 69
6.3 **Chemotherapy in the Treatment of Intraocular Retinoblastoma** 69

6.3.1 Unilateral Retinoblastoma 69
6.3.2 Bilateral Retinoblastoma 70
6.3.3 New Tumor Formation on Chemotherapy 72
6.3.4 Therapy-Related Leukemia 73
6.4 Periocular Administration of Chemotherapy 73
6.4.1 Mechanisms for Transscleral Drug Delivery 73
6.4.2 Periocular Chemotherapy in Retinoblastoma 75
6.5 Intravitreal and Intrarterial Chemotherapy for Intraocular Retinoblastoma 77
6.6 Treatment of Extraocular Retinoblastoma 77
6.6.1 Orbital and Locoregional Retinoblastoma 77
6.6.2 Metastatic Retinoblastoma 78
6.7 Translational Research and Emergent Therapies in Retinoblastoma 79
6.8 Specific Agents 81
6.8.1 Vincristine 81
6.8.2 Carboplatin 81
6.8.3 Etoposide (VP-16) 82
6.8.4 Doxorubicin 82
6.8.5 Cyclophosphamide 83
6.8.6 Cisplatin 84
6.8.7 Topotecan 85
6.8.8 Thiotepa 85
References 86

7 Treatment of Intraocular Retinoblastoma

M. W. Wilson

7.1 Introduction 91
7.2 Primary Treatments 91
7.3 Focal Therapies 94
7.4 Emerging Treatments 99
7.5 Conclusion 99
References 99

8 Treatment of Extraocular and Metastatic Retinoblastoma

G. L. Chantada · I. J. Dunkel

8.1 Introduction 103
8.2 Patients with High Risk Intraocular Disease .. 104
8.2.1 Choroidal Invasion 105
8.2.2 Optic Nerve Invasion 105
8.3 Patients with Microscopic Residual Disease after Enucleation 106
8.3.1 Trans-Scleral Invasion 107
8.3.2 Future Directions 108
8.4 Orbital and Locoregional Disease 108
8.4.1 Orbital Relapse 109
8.4.2 Special Situations 110
8.5 Metastatic Disease 111
8.5.1 Stage 4a: Metastatic Disease Without CNS Involvement 111
8.5.2 Stage 4b: Distant Metastatic Disease with CNS Involvement 112
8.5.3 Future Research 112
References 113

9 Second Malignancies and Other Long Term Effects in Retinoblastoma Survivors

C. Rodriguez-Galindo

9.1 Introduction 115
9.2 Second Malignancies 115
9.2.1 Osteosarcoma 117
9.2.2 Soft Tissue Sarcomas 119
9.2.3 Skin Cancers 120
9.2.4 Lung Cancer and Other Common Cancers of Adulthood 120
9.2.5 Hematologic Malignancies 121
9.2.6 Trilateral Retinoblastoma 121
9.3 Other Long Term effects 123
9.3.1 Orbital Growth and Facial Asymmetry .. 123
9.3.2 Visual Outcome 123
9.3.3 Cognitive and Functional Development of Patients with Retinoblastoma 123
9.3.4 Other Late Effects 124
References 124

10 Visual Rehabilitation
M.E. Hoehn

10.1 Introduction 127
10.2 Spectacles 127
10.3 Patching or Pharmacologic Penalization 129
10.4 Cataract Surgery 129
10.5 Strabismus Surgery 131
10.6 Low Vision 131
10.7 Conclusion 132
References 132

11 Retinoblastoma in Developing Countries
G.L. Chantada · S. Luna-Fineman
I. Qaddoumi · A. Furmanchuk · J. Wilimas

11.1 Introduction 133
11.2 Delayed Diagnosis 134
11.2.1 Causes of Delayed Diagnosis 135
11.2.2 Preventing Late Diagnosis 135
11.3 Special Problems in the Treatment of Retinoblastoma in Less Developed Countries 137
11.4 Resources to Address this Global Problem 138
References 140

Appendix 143

Subject Index 153

Biology of Retinoblastoma

M.A. Dyer

Contents

1.1 Landmark Discoveries in Cancer Genetics 1
1.2 The Retinoblastoma Paradox 2
1.3 Secondary Genetic Lesions in Retinoblastoma. 3
1.4 Preclinical Models of Retinoblastoma 5
1.5 Improving Retinoblastoma Treatment with Preclinical Studies 7
1.6 Cell of Origin for Retinoblastoma. 7
1.7 Conclusions. 8
References. 8

1.1 Landmark Discoveries in Cancer Genetics

Studies on retinoblastoma have led to several landmark studies in cancer genetics over the past 4 decades. In 1971, Knudson proposed that retinoblastoma might initiate by biallelic inactivation of a putative tumor suppressor gene (Knudson 1971). This "two-hit hypothesis" was based on the observation that there were two distinct forms of retinoblastoma seen in the clinic. Children with a family history of retinoblastoma often had bilateral multifocal retinoblastoma. In contrast, children with unilateral retinoblastoma rarely had any family history of the disease. Knudson proposed that for retinoblastoma to form, both copies of a putative tumor suppressor gene had to be inactivated. Children with a family history of retinoblastoma inherited a defective copy of this tumor suppressor gene and were likely to have retinal cells that sustained mutations in the second allele, leading to multifocal bilateral retinoblastoma. In contrast, children who have two intact copies of the retinoblastoma susceptibility gene develop retinoblastoma only when a single cell sustains two independent mutations that inactivate both copies of the gene. The lower probability of two inactivating mutations in the retinoblastoma susceptibility gene could account for the observation that these children often had unilateral retinoblastoma with fewer tumor foci.

Several years later, Weinberg's lab cloned Knudson's putative tumor suppressor gene by studying genetic lesions and chromosomal aberrations in families with a history of retinoblastoma (Friend et al. 1986). This was the first human tumor suppressor gene to be cloned and it was named *RB1* (Friend et al. 1986). Initially, researchers believed that *RB1* was important

C. Rodriguez-Galindo and M.W. Wilson (eds.), *Retinoblastoma*, Pediatric Oncology,
DOI 10.1007/978-0-387-89072-2_1,

for retinoblastoma susceptibility, but its role in other human cancers was unknown until Harbour and colleagues found that the *RB1* gene was also mutated in lung cancer (Harbour et al. 1988). Today, it is widely held that most, if not all, tumors have sustained genetic lesions in their Rb pathway that contribute to deregulated cellular proliferation. These landmark studies on the genetics of retinoblastoma susceptibility have had a major impact on our understanding of tumor suppressor genes and have formed the framework for much of our current knowledge of genetic lesions associated with tumorigenesis.

1.2 The Retinoblastoma Paradox

Having established that mutations in the *RB1* gene led to retinoblastoma in children and that virtually every retinoblastoma initiated with *RB1* inactivation, three research teams set out to model retinoblastoma in mice by targeted mutagenesis of the mouse *Rb1* gene. In 1992, three labs simultaneously published their characterization of the *Rb*-deficient mice (Lee et al. 1992; Jacks et al. 1992; Clarke et al. 1992). Surprisingly, mice that inherit a defective copy of the *Rb1* gene never develop retinoblastoma. Importantly, *Rb1* is a tumor suppressor in mice because the $Rb^{+/-}$ mice have an increased incidence of pituitary tumors. In addition, the human *RB1* gene can rescue the embryonic lethality associated with germline inactivation of both copies of the *Rb1* gene, suggesting that much of Rb function in development is conserved across mammalian species (Maandag et al. 1994). Taken together, these observations suggest that the paradox surrounding the species-specific susceptibility to retinoblastoma following *Rb* gene inactivation is probably not due to divergent functions of the Rb protein in mice and humans.

The first clue to begin to explain why mice do not develop retinoblastoma came from a study using chimeric mice made from embryonic stem (ES) cells lacking both copies of *Rb1* alone or in combination with biallelic inactivation of another Rb family member called *p107* (Robanus-Maandag et al. 1998). Chimeric mice made with $Rb^{-/-}$ ES cells did not develop retinoblastoma suggesting that loss of heterozygosity at the *Rb1* locus was not the rate-limiting step to tumor initiation in mice. Importantly, chimeric mice made from $Rb^{-/-}$; $p107^{-/-}$ mice did develop retinoblastoma suggesting that p107 can suppress retinoblastoma in mice. Chimeric mice are technically challenging to generate, and this study was limited to a handful of animals with retinoblastoma. More importantly, chimeric mice are not feasible for testing new therapies to treat retinoblastoma, so this discovery had no impact on the clinical management of retinoblastoma. In addition, these studies did not explain why the *p107* gene had to be inactivated in addition to the *Rb* gene to form retinoblastoma in mice.

Several years after this important discovery, studies on the role of the Rb family in mouse and human retinal development offered an explanation to this longstanding paradox (Donovan et al. 2006). We found that when Rb is inactivated in the developing retina, the p107 gene is upregulated in a compensatory manner. Previous studies have shown that this is probably due to a direct role of Rb in suppressing p107 expression in the mouse through conserved E2F binding sites in the p107 promoter. We also found that p107 can compensate for Rb inactivation, which explains why p107-deficient mice do not develop retinoblastoma (Donovan et al. 2006; Zhang et al. 2004). Based on these data and the normal expression pattern of Rb and p107 in the developing mouse retina, we hypothesized that simultaneous inactivation of Rb and p107 in the developing mouse retina would lead to retinoblastoma. Using *Chx10-Cre*;$Rb^{Lox/Lox}$;$p107^{-/-}$ mice, we were able to produce the first knockout mouse model of retinoblastoma by inactivating the *Rb* gene in the retinal progenitor cells of $p107^{-/-}$ mice. Shortly after this study was published, two independent groups published similar findings (MacPherson et al. 2004; Chen et al. 2004). One of these groups extended our findings to show that simultaneous inactivation of *Rb* and *p130* could also lead to retinoblastoma (MacPherson et al. 2004). Our developmental studies have shown that there is no compensation by p130 when either Rb or p107 is inactivated (Donovan et al. 2006). However, there is redundant expression of Rb and p130 in a subset of retinal cells during postnatal mouse retinal development, and we have postulated that simultaneous inactivation of Rb and p130 can overcome this intrinsic genetic redundancy (Macpherson and Dyer 2007).

These data from genetic studies of the developing mouse retinae do not explain why human are susceptible to retinoblastoma following *RB1* gene inactivation. To address this question, we studied the expression of the Rb family (Rb, p107 and p130) at 8 stages of human retinal development (Donovan et al. 2006). The notable difference between humans and mice is the expression of p107. In mice, the primary family member expressed in retinal progenitor cells during embryonic development is the p107 gene. Around birth, p107 levels decrease and Rb takes its place as the major Rb family member in retinal progenitor cells. Human retinal progenitor cells do not express p107 at any stage of development. To test if p107 could compensate for RB1 loss in the human retina, we reduced RB1 protein levels in the developing human retina using an siRNA (Donovan et al. 2006). We could detect no compensatory increase in p107 following *RB1* gene inactivation in the human fetal retinae. Taken together, these data suggest that the species-specific difference in retinoblastoma susceptibility to Rb gene inactivation reflects this differential compensation by the p107 gene in mice and humans.

1.3 Secondary Genetic Lesions in Retinoblastoma

It has been well established that cancer progression involves sequential genetic lesions in tumor suppressor pathways that control proliferation, cell death, cell adhesion, telomere maintenance and growth factor dependence. As mentioned above, retinoblastoma initiates with inactivation of the *RB1* tumor suppressor gene. However, until recently, relatively little was known about the subsequent genetic lesions that contribute to retinoblastoma progression. In addition to the Rb pathway, one of the most important tumor suppressor pathways is the p53 pathway. The p53 pathway is responsible for inducing cell cycle exit and/or apoptosis when a cell encounters inappropriate deregulated proliferation or "oncogenic stress." It is important to note that the p53 pathway is directly connected to the Rb pathway through the *p14*^{ARF} tumor suppressor gene (Fig. 1.1). Jackie Lees and colleagues have shown that the *p14*^{ARF} gene is regulated by RB1 through E2F3a/b (Aslanian et al. 2004). Therefore, in a mature cell that exhibits oncogenic stress and deregulated RB1 function, the *p14*^{ARF} gene is activated and this leads to accumulation of p14^{ARF} protein, which in turn sequesters the MDM2 protein. The p53 protein is regulated by the combined activity of MDM2 and MDMX through distinct mechanisms (Marine et al. 2007). MDM2 regulates p53 protein stability, subcellular localization and binding to the promoters of p53 target genes. In contrast, MDMX is believed to regulate p53 transcriptional activity once it has bound the target genes involved in cell death and cell cycle exit. This well-established connection between the Rb and p53 tumor suppressor pathways led us to begin to explore the p53 pathway in retinoblastoma. Specifically, if *RB1* gene inactivation is the initiating genetic lesion in retinoblastoma, then according to the established dogma, the p53 pathway should be activated, and this should lead to rapid cell cycle exit and cell death through activation of *p14*^{ARF}. We found that the *p14*^{ARF} gene is expressed at very high levels in primary retinoblastomas suggesting that the *p14*^{ARF} gene is directly regulated by RB1 in retinoblasts (Laurie et al. 2006). Next, we explored the other genes in the p53 pathway including *MDM2, MDMX* and *p53*. We found that the *MDMX* gene was amplified in 65% of human retinoblastomas and *MDM2* was amplified in an additional 10% of cases (Laurie et al. 2006). The p53 gene was intact in all of the retinoblastomas analyzed and functional p53 protein was produced in retinoblastoma. These data led to a model in which retinoblastomas initiate with *RB1* gene inactivation producing deregulated proliferation of retinoblasts in the developing retina, and these cells subsequently sustain a genetic amplification of the *MDMX* gene (Fig. 1.1). Due to the connection between the Rb and p53 pathways, the ectopic proliferation of *RB1*-deficient retinoblasts is offset by p53-mediated cell death until the p53 pathway is suppressed by increased MDMX expression. MDMX can then bind and suppress p53-mediated transcriptional activation, and this is not reduced by p14^{ARF} because it is unable to bind to MDMX. To directly test this model, we performed a series of experiments in mouse models of retinoblastoma as well as primary human fetal retinae (Laurie et al. 2006). Data from these studies confirmed that

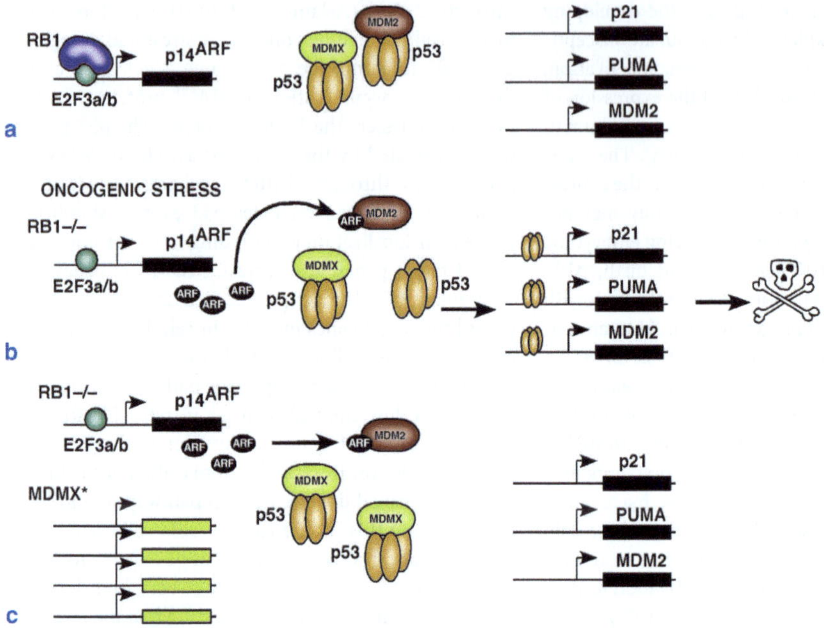

Figure 1.1

The Rb and p53 pathways are interconnected through the p14^{ARF} tumor suppressor. **a** In normal retinoblasts, the Rb protein binds the promoter of the *p14^{ARF}* gene and suppresses transcription. The low levels of p53 protein found in normal retinoblasts are bound to the two negative regulators of p53 called MDM2 and MDMX. As a result, the p53 target genes important for mediating cell cycle exit and cell death are silenced. **b** In a retinal cell lacking Rb, p14^{ARF} transcription is activated and this sequesters MDM2, freeing up p53 to activate the transcription of genes important for mediating cell cycle exit and cell death. In this way, cells undergoing oncogenic stress are eliminated and this helps to prevent tumor initiation. MDMX is not bound by p14^{ARF}. **c** We have found that in Rb-deficient retinoblasts, the *MDMX* gene is amplified and MDMX protein and mRNA accumulate. This leads to inactivation of p53, and the accumulated p14^{ARF} cannot suppress MDMX because it does not efficiently bind to the MDMX protein

ectopic expression of MDMX can indeed suppress p53-mediated cell death in *RB1*-deficient retinoblasts. More recently, we have generated a mouse strain with conditional Cre-mediated increased expression of the *MDMX* gene in *Rb;p107*-deficient retinoblasts (Dyer and Lozano, in preparation). As predicted, these mice develop aggressive, invasive retinoblastoma similar to those of *Chx10-Cre;Rb$^{Lox/Lox}$;p107$^{-/-}$;p53$^{Lox/Lox}$* mice (Fig. 1.2).

These data not only provided the first insight into the secondary genetic lesions of retinoblastoma but they also provided the first target for locally delivered chemotherapy. We found that a small molecule inhibitor of MDM2-p53 called nutlin-3a could also bind MDMX and prevent binding of MDMX to p53 (Laurie et al. 2006). In animal models of retinoblastoma, locally delivered subconjunctival nutlin-3a could induce p53-mediated cell death and provided a more effective and less toxic treatment for retinoblastoma than the conventional broad-spectrum systemic chemotherapy that is used to treat retinoblastoma throughout the world.

Having established the primary and secondary genetic lesions in retinoblastoma, one of the most

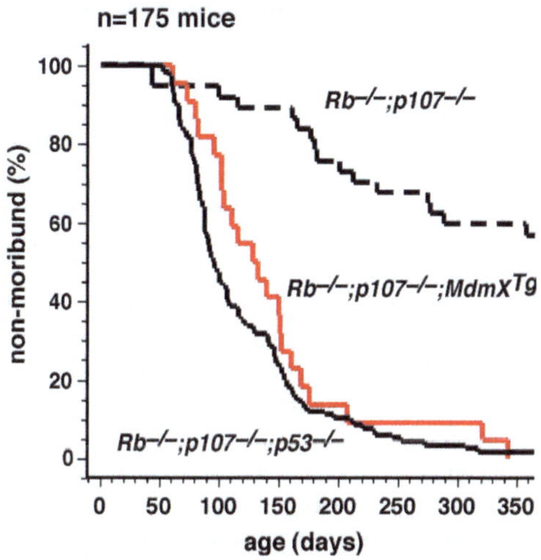

Figure 1.2

The p53 pathway suppresses retinoblastoma in mice. Conditional inactivation of *Rb* and *p107* in the developing mouse retina leads to retinoblastoma, but this is a mild form of the disease that tends to be unilateral and does not invade or metastasize efficiently. The majority of animals can live up to 1 year of age without requiring intervention due to tumor progression. In contrast, conditional inactivation of *Rb, p107* and *p53* leads to aggressive and invasive retinoblastoma that is typically bilateral and accompanied by local invasion and metastasis. Virtually, all animals must be euthanized due to tumor progression by the time they reach the age of 200–250 days. Previous studies have shown that the p53 gene is not mutated in human retinoblastomas and we have reported that MDMX gene amplification leads to suppression of the p53 pathway in human retinoblastoma. Based on these data, we predicted that conditional ectopic expression of MDMX in *Rb,p107*-deficient retinoblasts would lead to aggressive invasive retinoblastoma similar to that seen with *Rb, p107- and p53*-deficient retinoblasts. This is precisely what we found (*red line*)

important questions that remains is what are the genetic lesions that contribute to tumor cell invasion and metastasis. Virtually, nothing is known about the genetic lesions that follow Rb and p53 pathway inactivation and contribute to changes in cell adhesion and motility that allow retinoblastoma tumor cells to invade the anterior chamber, the choroid, the retina, and the optic nerve. The new preclinical models of retinoblastoma that develop aggressive metastatic disease combined with bioinformatics approaches to identify the critical molecular pathways should pave the way for major advances in this area of retinoblastoma research (Ajioka et al. 2007).

1.4 Preclinical Models of Retinoblastoma

Several different preclinical models of retinoblastoma have been developed over the past several years (Zhang et al. 2004; Laurie et al. 2005). As with any animal model of human disease, these models have inherent strengths and weaknesses and the best approaches focused on using preclinical models to assess the efficacy of new therapies combine complementary models. One of the first preclinical models of retinoblastoma was the SV40 T antigen model that was produced as an unintended consequence of efforts to produce a different type of model (O'Brien et al. 1990). The imprecise manner in which this model was generated, as well as the lack of subsequent characterization, makes it of little use for modeling human retinoblastoma. Moreover, it is now widely accepted in cancer biology that ectopic expression of potent viral oncogenes in mouse tissues rarely recapitulate the human cancers that form by inactivation of tumor suppressor pathways. Indeed, it is not even known when or where the viral oncogene is expressed in the T-antigen mouse model of retinoblastoma, making it virtually unusable for modeling human retinoblastoma.

As mentioned above, in 1992, three different laboratories characterized mice carrying a targeted deletion of the *Rb1* gene. Based on the genetics of the human disease, researchers predicted that the $Rb1^{+/-}$ mice would develop bilateral retinoblastoma just as children who inherit a defective copy of the *RB1* gene. Surprisingly, these mice never developed retinoblastoma. Our study showing that *p107* compensates for the loss of *Rb1* in the mouse retina suggested that simultaneous inactivation of both *Rb1* and *p107* may lead to retinoblastoma in mice. We were able to directly test this hypothesis using a conditional inactivation approach, which was required because *Rb*-deficient mice exhibit an embryonic lethal phenotype. We showed that *Chx10-Cre;Rb*$^{Lox/Lox}$*;p107*$^{-/-}$ mice develop retinoblastoma, and this was later confirmed by two other laboratories using different Cre transgenic lines (Zhang et al. 2004; MacPherson et al. 2004; Chen et al. 2004). The advantage of these models is that the tumors initiate during retinal development in utero just as in human retinoblastoma and they initiate with inactivation of the Rb pathway. Since these early studies, several other genetic combinations have been characterized that develop retinoblastoma. These include: *Chx10-Cre;Rb*$^{Lox/Lox}$*;p107*$^{-/-}$*;p53*$^{Lox/Lox}$, *Chx10-Cre;Rb*$^{Lox/Lox}$*;p130*$^{-/-}$, *Chx10-Cre;Rb*$^{Lox/Lox}$*;p130*$^{-/-}$*;p53*$^{Lox/Lox}$, *Chx10-Cre;Rb*$^{Lox/Lox}$*; p107*$^{+/-}$*,p130*$^{-/-}$, *Chx10-Cre;Rb*$^{Lox/Lox}$*;p107*$^{-/-}$*;MDMX*^{Tg} and similar genotypes with other Cre transgenes (Ajioka et al. 2007). A detailed comparison of each of these strains will be required to determine which most faithfully recapitulates the human disease and is therefore the best model for preclinical studies of new therapies to treat human retinoblastoma.

One of the limitations of these genetic murine models of retinoblastoma is that they are often multifocal originating from patches of cells lacking Rb pathway function. In contrast, it is believed that in the human retina, retinoblastoma forms from a small number of individual cells in isolated regions of the retina. Moreover, it has not been demonstrated that the mouse tumors recapitulate the subsequent genetic lesion found in human retinoblastoma, such as *MdmX* amplification.

In contrast, orthotopic xenograft models have several advantages that complement the deficiencies in the genetic models of retinoblastoma (Fig. 1.3) (Laurie et al. 2005). First, they are established in the developing

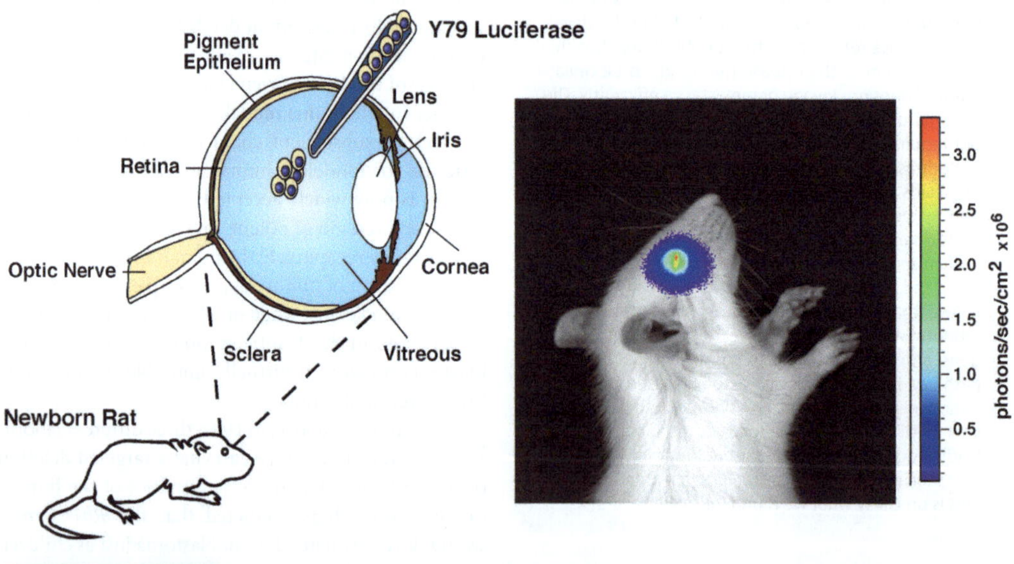

Figure 1.3

Orthotopic retinoblastoma xenograft using newborn rats and mice. To complement the genetic models of retinoblastoma, we have also developed and characterized an orthotopic xenograft model. A human retinoblastoma cell line expressing firefly luciferase was generated, and when 1,000 cells are injected into the vitreous of a newborn rat or mouse pup eye, they rapidly expand and form retinoblastoma in the subsequent 9–10 days. They reorganize the retinal vasculature and invade the surrounding tissue. Longitudinal studies with these animals can be carried out due to the noninvasive detection of tumor cell growth (and response) using the Xenogen imaging system

vitreous, which is precisely where the tumor forms normally. Second, they are formed from human tumor cell lines that were derived from enucleated retinoblastoma eyes. Third, they have well characterized genetic lesions that occur in the human disease and serve as a reasonable model for aggressive human retinoblastoma. Fourth, they grow in the vitreous and reorganize the retinal vasculature similar to that seen in human retinoblastoma. They are also much higher throughput than the mouse models and have well characterized tumor initiation and progression. These models have been extensively used in preclinical studies of chemotherapy for the treatment of retinoblastoma as well as other novel methods to stop retinoblastoma tumor progression. The limitation of xenograft models is that the tumor is formed by fully transformed retinoblastoma cell lines that may have undergone genetic changes that allow them to grow in culture and are not present in the primary tumor. In addition, they do not go through the process of tumor initiation and progression in situ and, in this regard, they do not recapitulate the human disease. The strengths and weaknesses of the knockout mouse models and the orthotopic xenograft models are complementary and, therefore, the best preclinical studies combine these two models to gain the most complete picture of treatment efficacy before moving into clinical trials.

1.5 Improving Retinoblastoma Treatment with Preclinical Studies

Preclinical models are required for rare childhood cancers, such as retinoblastoma, because there are not enough patients for large-scale multicenter clinical trials. A single clinical trial for retinoblastoma may take up to 5 years to complete. Preclinical models that faithfully recapitulate the human disease provide a unique opportunity to test a variety of different combinations of chemotherapy in a fraction of the time required for a human clinical trial. Moreover, preclinical studies allow researchers to optimize the timing and method of drug delivery and the relationship between pharmacokinetics and pharmacodynamics for each treatment.

The major challenges that we currently face for preclinical studies of retinoblastoma are related to the diagnosis of early stage tumors and monitoring tumor progression using imaging modalities that are used in the clinical management of retinoblastoma. It is also very important to monitor visual acuity in preclinical models of retinoblastoma because the ultimate goal of therapeutic intervention is to preserve vision without risking the child's life. A definitive diagnosis of retinoblastoma is made using a retinal camera, MRI, and ultrasound. Therefore, these modalities must be incorporated into preclinical studies of retinoblastoma. Intraocular pressure (IOP) must also be carefully monitored because, in some cases, elevated IOP can lead to optic nerve damage and secondary blindness. The most comprehensive preclinical studies of retinoblastoma would incorporate tumor diagnosis using a retinal camera combined with ultrasound and MRI, and visual acuity would be continuously monitored along with IOP over the course of treatment.

The other advantage offered by preclinical models is the opportunity to study alternative methods for drug delivery. In patients, clinicians have experimented with subconjunctival delivery of chemotherapy as well as intraocular delivery, but a careful side-by-side comparison of these different approaches.

1.6 Cell of Origin for Retinoblastoma

One of the most debated topics in the retinoblastoma field is the identification of the cell of origin (Macpherson and Dyer 2007; Dyer and Bremner 2005). Traditionally, pathologists have characterized the structure histopathological features of tumors and compared those to cell types found in the normal tissue to provide support for the cell of origin. More recently, scientists have used sophisticated molecular analyses and advanced imaging techniques to provide more detailed profiles of the differentiated features of tumor cells. However, the major limitation of this approach is that it assumes that tumor cells are somehow fixed in their developmental program and that this relates to the cell of origin. This view fails to take into account the evidence accumulated over the past decade that tumor suppressor genes can regulate cell fate specification and differentiation as well as proliferation and survival. Therefore, inactivation of one or more tumor suppressor pathways may lead to changes in the apparent fate of developing tumor cells in addition to changes in their proliferation and survival. This makes it difficult if not impossible to identify the cell of origin for a tumor by characterizing the tumor cells no matter what techniques are employed. It is much more informative to identify the precise genetic lesions that initiate and propagate the tumor and then study how those genetic changes affect different cell types in the tissue of origin. Using this approach, we can compare the tumor phenotype from different cells of origin with the genetic lesions seen in the human tumors to reconstruct the biology of tumor progression.

Another complicating factor in CNS tumors, such as retinoblastoma, is that the tumor may originate from a retinal progenitor cell. In the mammalian CNS, progenitor cells are multipotent, and therefore, when these cells become transformed, they may produce cells that express a variety of markers and further complicate efforts to infer the cell of origin.

For retinoblastoma, the evidence points to a retinal progenitor cell as the cell of origin and this has led to a general consensus in the field (Macpherson and Dyer 2007). Preclinical models were instrumental in making these advances in our understanding of the cell of origin. The first piece of evidence is that retinoblastoma mutations likely occur in dividing cells and these cells are the retinal progenitor cells. Moreover, efforts to model retinoblastoma in newly postmitotic cells or differentiated cells in the mouse retinae have been largely unsuccessful (Vooijs et al. 2002). Also, retinoblastomas have many features of retinal progenitor cells and produce differentiated cells with features of amacrine neurons and horizontal neurons (Zhang et al. 2004; Ajioka et al. 2007). It is not known if this is a default state or if this is the stage of development that initiated the tumor initiation mutation. The only piece of evidence that the cell of origin may not be a progenitor cell has come from recent studies showing that a differentiated horizontal neuron can give rise to retinoblastoma in one particular animal model (Ajioka et al. 2007). We think this reflects a unique aspect of horizontal neurons rather than the true cell of origin in human retinoblastoma.

1.7 Conclusions

Research on retinoblastoma has been at the center of many of the landmark discoveries in cancer genetics over the past 3 decades. However, despite these important advances in our understanding of cancer initiation and progression, research discoveries have had little impact on the clinical management of retinoblastoma until recently. By focusing on the role of the Rb family in retinal development, several research teams have gained insight into how the Rb family of proteins regulates retinal progenitor cell proliferation and differentiation in the retina. In just a few years, novel animal models of retinoblastoma have been developed that recapitulate the human disease and these models have now been used to test new combinations of chemotherapy and have contributed to innovative clinical trials. Moreover, mouse models were instrumental in identifying secondary genetic lesions in retinoblastoma and developing the first targeted chemotherapy for this disease. Finally, studies on genetically engineered mice have led to a better understanding of the retinoblastoma cell of origin and retinoblastoma progression. These advances and many others have set the stage for a new phase of retinoblastoma research in which preclinical studies will more directly impact clinical trials for this debilitating childhood cancer.

References

Ajioka I et al (2007) Differentiated horizontal interneurons clonally expand to form metastatic retinoblastoma in mice. Cell 131(2):378

Aslanian A, Iaquinta PJ, Verona R, Lees JA (2004) Repression of the Arf tumor suppressor by E2F3 is required for normal cell cycle kinetics. Genes Dev 18(12):1413

Chen D et al (2004) Cell-specific effects of RB or RB/p107 loss on retinal development implicate an intrinsically death-resistant cell-of-origin in retinoblastoma. Cancer Cell 5(6):539

Clarke AR et al (1992) Requirement for a functional Rb-1 gene in murine development. Nature 359(6393):328

Donovan SL et al (2006) Compensation by tumor suppressor genes during retinal development in mice and humans. BMC Biol 4:14

Dyer MA, Bremner R (2005) The search for the retinoblastoma cell of origin. Nat Rev Cancer 5(2):91

Friend SH et al (1986) A human DNA segment with properties of the gene that predisposes to retinoblastoma and osteosarcoma. Nature 323(6089):643

Harbour JW et al (1988) Abnormalities in structure and expression of the human retinoblastoma gene in SCLC. Science 241(4863):353

Jacks T et al (1992) Effects of an Rb mutation in the mouse. Nature 359(6393):295

Knudson AG (1971) Mutation and cancer: statistical study of retinoblastoma. PNAS 68:820

Laurie NA et al (2005) Topotecan combination chemotherapy in two new rodent models of retinoblastoma. Clin Cancer Res 11(20):7569

Laurie NA et al (2006) Inactivation of the p53 pathway in retinoblastoma. Nature 444(7115):61

Lee EY et al (1992) Mice deficient for Rb are nonviable and show defects in neurogenesis and haematopoiesis. Nature 359(6393):288

Maandag EC et al (1994) Developmental rescue of an embryonic-lethal mutation in the retinoblastoma gene in chimeric mice. EMBO J 13(18):4260

Macpherson D, Dyer MA (2007) Retinoblastoma: from the two-hit hypothesis to targeted chemotherapy. Cancer Res 67(16):7547

MacPherson D et al (2004) Cell type-specific effects of Rb deletion in the murine retina. Genes Dev 18(14):1681

Marine JC, Dyer MA, Jochemsen AG (2007) MDMX: from bench to bedside. J Cell Sci 120(Pt 3):371

O'Brien JM et al (1990) A transgenic mouse model for trilateral retinoblastoma. Arch Ophthalmol 108(8):1145

Robanus-Maandag E et al (1998) p107 is a suppressor of retinoblastoma development in pRb-deficient mice. Genes Dev 12(11):1599

Vooijs M, te Riele H, van der Valk M, Berns A (2002) Tumor formation in mice with somatic inactivation of the retinoblastoma gene in interphotoreceptor retinol binding protein-expressing cells. Oncogene 21(30):4635

Zhang J, Schweers B, Dyer MA (2004) The first knockout mouse model of retinoblastoma. Cell Cycle 3(7):952

Epidemiology

M. Orjuela

Contents

2.1 **Introduction** 11
2.2 **Incidence** 12
2.2.1 Population Differences in Incidence 12
2.2.2 Variation Within Countries: Subpopulations with Higher Incidence 14
2.2.3 Gender Differences 15
2.2.4 Biologic Underpinnings of Epidemiologic Studies on Retinoblastoma 15
2.3 **Potential Hypotheses** 16
2.3.1 Parental Occupations 16
2.3.2 Parental Age 16
2.3.3 In Vitro Fertilization (IVF) 17
2.3.4 UV Exposure 17
2.3.5 Nonoccupational Parental Exposures 18
2.3.6 Diet 18
2.3.7 Viral Agents 19
2.3.8 Diagnostic Interval 19
2.3.9 Screening and Media Campaigns 20
2.4 **Summary** 20
References 21

2.1 Introduction

From an epidemiologic perspective, retinoblastoma is one of the most interesting childhood tumors to study. Retinoblastoma is a primitive neuroectodermal tumor, and its occurrence in early childhood suggests that incidence can be associated with events affecting development of neuroectodermal tissues during the fetal period. Furthermore, it exists in two genetically distinct forms associated with differing (though not mutually exclusive) clinical presentations (see chapters 3 and 4). This allows the formulation of two distinct, though parallel, mechanisms for disease development. Additionally, there is considerable geographic variation in incidence, suggesting differential genetic susceptibility or environmental exposure(s). The combination of these three factors: a defined and relatively limited temporal window for development; two genetically distinct forms arriving, via different genetic pathways, to essentially identical histologic presentations; and the geographic variation in incidence suggest several handles/angles through which one could examine associations and risk factors for development of this disease. Despite these facts, and due in large part to the rarity of the disease, little is understood about the factors that culminate in the relatively well understood cell cycle and apoptotic pathway defects that define retinoblastoma at a molecular level.

Much has been published regarding the molecular changes that occur during the development of retinoblastoma, and recently, more reports have become available regarding incidence, survival, and treatment in countries outside of northern North America and Europe. Results from these studies point to some potential risk factors underlying disease development;

C. Rodriguez-Galindo and M.W. Wilson (eds.), *Retinoblastoma*, Pediatric Oncology, DOI 10.1007/978-0-387-89072-2_2, © Springer Science+Business Media, LLC 2010

however, few studies have been done to specifically elucidate these factors. Thus, this discussion of the epidemiology of retinoblastoma will, out of necessity, focus on disease incidence and on those few hypotheses that have been explored using population based study methodology.

2.2 Incidence

2.2.1 Population Differences in Incidence

Global incidence data for retinoblastoma show an approximate 50-fold variation, which is highly atypical for a pediatric tumor. This degree of variation is comparable to that seen in adult malignancy, such as cervical, gastric, and colon cancer, in which variations in environmental exposures – such as infectious agents and diet – are known to play a role. Other pediatric tumors with widely varying incidence rates, such as Hodgkin and non-Hodgkin Lymphomas, are tumors in which infectious agents are known to play a role. For retinoblastoma, when incidence data show separate rates for unilateral and bilateral disease, variation in incidence appears largely restricted to unilateral disease (Stiller and Parkin 1996). The incidence of unilateral retinoblastoma appears to be higher in several less affluent regions of the world, suggesting that environmental factors associated with poor living conditions may increase the risk of mutagenesis in retinal cells (Stiller and Parkin 1996); however, many of the rates that suggest increased incidence in less affluent countries are based on small numbers of cases and thus, need to be interpreted with caution.

Retinoblastoma occurs primarily in children under the age of 5 years, with a median age of diagnosis of 24 months in children with unilateral disease and 9–12 months in children with bilateral disease (Goddard et al. 1999; Butros et al. 2002). Later age at diagnosis is generally reported in areas where there is decreased access to medical care, but diagnosis in children older than 5 years of age is rare. One group in Sao Paulo, Brazil, examined the incidence of retinoblastoma in older children and found that of 453 cases of retinoblastoma, only 3.5% (16) were diagnosed after 60 months of age (Aguirre Neto et al. 2007). Incidence rates are thus frequently expressed as "per million children 0–4 years of age," rather than as "per million children 0–14 years of age," as is common for other childhood cancers.

According to population-based registry data compiled and published by the International Agency for Research in Cancer (IARC), incidence rates are generally similar in North America, Europe, and Australia; somewhat higher rates are observed in Central and South America; a wide range of rates are reported in Asia with the highest in one region in India (Chennai); and generally higher rates are observed in Africa (Parkin et al. 1998). This pattern supports the hypothesis of higher retinoblastoma incidence in less industrialized countries, though the highest rates are clearly in Africa and a range of rates are observed in other less industrialized countries. A comparison of the incidence rates for those registries with incidence greater than 15 per million children less than 5 years, using the registry data compiled by IARC, is shown in Table 2.1 (Parkin et al. 1998). Large variation within geographic regions and even within countries is evident within both more and less industrialized regions (comparisons are limited to those countries with multiple registries). Variation within the US is described below. In Europe, although most countries have incidences in the range of 6–12 per million less than 5 years, much lower rates are noted in Bulgaria, and higher rates are noted for several countries (see Table 2.1).

There is marked variation in rates within Latin America, though data is limited to those countries or cities with registries. Incidence rates cluster into two groups: less than 9.5 per million in countries such as Cuba and Uruguay with the lowest rates, and greater than 15 per million children <5 years in others. Some of this variation appears to correlate with variation in development indices, such as Gross National Product, literacy, and degree of health care system infrastructure. Within countries, there is also a suggestion of variation by economic development, with higher rates in poorer regions of countries such as Mexico (see below) and Brazil, where incidence in Goiania is 1.6 times that of Belem. The regions with higher incidence may differ from those with lower incidences in many other factors including ethnic origin and environmental exposures.

Table 2.1. Registries with the highest incidence of retinoblastoma

Rates per million children ages 0–4	Registry/Ethnicity	Country	Incidence[a]	Total cases (N < 1 yr) + (N age 1-4)	Ratio M:F
Registries with rates >20.0	Bamako	Mali	42.5	2+46	1.5
	Kampala	Uganda	24.0	4+15	1.4
	Zimbabwe (African ancestry)	Zimbabwe	23.3	1+17	1.3
	Hawaii (native Hawaiians)[b]	US	22.5	4+7	0.2
	IMSS Chiapas[b,e]	Mexico	21.8	12	0.5
	Alaska (natives)[b]	US	[c]	8	0.33
Registries with rates 17.5–20.0	Chennai/Madras	India	19.6[d] (15.9–16.1)	10+68	1.0
	Hanoi	Vietnam	18.9	3+14	2.3
	Singapore (Chinese)	Singapore	18.8	5+24	1.5
	New Zealand (non-Maori)	NZ	18.6	18+36	1.2
	New Zealand (Maori)[b]	NZ	17.8	4+11	0.9
	Valencia	Spain	17.8	6+12	1.4
Registries with rates 15.0–17.4	Philippines	Philippines	17.4	22+155	1.3
	Cali[b]	Colombia	17.1	4+20	0.5
	Quito[b]	Ecuador	16.6	2+15	0.7
	Ibadan	Nigeria	16.1	4+26	1.5
	Costa Rica[b]	Costa Rica	15.7	17+35	0.8
	Lima	Peru	15.5	4+15	1.0
	Norway	Norway	15.4	11+29	1.3
	Belem[b]	Brazil	15.4	0+10	0.6
	Denmark	Denmark	15.3	14+24	1.8

[a] Annual incidence per million children ages 0–4 years. From Parkin et al 1998 except as otherwise noted
[b] Populations with F:M >1.0
[c] The rate was 7.4 per million children under 14 years. If their rate were calculated based on children under age 5, their rate would likely surpass 20 per million, though this rate was based on a small number of children
[d] Incidence decreased in follow up report based on data from later years
[e] From Fajardo Gutierrez et al. 2007

In Asia and Oceania, some registries have documented incidence by ethnic origin, and this has further highlighted populational differences in incidence; for example, in New Zealand, rates differ between Maoris and non-Maoris (see Table 2.1), and in Singapore, where incidence in Malays is one third that of ethnic Chinese. Regional variations in incidence are also present. Notably, incidence in India is markedly higher in Chennai (formerly Madras) than in Delhi, Bombay, Bangalore, or Poona. Incidence in New Zealand is far higher than incidence in Australia. Incidence in Africa also varies greatly, with population based registries in Algeria and Egypt documenting rates of 4–6 per million <5 years, while incidence rates for some sub-Saharan African countries, such as Mali, Uganda, and Zimbabwe, are amongst the highest worldwide. These incidence variations suggest that environmental factors may be playing a role, though genetic susceptibility to particular environmental exposures may explain some of these differences.

Recent articles have further delineated population differences. In Europe, a recent evaluation of incidence of retinoblastoma in European children (1978–1997) using data collected through the Automated Childhood Cancer Information System project and including data from 60 registries demonstrated an overall incidence that increased by 1% per year over the 20-year period beginning in 1978. The age-standardized incidence rate for the age range 0–14 years was 4.1 per million children, with one third of cases affected with bilateral disease (MacCarthy et al. 2006). In contrast, a recent study by Seregard et al., in Sweden and Finland, where birth cohort analysis was possible, demonstrated that incidence was stable from 1990 to 1998, with a mean incidence rate of 11.8 (95% CI 10.5–13.1) and 11.2 (95% CI 9.4–13.0) per 1 million children less than 5 years of age in Sweden and Finland, respectively, despite the fact that analysis looking at annual incidence rates suggested an increase during that period (Seregard et al. 2004). Similarly, in a study examining incidence rates in Germany over the 20-year period beginning in 1987, incidence based on 732 retinoblastoma cases registered in German Children's Cancer Registry (one third were bilateral), demonstrated an age-standardized incidence rate/year for all children <15 years of 4.0 per million with stable rates throughout this period (D. Debling, personal communication).

Some registries have published follow up reports after the compilation of the 1998 IARC monograph. For India, a follow up study done in Chennai showed a slight decrease in incidence of retinoblastoma. From 1990 to 2001 in children <5 years, incidence was 15.9 (males)–16.1 (females) per million, a decrease from that reported earlier, suggesting a change in underlying risk factors. Interestingly, survival in Chennai is noted to be far less than in other parts of the world at 48%; thus, the overall elevated incidence is not likely to result from an increase in inherited familial cases (Swaminathan et al. 2008). In Karachi, Pakistan, registry data also suggests elevated incidence (Bhurgri et al. 2004). Incidence from this registry, however, was reported only as frequency in the IARC compilation because of a lack of actual population estimates (the last census was in 1981). After the data was compiled by IARC, the registry itself published data on cases reported in the 5 years following the IARC publication. They calculated the Age Standardized Incidence for Karachi itself at 5.3 per 100,000 children (or 53 per million) <5 years, which would place its incidence as the highest in the IARC reports. However, given concerns regarding underestimation of the actual source population, it is likely that this incidence is much lower. This group also reports a predominance of males to females (M:F 1.5), but as noted by IARC, this is true for all cancers in Karachi and is thought to represent a relative neglect of illness in girls. Reliable incidence data for Islamabad are also not available, but frequency data there also demonstrates an elevated M:F ratio (1.9) (Parkin et al. 1998). Although incidence estimates for Pakistan are not reliable, there is a suggestion of increased incidence, as the relative frequency of retinoblastoma compared with other pediatric malignancies is 7.4% (compared with 3% in US White populations) (Parkin et al. 1998).

2.2.2 Variation Within Countries: Subpopulations with Higher Incidence

The overall incidence of retinoblastoma in the U.S. has been stable over the 20-year period ending in 1995, ranging from 10 to 14 per million children <5 years, with retinoblastoma comprising 3–4% of childhood cancer. However, incidence within the US is not uniformly distributed and there appears to be variation by ethnicity, gender, and geographic region. Within the US, particular subpopulations have unusually elevated incidence. In most of the US registries, the rates amongst African American children are higher than those in "non-black" or "white" children. The difference in rates between ethnic groups is quite variable, with the ratio of incidence of "black" to "white" ranging from 1.43 in the Greater Delaware Valley, to 1.17 in New York State and 1.15 in the combined SEER registries, and 0.47 in Los Angeles. In the Hawaii SEER registry data (see Table 2.1), native Hawaiians appear to have an increased incidence of retinoblastoma. Similarly, Alaska natives had a rate significantly higher than US whites in SEER data (Odds Ratio [OR] 2.8; 95% CI 1.3–5.3). Like the Alaskan Native children, the rate in the New Mexico SEER registry Native Americans was higher (6.8 per million <14 years) compared with "white" children from the combined SEER registries (2.7 < 14 years) (OR 2.5; 95% CI 1.4–4.5). Interestingly, the overall rates for childhood cancer in Alaskan Natives and

New Mexico Native Americans were lower than those in SEER registry data for white children, though the rate for osteosarcoma (but not other bone tumors) was also higher among New Mexico Native Americans when compared with US whites (SEER) (OR 1.8; 95% CI 1.0–3.4) (Lanier et al 2003). Given the biological overlap between osteosarcoma and retinoblastoma, this finding is particularly intriguing. Interpretation of these variations based on data from regional US subpopulations is limited by the small number of cases upon which the incidence rates are based.

In a recent population-based study by Fajardo-Guttierez et al in Mexico, in which it was possible to examine regional differences in the incidence of retinoblastoma within the Mexican Social Security system (IMSS), the highest incidence of retinoblastoma occurred in the state with the highest incidence for central nervous system tumors (Chiapas, see Table 2.1) (Fajardo Gutierrez 2007). Although the incidence of retinoblastoma was highest in Chiapas – the poorest state in Mexico and a state in which a high proportion of the population is indigenous – the number of cases on which incidence was calculated is very small.

Some populations with apparent excess of retinoblastoma have a relative paucity of neuroblastoma (Alaskan natives, New Mexico American Indians, Chiapas) as if one occurred in greater numbers at the expense of development of the other. This may indicate a possible shared underlying mechanism of tumor formation in which different factors lead to a bifurcation in the formation of a primitive neuroectodermal tumors (PNET) leading to development of neuroblastoma in one population, and retinoblastoma in another. Alternatively, the factors that lead to development of retinoblastoma may coexist with factors that protect against neuroblastoma.

2.2.3 Gender Differences

Comparing incidence worldwide, focusing on those countries with the higher incidence rates, we see some differences in the incidence by gender (Table 2.1). In some regions of the world, there appear to be slightly more male cases than female cases, while in other regions, the difference is markedly in the other direction. In some populations of Latin America and in native American populations of North America, the incidence in girls is much higher than in boys; for example, the Alaskan Native population had a 3:1 Female:Male incidence (Lanier et al. 2003), and in the states in Mexico, in which retinoblastoma figured amongst the five most common pediatric malignancies – Chiapas (where it was second) and Veracruz (where it was fifth) – there was a predominance of female cases, with M:F 0.5 and 0.7, respectively. In Oman, where the incidence is only 8.3 per million <5 years of age, the ratio of M:F is 0.7 as well (Khandekar et al. 2004). However, all of these data are the results of observations on small numbers of cases in each registry. Unfortunately we do not have data on laterality from the majority of these registries, thus it is not possible to see if the ratio of male to female cases varies by laterality.

2.2.4 Biologic Underpinnings of Epidemiologic Studies on Retinoblastoma

Hereditary retinoblastoma is characterized by the presence of a germline mutation, earlier clinical manifestation of disease with disease detectable in utero in children with known familial disease, and very elevated risk of developing secondary malignancies. All children with bilateral tumors and roughly 15% of children with unilateral tumors have this form of disease. There are no definitive clinical characteristics that differentiate the 15% of unilateral patients with germline mutations from the 85% who lack them. The ability to differentially examine risk factors for tumors involving germline mutations from those without them by using laterality as a proxy is thus hampered. Ongoing epidemiologic studies, such as one by the Children's Oncology Group, will be able to bypass this imprecision by evaluating tumor mutations directly.

Studies done to date have relied on the relative distinctiveness of the laterality phenotypes in order to analyze results. Although much is understood about the effects of the *RB1* mutations underlying the formation of retinoblastoma, little is known about the etiology of these mutations in germinal or retinal cells. New germline mutations are known to occur preferentially on the paternal allele, suggesting the implication of paternal preconception risk factors (Zhu et al. 1989; Kato et al. 1994; Dryja et al. 1989). However, there is no knowledge about the etiology of retinal cell mutations or their time of occurrence, and little is known about the causes of unilateral disease. The crucial period for mutation development in retinoblastoma may be during retinal formation occurring in early embryonal development between the 4th and 8th week of gestation, or during infancy as retinal cells continue to divide until about age 2 years. Although as stated earlier, the molecular changes leading to retinoblastoma are well characterized, the role of risk factors or contributing exposures has been studied only rarely. Below is a summary of studies that explore risk factors or characteristics hypothesized to play a role in disease development.

2.3 Potential Hypotheses

2.3.1 Parental Occupations

Because retinoblastoma occurs during infancy and early childhood, the examination of risk factors and environmental exposures has focused primarily on potential contributions from parental exposures. Given the low incidence of retinoblastoma, traditional epidemiologic studies have been limited to case-control and case-series studies. The largest and most extensively reported study has been a case-control telephone interview study conducted by the Children's Cancer Study Group in 67 bilateral and 115 unilateral cases who did not have a family history of the disease.(Bunin 1990) In this study, paternal employment in the military (OR 2.8; 95% 1.1–8.8, $p = 0.04$) or in the metal industry (OR infinity; 95% CI 1.4-infinity, $p = 0.02$) was associated with having a child with bilateral disease, and paternal employment as a welder or machinist was associated with having a child with unilateral disease (OR 4.0; 95% CI 1.1–22.1, $p = 0.04$). These findings are similar to those from studies done on other PNETs of childhood (Olshan et al. 1999). Interestingly, this study also examined potential transgenerational exposures and found that maternal grandparental employment in farming was also associated with unilateral disease (OR 10.0; 95% CI 1.4–433, $p = 0.02$).

One retrospective cohort study of Norwegian agricultural workers noted an increased incidence of retinoblastoma in children whose parents had worked with pesticides (Kristensen et al. 1996). This is particularly intriguing given the findings of the above noted association between unilateral retinoblastoma and maternal grandparent farm work (Bunin et al. 1990), as well as because work done earlier as part of a case-control study in Mexico found increased risk with paternal occupation as a farm worker (bilateral disease) (OR 2.7; 95% CI 1.1–6.5) (Orjuela et al. 2000a) and with maternal and infant exposure to chickens and pigs (unpublished data); these trends echo findings in epidemiologic studies of other PNETs. For example, maternal occupation as a farm worker has also been associated with development of neuroblastoma (Olshan et al. 1999). For brain tumors, increased risk has been found for agricultural workers, or for maternal exposure to farm animals or farm residence (Preston-Martin et al. 1993; Bunin et al. 1994; Holly et al. 1998; Kristensen et al. 1996; Cordier et al. 2001). In those studies of brain tumors in which farm animal exposure has been analyzed by species, exposure to chickens and pigs conferred increased risk of PNET (medulloblastoma) (Holly et al. 1998; Kristensen et al. 1996).

2.3.2 Parental Age

Increased parental age has been associated with greater risk for bilateral retinoblastoma. Advanced paternal age is hypothesized to be associated with an increased risk of new germ cell mutations by way of increased opportunity for mutation formation in dividing spermatocytes. Since new germline mutations occur preferentially on the paternal allele, this hypothesis has some biological plausibility. Earlier studies from the Dutch population based registries found that increased parental age (of both fathers and mothers) was significantly associated with increased Relative Risk of having a child with bilateral (but not unilateral) retinoblastoma (Moll et al. 1996). However, these studies were hampered by relatively small sample sizes. One case-series study from India found that fathers of children with nonfamilial bilateral disease were older than those of children with unilateral disease (Sivakumaran et al. 2000). Two recent European studies attempted to address this question using the case data available from larger national registries. One such study in the UK matched cases ascertained from the national registry (diagnosed from 1968–1986) with birth record controls matched on date of birth, sex and origin. The OR for retinoblastoma resulting from assumed new germ cell mutations among children of fathers who were at least 45 years old at the time of the child's birth was 3.0 (95% CI 0.2–41.7) (Dockerty et al. 2001). Although this finding was not significant, it was suggestive and consistent with results of earlier studies. The authors did not hypothesize an increased risk from advanced maternal age, nevertheless, the effect observed in women between 30 and 34 years of age was also elevated, with an OR 2.03 (95% CI 0.87–4.74) when compared with women 25–29 years of age. The authors were able to eliminate cases with family history and further restricted their analysis to bilateral cases. However, because of the high degree of correlation between maternal and paternal ages, the authors were unable to separate the effects of parental age. A more recent study done in Sweden is the only population-based cohort study thus far with the power to examine the independent effect of parental age on incidence of childhood cancer (Yip et al. 2006). In this study, the authors were able to separate the effects of maternal from paternal age and found that advanced *maternal* age is actually significantly predictive of increased risk of having a child with retinoblastoma. Although a modest increased risk associated with advanced paternal age was apparent, the effect disappeared after adjusting for maternal age. This Swedish study assessed parental ages via national registries by examining 4.3 million children (and their parents) born between 1961 and 2000, including 226 cases of retinoblastoma. Yip et al. found that for children <5 years of age, increased maternal age (after adjustment for paternal age) was associated with elevated risk of retinoblastoma (when women older than 40 years at age of childbirth were compared with women younger than 25 years at childbirth), the Incidence Rate Ratio was 2.39; 95% CI 1.17–4.85) (Yip et al. 2006) This finding suggests that maternal risk factors can contribute to likelihood of developing hereditary (bilateral) retinoblastoma despite the fact that new mutations were expected to occur on the paternal allele given prior findings. When comparing these results with those of the UK study, it is important to note that in the latter case, women younger than 25 years of age had lower incidences of having children with retinoblastoma than the designated reference group (25–29); thus, if these younger mothers had been used as a reference group, it is likely that results in the UK study might have been similar those from the Swedish study.

2.3.3 In Vitro Fertilization (IVF)

Recently, another risk factor has emerged, which may be closely linked to the risk factor of increased maternal/paternal age. A study done through the Dutch Retinoblastoma registry found that children conceived by means of in vitro fertilization (IVF) had a 5–7-fold increased risk of retinoblastoma (Moll et al. 2003); however, these results were based on only 5 cases (2 bilateral, 3 unilateral). Although studies done in birth cohorts of children born after IVF in the UK, Denmark, and Australia observed no increase in incidence of retinoblastoma (Bradbury and Jick 2004; Lidegaard et al. 2005; Bruinsma et al. 2000), it is possible that the increases in incidence found in Holland might in part be related to parental age. None of the birth cohort studies restricted analysis to a subpopulation with older parental ages in order to examine the effect on risk of retinoblastoma. Further examination of the incidence of retinoblastoma in children conceived through IVF will be essential to determine if the effect is indeed independent of parental age.

2.3.4 UV Exposure

One explanation posited for the geographic variations in retinoblastoma incidence has been the inherent geographic differences in ultraviolet (UV) radiation exposure. One group of investigators had suggested that the geographic differences that are found in the incidence of unilateral disease can be attributed to the annual environmental exposure to UV rays, but that the incidence of bilateral tumors is unrelated to UV exposure. Increased UV exposure to the retina would lead to increased probability of mutations and thus tumors in the retina. Hooper et al found that incidence of retinoblastoma falls significantly with increasing geographic latitude, and that increased incidence of unilateral disease (but not bilateral disease) is significantly associated with increased annual ambient exposure to UV rays (Hooper et al. 1999) However, a subsequent analysis by the NCI found that although incidence of retinoblastoma was significantly correlated with UV-B radiation exposure levels, this association disappeared after adjusting for climate, race, and socioeconomic development. As a result, they concluded that geographic variation is not explained by variations in UV exposure, but rather that tropical climate and exposure related to ethnic susceptibility and economic development may be confounding the association found with UV exposure (Jemal et al. 2000). Studies done on this topic have only looked at the UV exposure of a given geographic region but have not taken into account individual differences in duration of exposure.

2.3.5 Nonoccupational Parental Exposures

Other parental exposures have been examined as potential risk factors for retinoblastoma. In a study by Bunin et al., gestational exposure to X-ray OR 2.3; $p=0.08$), a morning sickness medication (which is no longer available) (OR 2.8; $p=0.02$), and low maternal educational level (not finishing high school) (OR 5.5; $p=0.03$) were associated with increased risk for having a child with unilateral disease. Two other exposures were found to be significantly protective: multivitamin use during pregnancy (for both unilateral and bilateral forms of the disease) and periconceptional use of barrier contraceptive (OR 0.1; $p=0.02$) or spermicide (OR 0.2; $p=0.02$. The protective effects of these two factors were further explored in the context of another study (see below).

In a later study of 106 children with retinoblastoma and 198 hospital-based controls at the Instituto Nacional de Pediatria (INP), a public tertiary care hospital in Mexico City, a significantly increased risk for the development of unilateral retinoblastoma was associated with factors related to maternal poverty during pregnancy, including poor nutrition (OR 2.3; 95% CI 1.2–2.4), lack of prenatal care (OR 2.6; 95% CI 1.1–5.9), delivery at home (OR 4.8; 95% CI 2.1–11.0), low level of maternal education (not finishing secondary school) (OR 3.7; 95% CI 1.4–9.5), birth outside of the capital (OR 2.5; 95% CI 1.3–5.0), and breast feeding for longer than 6 months (OR 2.4; 95% CI 1.3–4.3) (Orjuela et al. 2000a). None of these risk factors appeared to play a role in development of bilateral disease, although analysis was hampered by the small number of cases with bilateral disease. *Per capita* and household income did not appear to contribute to risk. These factors echoed in part the findings from the US study. Together, these socioeconomic indicators are more suggestive of an underlying mechanism that could be correlated with lower maternal socioeconomic status in Mexico rather than suggesting that a lower socioeconomic status per se increases risk. Among the potential underlying factors that could contribute risk, nutrient intake is one of the mechanistically more interesting possibilities.

2.3.6 Diet

Recent studies have suggested that gestational nutrient intake may be relevant to the development of PNET tumors, such as neuroblastoma, medulloblastoma, and retinoblastoma. The case-control study by Bunin et al in the US found a significantly protective effect against both unilateral (OR 0.4; $p = 0.02$) and bilateral disease (OR 0.2, $p = 0.02$) for mothers who consumed multivitamins during pregnancy (Bunin et al. 1989). The case-control study in Mexico found that maternal diets low in vegetables, folate, lutein, and vitamin B6 intake during pregnancy were associated with a 2–4-fold increased risk of having a child with sporadic retinoblastoma (Orjuela et al. 2005). The significantly increased risk for developing unilateral disease that was associated with breast feeding for longer than 6 months also suggests an increased risk associated with prolonged dependence on breast milk for nutrients, and possibly a protective effect of substituting formula (which has synthetic vitamins added) or other foods. Breast fed infants receive folate and other B vitamins in breast milk, however, the levels of these in breast milk necessarily depend on maternal diet. Decreased intake of these nutrients, necessary for DNA methylation and synthesis, as well as retinal function, may increase risk for having a child with sporadic retinoblastoma. Other studies have found similar increased risk for development of neuroblastoma and medulloblastoma associated with lower maternal micronutrient intake during pregnancy (Bunin et al. 1993; Olshan et al. 2002; French et al. 2003).

2.3.7 Viral Agents

The geographic variations in patterns of incidence of retinoblastoma have led investigators to wonder about the possibility of involvement by an infectious agent. The retinoblastoma protein, pRb, which is generally absent or truncated and ineffective in retinoblastoma as a result of *RB1* mutations, can be inactivated by three viral proteins, which share sequence homology for a region that binds and inactivates pRb. These three viral proteins are the E7 protein of the human papilloma virus (HPV), the T antigen of the SV40 virus, and the E1A antigen of adenovirus. Their potential to inactivate pRb suggested a possible role for these viruses in development of a subset of retinoblastoma. The distribution of areas of increased incidence of retinoblastoma shared some similarity with areas of increased incidence of cervical carcinoma known to be causally associated with HPV. The US-based study's finding of the tenfold protective effect of periconceptional use of barrier contraceptives also suggested the possible involvement of a sexually transmitted agent.

DNA sequences from oncogenic HPV subtypes (16 and 18) were detected in about one third of fresh frozen retinoblastoma tumor samples studied in central Mexico, suggesting a role for HPV infection (Orjuela et al. 2000b). Tumors containing HPV had significantly lower proliferative indexes and clinically less invasive behavior. Similarly, in Brazil, Palazzi, Villa et al examined paraffin-embedded tumor tissue from 43 children with unilateral retinoblastoma for HPV DNA using PCR/ dot blot hybridization and also found high risk oncogenic HPV DNA types 16 and 35 in 12 (27.9%). A higher frequency of differentiated tumors (63.3%) was observed among the HPV-positive tumors (Palazzi et al. 2003). Montoya Fuentes in Northern Mexico examined 51 paraffin embedded samples (collected between 1985 and 1997) and found that 35% of tumors contained oncogenic HPV subtypes (by PCR and immunohistochemistry); 31.4% (16 cases) with HPV 33 and 5.9% (3) with HPV 31,35, or 51. Interestingly, no tumors with HPV 16 or 18 were found, and 2 of the 18 cases with High Risk HPV were bilateral. Their study found a slightly higher proportion of advanced stage disease at diagnosis (St. Jude stage 3 or greater) in children whose tumors were HPV negative when compared with those that were HPV positive (18% vs. 13%) (Montoya-Fuentes et al. 2003). More recently, a study in India has found HPV16 in 27% of 44 tumors. Tumors that were HPV positive were more likely to have detectable pRb and to have occurred in children diagnosed before 18 months of age (Krishnakumar 2008). Oncogenic HPV subtypes found in various studies are among those causally associated with the development of cervical cancer; however, one study has not found presence of HPV or other possible causal viruses in retinoblastoma tumors from the US and Canada (Gillison et al. 2007). Thus, the evidence for a role of HPV is not conclusive. More molecular evidence of a possible role for HPV in development of retinoblastoma has recently been published by Ponce-Castaneda et al who have found that gene expression profiles made from tumor tissue from retinoblastoma differ by HPV status. Tumors with differing HPV status (presence versus absence by PCR) differ significantly in their expression of certain genes involved in inflammatory responses, while their gene expression profiles do not differ as clearly when comparing unilateral and bilateral tumors (Ponce-Castaneda et al. 2008). Together, these studies suggest an intriguing possible mechanism that may contribute as a cofactor for incidence of retinoblastoma in some areas of the world, but further work to better elucidate a potential infectious etiology is needed.

2.3.8 Diagnostic Interval

Most reports on incidence of retinoblastoma have not discussed disease stage, in large part because registries generally do not collect these data. Relative prevalence of metastatic disease is limited to reports originating from clinical treatment centers: For example, in a report of 141 children with retinoblastoma followed in Istanbul, 9.9% presented with metastatic disease (Ozkan et al. 2006), while in Ankara, 20.9% of 91 children had metastatic disease (Ozdemir et al. 2007). A report on the incidence amongst Swiss children recorded over a period of 42 years showed that the incidence of more advanced intraocular disease, group E, has decreased. The authors noted an association with decreasing interval of time between the first symptoms (usually by parents) and retinoblastoma diagnosis. Over the 42-year period, this time interval decreased significantly only for unilateral disease (Wallach et al. 2006). Other reports from Argentina and Brazil have noted that children with a longer period of time between noting of symptoms and diagnosis of disease were also more likely to have more clinically advanced disease (Erwenne and Franco 1989; Chantada et al. 1999). These findings suggest a benefit of diagnosing disease closer to the time that symptoms are first noted, implying a linear relationship between this interval and disease progression. However, more recent work in a public hospital serving uninsured patients from central Mexico has not demonstrated a significant association between longer diagnostic delay and more advanced clinical stage (by either ABC or St Jude's staging) for 125 newly diagnosed patients without a family history who had either bilateral or unilateral disease (Orjuela et al. unpublished data). It is thus less certain that increased delay in diagnosis necessarily leads to progression and development of more advanced disease.

2.3.9 Screening and Media Campaigns

Some experts have advocated the importance of establishing retinoblastoma screening programs, as well as media campaigns to increase public awareness and thus empower parents to seek medical attention earlier. Given retinoblastoma's incidence of 1 in approximately 16,000 live births, campaigns for public awareness will need to weigh its incidence and potential public health impact when prioritizing time for retinoblastoma in public service announcements. Screening campaigns will also need to proceed with caution, given the inherent difficulties of mounting effective screening for rare diseases. The screening campaigns mounted for neuroblastoma, another primitive neuroectodermal tumor of early childhood, have not been successful in decreasing disease related mortality nor in decreasing incidence of clinically more advanced disease (Schilling et al. 2002; Woods et al. 2002; Yamamoto et al. 2002; Maris and Woods 2008). This lack of success may in part be ascribed to inherent biologic differences between more invasive and less invasive forms of neuroblastoma (Maris 2007). During the intervening time since the screening programs for neuroblastoma were first created, investigators have developed a better understanding of the biology of neuroblastoma (Hiyama et al. 2008). The underlying assumption, that the degree of invasiveness is linearly related to the amount of time that the disease remains untreated, now appears to underestimate the true biologic complexity of the disease. Advances in the understanding of the biology of retinoblastoma may help better elucidate the potential benefit derived from a screening program for retinoblastoma. For this disease, the question remains: is more aggressive disease biologically distinct from less aggressive or invasive disease? And, from the epidemiologic perspective, are risk factors the same for more invasive and less invasive disease?

2.4 Summary

Risk factors for development of sporadic (without family history of this disease, either laterality) retinoblastoma are poorly understood. Here, we have presented variations in incidence of retinoblastoma and risk factors that have been proposed as potentially important for development of retinoblastoma. In aggregate, the geographic and ethnic variations in incidence in retinoblastoma are suggestive of underlying risk factors for development of disease. Closer examination of factors that may differ between populations with different rates could improve our understanding of disease development. Studies that focus on the likely windows of susceptibility and utilize information from genetic analysis in order to differentiate forms of the disease will inform our understanding of retinoblastoma and may potentially inform therapy and strategies for earlier detection. Future epidemiologic studies may help elucidate whether more aggressive disease is associated with the same risk factors as less aggressive disease. Such an understanding would inform efforts aimed at earlier disease detection.

Acknowledgments. The author gratefully acknowledges the assistance of Aisha Siebert, MPH, and of Drs M. Veronica Ponce, Arturo Fajardo Gutierrez, A. Krishnakumar, and Desiree Debling, who generously shared data in advance of publication. In addition, the author is appreciative for assistance from Dr M. Ramirez Ortiz, and Dr W. Gauss. This work was supported in part by NIH 1 R01 CA98180 and ACS RSG CNE-104953.

References

Bhurgri Y, Muzaffar S, Ahmed R, Ahmed N, Bhurgri H, Usman A, Faridi N, Malik J, Kazi LA, Bashir I, Kayani N, Bhurgri A, Pervez S, Hasan SH, Soomro AH (2004) Retinoblastoma in Karachi, Pakistan. Asian Pac J Cancer Prev5 :159–163

Bradbury BD, Jick H (2004) In-vitro fertilization and childhood retinoblastoma. Br J Clin Pharmacol 58: 209–211

Bruinsma F, Venn A, Lancaster P, Speirs A, Healy D (2000) Incidence of cancer in children born after in-vitro fertilization. Hum Reprod 15:604–607

Bunin GR, Buckley JD, Boesel CP, Rorke LB, Meadows AT (1994) Risk factors for astrocytic glioma and primitive neuroectodermal tumor of the brain in young children: a report from the Children's Cancer Group. Cancer Epidemiol Biomarkers Prev 3:197–204

Bunin GR, Kuitjen RR, Buckley JD, Rorke LB, Meadows AT (1993) Relation between maternal diet and subsequent primitive neuroectodermal brain tumors in young children. N Engl J Med 329:536–541

Bunin GR, Meadows AT, Emanuel BS, Bucly JD, Woods WG, Hammond GD (1989) Pre- and post-conception factors associated with heritable and non-heritable retinoblastoma. Cancer Res 49:5730–5735

Bunin GR, Petrakova A, Meadows AT, Emanuel BS, Buckley JD, Woods WG, Hammond GD (1990) Occupations of parents of the children with retinoblastoma: a report from the Children's Cancer Study Group. Cancer Res 50:7129–7133

Butros LJ, Abramson DH, Dunkel IJ (2002) Delayed diagnosis of the retinoblastoma: analysis of degree, cause, and potential consequences. Pediatrics 109:e45

Chantada G, Fandino A, Manzitti J, Urrutia L, Schvartzman E (1999) Late diagnosis of retinoblastoma in a developing country. Arch Dis Child 80:171–174

Cordier S, Mandereau L, Preston-Martin S, Little J, Lubin F, Mueller B, Holly E, Filippini G, Peris-Bonet R, McCredie M, Choi NW, Arsla A (2001) Parental occupations and childhood brain tumors: result of an international case-control study. Cancer Causes Control 12:865–874

de Aguirre Neto JC, Antoneli CB, Ribeiro KB, Castilho MS, Novaes PE, Chojniak MM, Arias V (2007) Retinoblastoma in children older than 5 years of age. Pediatr Blood Cancer 48:292–295

Dockerty JD, Draper G, Vincent T, Rowan SD, Bunch KJ (2001) Case–Control study of parental age, parity and socioeconomic level in relation to childhood cancers. Int J Epidemiol 30:1428–1437

Dryja TP, Mukai S, Rapaport JM, Yandell DW (1989) Parental origin of mutations of the retinoblastoma gene. Nature 339:556–558

Erwenne CM, Franco EL (1989) Age and lateness of referral as determinant of extra ocular retinoblastoma. Ophthalmic Paediatr Genet 10:179–184

Fajardo-Gutiérrez A, Juárez-Ocaña S, González-Miranda G, Palma-Padilla V, Carreón-Cruz R, Ortega-Álvarez MC, Mejía-Arangure JM (2007) Incidence of cancer in children residing in ten jurisdictions of the Mexican republic: Importance of the Cancer registry (a population-based study). BMC Cancer 19:7–68

French AE, Grant R, Weitzman S, Ray JG, Vermeulen MJ, Sung L, Greenberg M, Koren G (2003) Folic acid food fortification is associated with a decline in neuroblastoma. Clin Pharmacol Ther 74:288–294

Gillison ML, Chen R, Goshu E, Rushlow D, Chen N, Banister C, Creek KE, Gallie BL (2007) Human retinoblastoma is not caused by known pRb-inactivating human DNA tumor viruses. Int J Cancer 120:1482–1490

Goddard A, Kingston JE, Hungerford JL (1999) Delay in diagnosis of retinoblastoma: risk factors and treatment outcome. Br J Ophthalmol 832:1320–1323

Hiyama E, Iehara T, Sugimoto T, Fukuzawa M, Hayashi Y, Sasaki F, Sugiyama M, Kondo S, Yoneda A, Yamaoka H, Tajiri T, Akazawa K, Ohtaki M (2008) Effectiveness of screening for neuroblastoma at 6 months of age: a retrospective population-based cohort study. Lancet 371:1173–1180

Holly EA, Bracci PM, Mueller BA, Preston-Martin S (1998) Farm and animal exposures and pediatric brain tumors. Cancer Epidemiol Biomarkers Prev 7:797–802

Hooper ML (1999) Is sunlight an aetiological agent in the genesis of retinoblastoma? Br J Cancer 79:1273–1276

Jemal A, Devesa SS, Fears TE, Fraumeni JF Jr (2000) Retinoblastoma incidence and sunlight exposure. Br J Cancer 82:1875–1878

Kato MV, Ishizaki K, Shimizu T, Ejima Y, Tanooka H, Takayama J, Kaneko A, Toguchida J, Sasaki MS (1994)

Parental origin of germ-line and somatic mutations in the retinoblastoma gene. Hum Genet 94:31–38

Khandekar R, Ganesh A, Lawati J (2004) A 12-year epidemiological review of retinoblastoma in Omani children. Ophthalmic Epidemiol 11:151–159

Kristensen P, Andersen A, Irgens LM, Bye AS, Sundheim L (1996) Cancer in offspring of parents engaged in agricultural activities in Norway: incidence and risk factors in the farm environment. Int J Cancer 65:39–50

Lanier AP, Holck P, Ehrsam Day G, Key C (2003) Childhood cancer among Alaska Natives. Pediatrics 112:e369

Lidegaard O, Pinbrog A, Andersen AN (2005) Imprinting diseases and IVF: Danish National IVF cohort study. Hum Reprod 20:950–954

MacCarthy A, Draper GJ, Steliarova-Foucher E, Kingston JE (2006) Retinoblastoma incidence and survival in European children (1978–1997). Report from the Automated Childhood Cancer Information System project. Eur J Cancer4 2:2092–2102

Maris JM (2007) Neuroblastoma. Lancet 369:2106–2120

Maris JM, Woods WG (2008) Screening for neuroblastoma: a resurrected idea? Lancet 371:1142–1143

Mohan A, Venkatesan N, Kandalam M, Pasricha G, Acharya P, Khetan V, Gopal L, Sharma T, Biswas J, Krishnakumar S (2009) Detection of human papillomavirus DNA in retinoblastoma samples: a preliminary study. J Pediatr Hematol Oncol 31:8–13

Moll AC, Imhof SM, Kuik DJ, Bouter LM, Den Otter W, Bezemer PD, Koten JW, Tan KE (1996) High parental age is associated with sporadic hereditary retinoblastoma: the Dutch Retinoblastoma Register 1862–1994. Hum Genet9 8:109–112

Moll AC, Imhof SM, Cruysberg JR, Shouten-Van Meeteren AY, Boers M, Van Leeuwen FE (2003) Incidence of retinoblastoma in children born after in-vitro fertilization. Lancet3 61:309–310

Montoya-Fuentes H, de la Paz Ramirez-Munoz M, Villar-Calvo V, Suarez-Rincon AE, Ornelas-Aguirre JM, Vazquez-Camacho G, Orbach-Arbouys S, Bravo-Cuellar A, Sanchez-Corona J (2003) Identification of DNA sequences and viral proteins of 6 human papilloma virus types in retinoblastoma tissue. Anticancer Res 23:2853–2862

Olshan AF, De Roos AJ, Teschke K, Neglia JP, Stram DO, Pollock BH, Castleberry RP (1999) Neuroblastoma and parental occupation. Cancer Causes Control 10:539–549

Olshan AF, Smith JC, Bondy ML, Neglia JP, Pollock BH (2002) Maternal vitamin use and reduced risk of neuroblastoma. Epidemiology 13:575–580

Orjuela M, Castaneda VP, Ridaura C, Lecona E, Leal C, Abramson DH, Orlow I, Gerald W, Cordon-Cardo C (2000a) Presence of human papilloma virus in tumor tissue from children with retinoblastoma: an alternative mechanism for tumor development. Clin Cancer Res 6:4010–4016

Orjuela M, Lecona E, Salazar A, Leal C, Abramson D, Mueller N (2000) Risk factors for the development of sporadic retinoblastoma in Mexico. In: Proceedings of the 91st annual meeting of the American association for cancer research, 2298

Orjuela MA, Titievsky L, Liu X, Ramirez-Ortiz M, Ponce-Castaneda V, Lecona E, Molina E, Beaverson K, Abramson DH, Mueller NE (2005) Fruit and vegetable intake during pregnancy and risk for development of sporadic retinoblastoma. Cancer Epidemiol Biomarkers Prev 14:1433–1440

Ozdemir H, Tacyildiz N, Unal E, Yavuz G, Ugur H, Gunduz K (2007) Clinical and epidemiological characteristics of retinoblastoma: correlation with Prognosis in a Turkish pediatric oncology center. Pediatr Hematol Oncol 24:221–231

Ozkan A, Pazarli H, Celkan T, Karaman S, Apak H, Kaner G, Uzel O, Yildiz I (2006) Retinoblastoma in Turkey: survival and clinical characteristics 1981–2004. Pediatr Int 48:369–373

Palazzi MA, Yunes JA, Cardinalli IA, Stangehaus GP, Brandalise SR, Ferriera SA, Sobrinho JSP, Villa LL (2003) Detection of oncogenic human papillomavirus in sporadic retinoblastoma. Acta Ophthalmol Scand 81:396–398

Parkin DM, Kramarova E, Draper GJ, Masuyer E, Michaelis J, Neglia JP, Qureshi S, Stiller CA (1998) International incidence of childhood cancer. International Agency for Research on Cancer, Lyon, France

Preston-Martin S, Lewis S, Winkelmann R, Borman B, Auld J, Pearce N (1993) Descriptive epidemiology of primary cancer of the brain, cranial nerves, and cranial meninges in New Zealand 1948–1988. Cancer Causes Control 4:529–538

Ponce-Castneda MV, Torres-Lopez J, Burgueno-Ferreira J, Bravo JC, Ramon G, Hernandez-Angeles A, Fernandez-Mendez K, Leon-Garcia D, Bautista-DeLucio VM, Ramierz-Ortiz M, Cabrera-Munoz ML, Sadowinky-Pine S, Ramirez J, Coello G, Mendoza-Rodriguez V, Lopez-Casillas F, Orjuela M (2008) Molecular evidence implicating HPV involvement in human retinoblastoma pathogenesis. In: Proceedings of ISGEDR 2008

Schilling FH, Spix C, Berthold F, Erttmann R, Fehse N, Hero B, Klein G, Sander J, Schwarz K, Treuner J, Zorn U, Michaelis J (2002) Neuroblastoma screening at one year of age. N Engl J Med 346:1047–1053

Seregard S, Lundell G, Svedberg H, Kivela T (2004) Incidence of retinoblastoma from 1958 to 1998 in Northern Europe: advantages of birth control analysis. Ophthalmology 111:1228–1232

Sivakumaran TA, Ghose S, Kumar HAS, Kucheria K (2000) Parental age in Indian patients with sporadic hereditary retinoblastoma. Ophthalmic Epidemiol 7:285–291

Stiller CA, Parkin DM (1996) Geographic and ethnic variations in the incidence of childhood cancer. Br Med Bull 52:682–703

Swaminathan R, Rama R, Shanta V (2008) Childhood Cancer in Chennai, India, 1990–2001: incidence and survival. Int J Cancer 122:2607–2611

Wallach M, Balmer A, Munier F, Houghton S, Pampallona S, von der Weid N, Beck-Popovic M (2006) Shorter Time to Diagnosis and Improved Stage at Presentation in Swiss Patients With Retinoblastoma Treated From 1963 to 2004. Pediatrics 118:e1493–e1498

Woods WG, Gao RN, Shuster JJ, Robison LL, Bernstein M, Weitzman S, Bunin G, Levy I, Brossard J, Dougherty G, Tuchman M, Lemieux B (2002) Screening of infants and mortality due to neuroblastoma. N Engl J Med 346:1041–1046

Yamamoto K, Ohta S, Ito E, Hayashi Y, Asami T, Mabuchi O, Higashigawa M, Tanimura M (2002) Marginal decrease in mortality and marked increase in incidence as a result of neuroblastoma screening at 6 months of age: cohort study in seven prefectures in Japan. J Clin Oncol 20:1209–1214

Yip BH, Pawitan Y, Czene K (2006) Parental age and risk of childhood cancers: a population-based cohort study from Sweden. Int J Epidemiol 35:1495–1503

Zhu X, Dunn J, Philips R, Goddard A, Paton K, Becker A, Gallie B (1989) Preferential germ line mutation of the paternal alley in retinoblastoma. Nature 340:312–313

Clinical Features, Diagnosis, Pathology

P. Chévez-Barrios · D. S. Gombos

Contents

3.1 Introduction 25
3.2 Initial Presentation 25
3.3 Clinical History 26
3.4 Initial Examination 27
3.5 Differential Diagnosis 27
3.6 Examination Under Anesthesia 28
3.7 Fine Needle Aspiration Biopsy 30
3.8 Grouping and Staging of Retinoblastoma 30
3.9 Pathology 30
3.10 Histologic Features 32
3.11 Extraocular Extension, Metastasis, and Prognostic Factors 33
3.12 Metastasis 36
3.13 Prognostic Factors for Metastasis 37
3.14 Trilateral Retinoblastoma and Other Tumors 37
3.15 Processing of Eyes with Retinoblastoma for Histopathologic Examination 38
References 39

3.1 Introduction

This chapter will review the clinical and histopathologic features associated with the presentation and diagnosis of retinoblastoma. A thorough appreciation of the differential and a detailed clinical assessments is the cornerstone of arriving at the proper diagnosis. Unlike most cancers, retinoblastoma is unique, as tissue is generally not necessary for diagnostic and treatment purposes. However, once the eye is enucleated, the histopathologic features guide therapy and prognosis. We will review ancillary testing that can assist the clinician and address pathologic features that can affect patient prognosis.

3.2 Initial Presentation

The vast majority of patients with retinoblastoma are referred with no known familial history or predisposition. The most common finding on presentation in North America and Western Europe is leukocoria, a white pupil (Fig. 3.1) that is generally detected by parents or family members (Wallach et al. 2006; Imhof et al. 2006; Balmer and Munier 1999). These findings may be intermittent depending upon the child's field of gaze. Photographs are helpful as they can demonstrate the presence of an abnormal white reflex retrospectively. Alternatively, leukocoria may be detected by the child's pediatrician on routine red reflex testing. Such findings should always confer an immediate referral to an ophthalmologist. Similarly, children who are unable to maintain orthophoria should be referred for a dilated funduscopic examination.

C. Rodriguez-Galindo and M.W. Wilson (eds.), *Retinoblastoma*, Pediatric Oncology,
DOI 10.1007/978-0-387-89072-2_3, © Springer Science+Business Media, LLC 2010

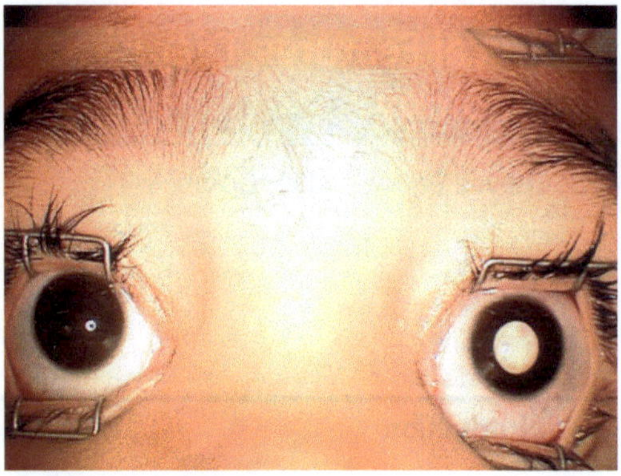

Figure 3.1

Clinical photograph of a child undergoing examination under anesthesia with leukocoria of the left eye. Notice the white pupillary reflex

Less common types of presentation occur and include redness, injection, and pain (Balasubramanya et al. 2004). These findings may present in an eye that has developed advanced disease with inflammation, increased intraocular pressure, and/or neovascular glaucoma. Blood (hyphema) or white cellular tumor deposits (pseudohypopyon) simulating inflammation in the anterior chamber of the eye may to also be signs at presentation. While trauma is not an uncommon finding in infants who develop hyphema, all children with this presentation should have retinoblastoma excluded prior to any invasive treatments (such as anterior chamber paracentesis) (Balasubramanya et al. 2004).

Orbital cellulitis is a less common means of presentation. Generally, this occurs in cases where there is significant intraocular necrosis; the cellulitis represents a secondary inflammatory response. Retinoblastoma may present in a more advanced stage with extraocular involvement. Massive proptosis with injection, swelling, and lymphadenopathy is the most common presentation in the developing world, but rare in North America or Europe (Bowman et al. 2008; Ajaiyeoba et al. 2007; Gündüz et al. 2006; Badhu et al. 2005).

Those with a known familial predisposition for retinoblastoma are generally diagnosed early in their course. These children are screened with exams under anesthesia (EUA) following birth. Small tumors are diagnosed before any clinical symptoms develop. Patients at high risk can be screened in utero with echography or imaging (MRI) (Maat-Kievit et al. 1993). Abnormal hyperechogenicity in the periocular region of the fetus may suggest development of the malignancy. Amniotic fluid can also be obtained for genetic testing (Rao et al. 2008; Pierro et al. 1993). Preterm delivery has been reported in patients diagnosed with retinoblastoma in utero in order to treat the tumor promptly.

3.3 Clinical History

A thorough and detailed clinical history is the first step in working through the differential diagnosis. One should inquire about the onset of symptoms, specifically, the timing and onset of leukocoria or strabismus. This may be supplemented with review of old photographs. The child's systemic health should be reviewed. Any recent changes in weight or appetite should be recorded. Of the ophthalmologic questions, the following should be asked has the child had any difficulties with vision, ocular preference between one eye and the other, any difficulty grasping for objects or recognizing individuals, and abnormal motility of the eye or nystagmus. In review of the child's recent medical history, it is important to record any recent trauma or illnesses, including fever or diarrhea. One should obtain an accurate birth history, including the weeks of pregnancy and any abnormalities associated with the pregnancy and/or delivery. One should inquire about any abnormal infections suffered by the mother or fetus. Postdelivery hospitalization and their course should be reviewed.

The differential diagnosis for retinoblastoma includes a number of conditions with genetic predisposition; thus, a detailed family history should be obtained (Field et al. 2007). One should review all malignancies developed in the family and inquire if any other members have had their eye removed or are known to be visually disabled or blind. In some cultures, the diagnosis of cancer may not be disclosed to other family members or the patient. Thus, it is important to inquire as to the etiology of those who are blind or who may have lost vision. It is also helpful to review any cancer syndromes or those who seem predisposed to cancer.

Ocular abnormalities that have a familial predisposition should be reviewed such as strabismus, cataracts, or visual disability. In some instances, a pedigree may be helpful in documenting abnormalities affecting siblings and distant relatives. It is important given the complexity of our modern family unit to review the family history of any birth parents and/or step children in cases where patients and siblings have different parents.

Given the differential diagnosis that includes potential exposure to infectious agents, a thorough social history should also be obtained. Any exposure to birds, cats, and dogs should be documented. In particular, one should inquire if the patient in question has been exposed to puppies and/or puppy feces. Finally, one should completely review the patient's medications and allergies.

3.4 Initial Examination

The initial clinical assessment of the child can be performed in the office setting. The child's mental status should be reviewed for an age appropriate response. Periocularly, one should assess the facial region for a normocephalic appearance. Low-set ears or a broad flat nasal bridge should be noted (due to its association with 13q deletion syndrome). The child's vision should be assessed – central steady and maintained vision and/or any strabismus should be documented. Cover/uncover testing is helpful in documenting ocular preference. The periocular area should be reviewed for any asymmetrical swelling or injection; any proptosis should be measured. If cooperative, a pupillary response should be assessed for an afferent defect. An obvious hyphema or hypopyon should be documented. In some instances, a cooperative child can be seen at the slit lamp, allowing for review of the anterior segment and iris. The intraocular pressure should be assessed by palpation and any asymmetry documented. A dilated funduscopic examination should be attempted in the office in order to confirm presence of any posterior pole masses. An initial ultrasound can be also performed to confirm an intraocular mass with findings suggestive of retinoblastoma (see echographic features of retinoblastoma under the section entitled, Examination Under Anesthesia).

Parents and siblings of the affected child should also have a dilated fundus examination to exclude any retinocytomas or spontaneously regressed retinoblastomas, which would suggest an inhereditable disease (Field et al. 2007; Smith et al. 2000).

3.5 Differential Diagnosis

There are many benign ocular conditions that can simulate retinoblastoma. Most can be differentiated with an appropriate assessment and ancillary testing (seeT able 3.1a nd Appendix).

Among the most common conditions that mimic retinoblastoma is Coats' Disease. This is an abnormality of the retinal vasculature of uncertain etiology. Patients are slightly older than most children with retinoblastoma (ages 4–10 years). Cases are usually unilateral with a predisposition in males. The lesions are associated with yellow exudative material and retinal telangiectasia. In advanced cases, massive exudation mimics a mass and the eyes develop neovascular glaucoma requiring enucleation.

Table 3.1. Differential diagnosis of retinoblastoma

Coats' disease
Persistent fetal vasculature (PFV)
Toxocariasis
Cellulitis
Metastasis
Cataract
Coloboma
Norrie's Disease
Herpes Simplex Retinitis
Cytomegalovirus Retinitis
Toxoplasmosis
Astrocytic hamartoma
Retinopathy of prematurity
Retinal detachment
Combined hamartoma of the retinal pigment epithelium
Myelinated nerve fiber

Angiography, echography, and neuroimaging can assist in distinguishing retinoblastoma from Coats' disease (Fernandes et al. 2006; Shields et al. 2001a).

Persistent fetal vasculature (PFV), also known as persistent hyperplastic primary vitreous (PHPV), is generally a unilateral condition associated with maldevelopment of the eye. These eyes present with an abnormal white reflex and associated cataract in an eye with reduced axial length. Advanced cases demonstrate ciliary processes dragged into the anterior segment. Echography can assist in measuring the axial length and demonstrating a hyaloid remnant or stalk emanating from the lens toward the optic nerve (Sun et al. 2003).

Retinopathy of prematurity (ROP), in its advanced state, can also be confused with retinoblastoma when severe neovascularization leads to retinal detachment and abnormal pupillary reflex. Today, many of these cases are indentified through routine ROP screening of at risk newborns. Infectious causes also need to be considered including toxocariasis, toxoplasmosis, congenital cytomegalovirus, and herpes simplex retinitis (Wolach et al. 1995). A metastatic neoplasm, such as leukemia, may present with a pseudohypopyon. Congenital abnormalities, such as retinoschisis, cataracts, and colobomas, can lead to an abnormal white pupillary reflex, but are generally easily distinguished from retinoblastoma under anesthetic exam. Norries' disease is a rare X-linked recessive abnormality associated with bilateral posterior pole masses. Retinal astrocytic hamartomas can appear similar to retinoblastoma foci, but are generally associated with syndromes such as tuberous sclerosis or neurofibromatosis.

3.6 Examination Under Anesthesia

One of the most critical aspects in the diagnosis of retinoblastoma is a careful funduscopic examination. Although not universal, the vast majority of retinoblastoma centers perform this under anesthesia. This includes a formal assessment of intraocular pressure (with Schiotz/Perkins tonometry or similar method). The patient is then examined for any abnormalities, such as cleft pallet or cleft lip, which may be associated with genetic syndromes. The anterior segment of the eye is assessed with microscopy. The conjunctiva and sclera should be assessed for any abnormal hyperpigmentation, mass, or injection. The cornea is reviewed for edema and its diameters are measured with calipers to assess for enlarged dimensions. The anterior chamber should be checked for signs of inflammation and the iris for nodularity or rubeosis. The lens should be assessed for any opacity, and ciliary processes should be documented if appreciated.

A funduscopic examination is performed with indirect ophthalmoscopy and gentle scleral depression to the ora serrata. Small retinoblastoma lesions may appear as translucent flat or dome shaped lesions. Associated lens opacity is rare, and the eyes are of normal axial length. As the tumors increase in size, they often take on a white or off-white, chalky color. Vascular dilatation and tortuosity is often associated in the form of a feeder vessel. Frank calcification can occasionally be seen and is highly suggestive of retinoblastoma (Figs. 3.2 and 3.3). Classically, the tumors are subdivided depending upon their growth pattern. The endophytic tumor grows into the vitreous cavity, while the exophytic form grows into the subretinal space elevating the retina. A third, albeit rare, subtype, is the diffuse infiltrating retinoblastoma, which can be the most challenging to diagnose, as a frank mass is not appreciated. Most often these cases occur unilaterally

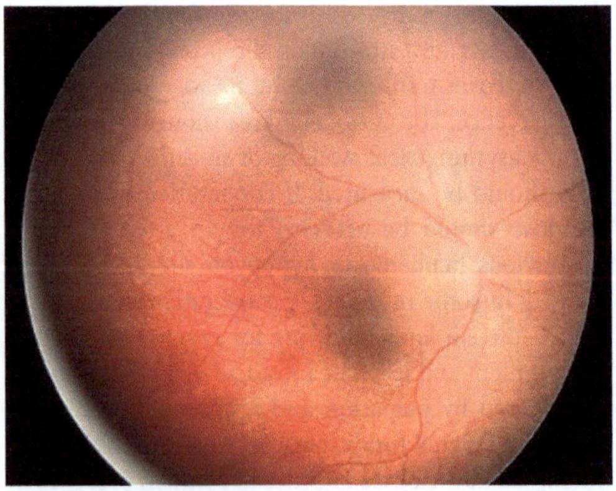

Figure 3.2

Fundus photograph of the right eye with a small- to medium-size superior temporal tan white retinal tumor

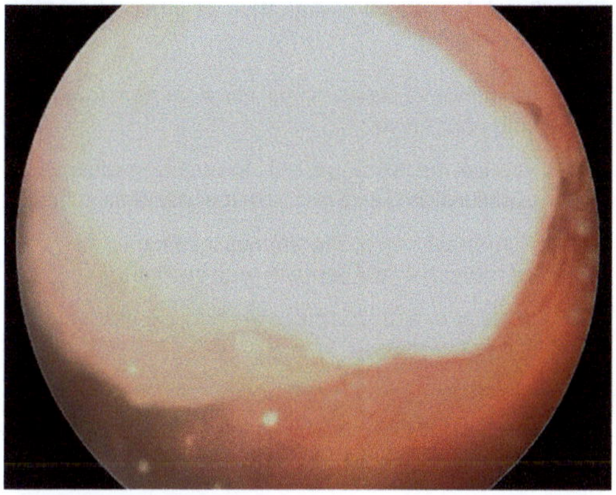

Figure 3.3

Fundus photograph of an eye with a large retinal and vitreous tumor with vitreous seeds. Notice the bright white color of the large mass and the small inferiorly located tumors floating in the vitreous

in older children and are sometimes mistaken for Coats' disease or inflammatory process with pseudo-hypopyon (Shields et al. 1991, 2001a).

In addition to a careful and thorough assessment of all lesions, the vitreous should be assessed for any signs of vitreous debris. Findings, such as retinal exudates and telangiectasia, are often associated with pseudoretinoblastoma such as Coats' disease. These lesions generally take on a more yellow color. Vitritis or tractional abnormalities are associated with inflammatory conditions such as toxocariasis (Wolach et al. 1995). In addition to retinal drawings, most centers obtain baseline fundus photography with use of a contact camera (RetCam® Clarity Medical Systems, Pleasanton, CA, USA). This instrument allows for photography and angiography throughout the posterior pole.

Ancillary testing should be obtained during the initial EUA. Ophthalmic echography is a critical tool in the diagnosis of retinoblastoma. Typically, on A-scan retinoblastoma foci demonstrate high internal echoes. On B-scan, calcified lesions demonstrate areas of high echogenicity with a characteristic loss of tissue echoes directly behind the tumor. While the diagnosis of retinoblastoma can be performed without fluorescein angiography, a number of centers perform this at baseline. Angiogram testing generally demonstrates an intense hyperfluorescence and a fine vascular network within moderately sized tumors. Late phases of the angiogram show marked staining and leakage.

Neuroimaging of the brain and orbit must always be performed at baseline. Neuroimaging should encompass the globe, orbit, central nervous system, and pineal region. The scans noninvasively demonstrate features supportive of a retinoblastoma diagnosis and can further assess the orbit for features of extraocular disease (Amoaku et al. 1996). In addition, imaging of the brain helps to rule out metastatic disease and so-called "trilateral retinoblastoma" of the pineal region (Gündüz et al. 2006; Amoaku et al. 1996; Bagley et al. 1996; Duncan et al. 2001).

Historically, the preferred imaging modality was the computed tomography (CT) scan. The significant calcification associated with retinoblastoma is easily visualized and its presence is highly correlative of retinoblastoma. However, lack of calcification does not rule out the malignancy. In recent years, spiral CT has gained interest in some centers due to the shortened acquisition time and limited need for general anesthesia. A number of experts have raised concern regarding the routine use of CT scans in patients at risk for retinoblastoma due radiation exposure. As a result, some oncologists prefer Magnetic Resonance Imaging (MRI) of the brain and orbit instead of CT. The advantages of this approach include limiting radiation exposure as well as improved visualization of the periorbital structures and orbital portion of the optic nerve (Apushkin et al. 2005; Bagley et al. 1996; O'Brien 2001; Brisse et al. 2007). Some reports have suggested MRI as a helpful adjunct in distinguishing Coats' disease from retinoblastoma.

Historically, lumbar puncture and bone marrow biopsy were performed at the time of diagnosis of retinoblastoma. In most centers, this approach has been abandoned unless the patient has altered complete blood counts, high-risk features such as extraocular orbital/CNS disease or massive choroidal involvement on histopathologic review (Azar et al. 2003). In cases where there exists continued ambiguity regarding the diagnosis, serology can be helpful in detecting elevated antibodies for select infectious etiologies including toxoplasmosis, toxocara canis, cytomegalovirus virus, and herpes infection.

3.7 Fine Needle Aspiration Biopsy

Under the vast majority of circumstances, the diagnosis of retinoblastoma can be performed without the need for cytopathologic confirmation. There have been a number of case reports citing extraocular extension and seeding of the tumor in the orbit, following vitrectomy of eyes with unexpected retinoblastoma or needle biopsy. Most experts do not recommend such an approach. However, under very select circumstances and only under the care of experienced ocular oncologists and ocular pathologists, needle biopsy has been described using a transcorneal method through the peripheral iris. Under all circumstances, a pars plana approach should be avoided (Shanmugam and Biswas 1997; Karcioglu 2002; Robertson 1997).

3.8 Grouping and Staging of Retinoblastoma

Generally, staging of the patient is performed by the pediatric oncologist while the grouping of the eye is performed by the ocular oncologist. Historically, the Reese–Ellsworth classification has been used to group eyes with intraocular retinoblastoma (see Table 3.2) (Kiss et al. 2008). The classification progresses from group Ia to Group Vb with more advanced grouping harboring a worse prognosis when treated with primary external beam radiation therapy. In recent years, a new system has been devised, referred to as the ABC system also known as the International Classification for Intraocular Retinoblastoma (see Table 3.3 and Appendix) (Kiss et al. 2008). The system groups the eye from A through E and is generally associated with best to worst prognosis associated with treatment including focal modalities and systemic chemotherapy. Eyes that are not felt to be salvageable including those with neovascular glaucoma, massive intraocular hemorrhage, and involvement of the anterior segment are generally classified as unsalvageable, group E.

Table 3.2. Reese–Ellsworth grouping

Ia	Solitary tumor <4 dd in size at or behind the equator
Ib	Multiple tumors, none >4 dd in size at or behind the equator
IIa	Solitary tumor 4–10 dd in size at or behind the equator
IIb	Multiple tumors 4–10 dd in size behind the equator
IIIa	Any lesion anterior to the equator
IIIb	Solitary tumor >10 dd in size behind the equator
IVa	Multiple tumors some >10 dd in size
IVb	Any lesion anterior to the ora serrata
Va	Massive tumor involving >50% of retina
Vb	Vitreous seeding

dd = disc diameters

Table 3.3. International classification of intraocular retinoblastoma grouping

A	No tumor >3 mm in dimension; away from fovea and optic nerve
B	Any eye not in Group A with no vitreous seeding, subretinal fluid is <5 mm from the base of the tumor
C	Tumors with focal fine vitreous seeding or subretinal fluid (less than one quadrant)
D	Massive or diffuse vitreous seeding, extensive subretinal masses
E	Unsalvageable eyes; neovascular glaucoma, tumor touching the lens, anterior segment tumor, phthisis, diffuse infiltrating retinoblastoma

A committee of retinoblastoma experts from large centers worldwide has developed a consensus classification for systemic staging. Patients are classified according to extent of disease and the presence of overt extraocular extension. In addition, a proposal for substaging considering histopathological features of enucleated specimens is presented to further discriminate between Stage I and II patients. Table 3.4 shows a summary of the classification system (Chantada and Doz 2006).

3.9 Pathology

Retinoblastoma originates in the sensory retina, expanding the retina and involving the vitreous cavity. The cell of origin of retinoblastoma is still unknown, but it represents a retinoblast with high mitotic activity and apoptotic rate (Nork et al. 1995). Gross features of retinoblastoma include a white-gray tumor with a chalky appearance and a soft, friable consistency.

Table 3.4. International staging system for retinoblastoma

Stage 0: Patients treated conservatively (subject to presurgical ophthalmologic classifications)
Stage I: Eye enucleated, completely resected histologically
Stage II: Eye enucleated, microscopic residual tumor
Stage III: Regional extension (a) overt orbital disease (b) preauricular or cervical lymph node extension
Stage IV: Metastatic disease (a) hematogenous metastasis: (1) single lesion (2) multiple lesions (b) CNS extension: (1) prechiasmatic lesion (2) CNS mass (3) leptomeningeal disease

Bright white speckles corresponding to calcifications are found throughout the tumor (Fig. 3.4). The gross features of retinoblastoma depend on the growth pattern of the tumor (McLean et al. 1994; Hurwitz et al. 2002). Some of these patterns correlate with clinical presentations and differences in biological behavior.

Tumors with endophytic growth pattern arise from the retina and grow into the vitreous cavity (Fig. 3.5). These tumors tend to entirely fill the cavity and produce floating tumor spheres called vitreous seeds. If tumor is left untreated, it eventually invades the anterior portion of the eye reaching the conjunctiva. From there, the tumor can permeate the lymphatic vessels and metastasize to regional lymph nodes (McLean et al. 1994; Hurwitz et al. 2002; Chévez-Barrios et al. 2007).

Exophytic retinoblastomas grow from the retina into the subretinal space and often cause serous

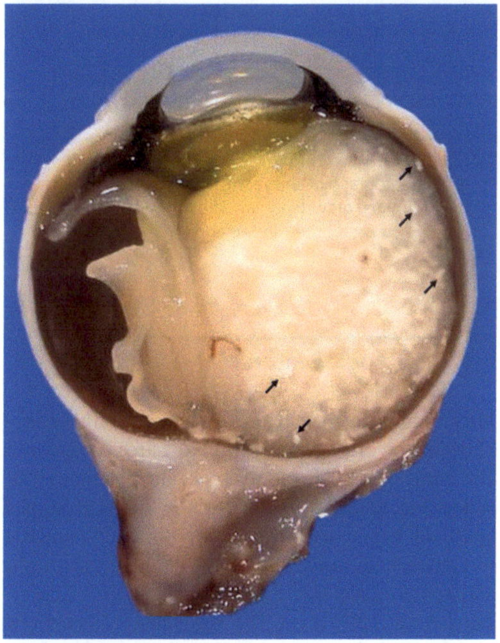

Figure 3.4

Gross photograph of an eye with retinoblastoma after initial removal of the superior calotte. Notice the tan white color of the tumor with small brighter white speckles that represent calcifications (*arrows*)

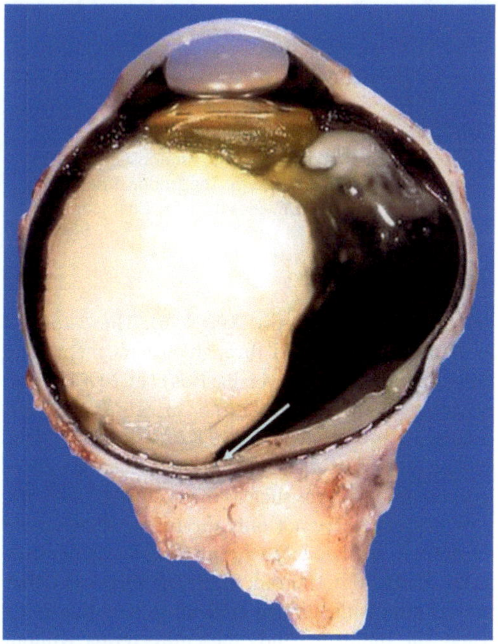

Figure 3.5

Gross photograph of an eye with retinoblastoma with an endophytic growth pattern. The tumor arises from the retina (*arrow*) and grows into the vitreous

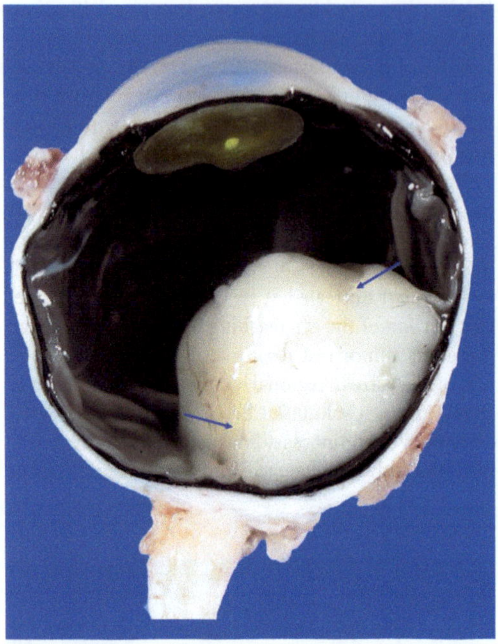

Figure 3.6

Gross photograph of an eye with retinoblastoma with an exophytic growth pattern. The tumor arises from the retina (*arrow*) and invades the subretinal space

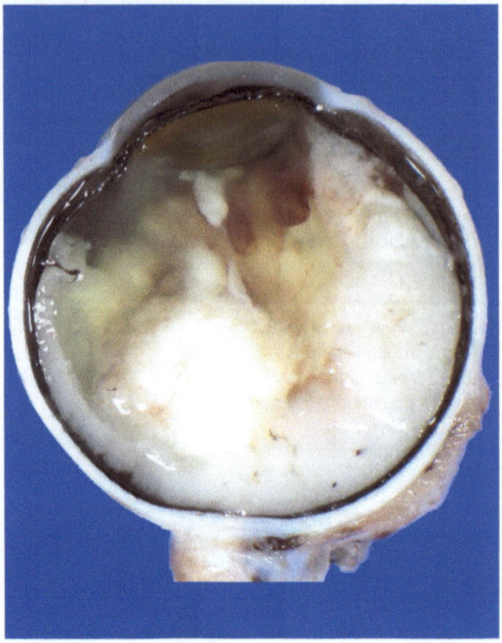

Figure 3.7

Gross photograph of an eye with retinoblastoma with an undetermined growth pattern. The tumor obliterates the retina and invades the vitreous and the subretinal space

detachments of the retina (Fig. 3.6). These tumors may invade the choroid through Bruch's membrane (Hurwitz et al. 2002; Chévez-Barrios et al. 2007). Mixed endophytic and exophytic tumor growth is the most common pattern encountered (Hurwitz et al. 2002; Chévez-Barrios et al. 2007) (Fig. 3.7). There are other less common patterns such as the extensively necrotic presentation, where not only the tumor shows more than 90% necrosis but also the intra-ocular tissues such as the ciliary body, choroid, and retina (Fig. 3.8). Other presentation is the diffuse infiltrating retinoblastoma where the tumor expands the entire retina without forming a discrete tumor mass and it tends to invade the anterior segment with a pseudohypopyon (McLean et al. 1994; Hurwitz et al. 2002; Chévez-Barrios et al. 2007; Croxatto et al. 1983; Shields et al. 1988).

3.10 Histologic Features

Microscopic examination of the eye with retinoblastoma reveals a tumor with large areas of necrosis and multifocal calcifications replacing portions of the retina (Fig. 3.9a). The majority of the tumor is formed by small hyperchromatic cells with a high nuclear to cytoplasmic ratio. The tumor cells are mitotically and apoptotically active (Hurwitz et al. 2002; Chévez-Barrios et al. 2007) (Fig. 3.9b). The viable cells surround blood vessels in a range of 90–110 micro forming a collarette (pseudorosettes) (Fig. 3.9c). Viability of the tumor cells depends on the intrinsic tumor blood supply. Areas of coagulative necrosis contain multiple foci of dystrophic calcification.

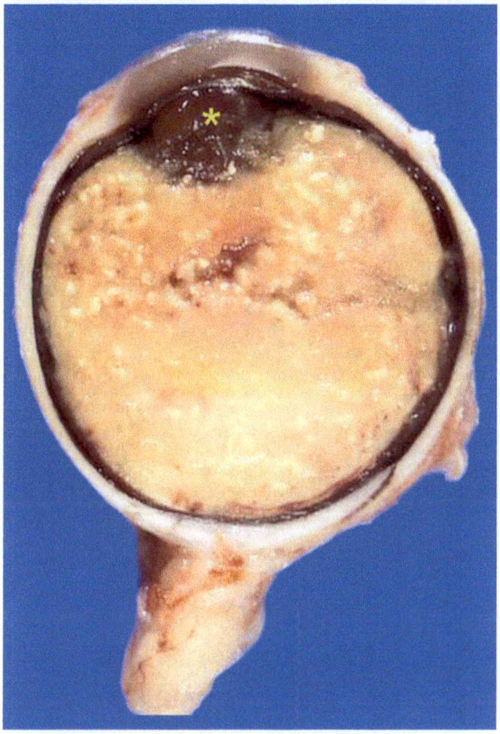

Figure 3.8

Gross photograph of an eye with extensively necrotic retinoblastoma. The tumor is tan with areas of hemorrhages and mostly necrotic. The intraocular structures are also necrotic. The lens (*) is cataractous

Some retinoblastomas show large areas of undifferentiated or poorly differentiated tumor; other tumors show a certain degree of differentiation represented by formation of rosettes. Flexner-Wintersteiner rosettes are highly characteristic of retinoblastoma, although they are also seen in pinealoblastomas and medulloepitheliomas. Flexner-Wintersteiner rosettes are lined by tall cuboidal cells that circumscribe an apical lumen. The apical ends attach to each other by terminal bars, and the cells may have apical cytoplasmic projections into the lumen of the rosette (Fig. 3.10a) (McLean et al. 1994; Hurwitz et al. 2002; Chévez-Barrios et al. 2007). Homer Wright rosettes are less common than Flexner-Wintersteiner rosettes, and they are found in a variety of neuroblastic tumors in addition to retinoblastoma. These rosettes do not surround a lumen, but rather extend cytoplasmic processes that fill the center of the rosette. Homer Wright rosettes may be incomplete and admixed with well-formed Flexner-Wintersteiner rosettes (Fig. 3.10b).

About 6–10% of tumors show benign photoreceptor differentiation into groups of cells with short cytoplasmic processes, abundant cytoplasm, and small round nuclei similar to photoreceptors. These groups of cells, which resemble a bouquet of flowers, are called "fleurettes" (Ts'o et al. 1970a; Ts'o et al. 1970b). Neither significant mitotic activity nor necrosis is observed within the fleurettes (Fig. 3.10c).

A benign counterpart of retinoblastoma called retinocytoma (also retinoma) that solely contains well-differentiated glial cells and fleurettes has been described. These benign tumors contain areas of abrupt calcification associated with retinal pigment epithelium proliferation. These tumors also contain the *RB1* mutations similar to their malignant counterpart (Singh et al. 2000; Dimaras et al. 2008; Margo et al. 1983).

3.11 Extraocular Extension, Metastasis, and Prognostic Factors

Optic nerve invasion: If left untreated, retinoblastoma usually fills the eye and completely destroys the internal architecture of the globe. The most common route of spread is by invasion through the optic nerve. However, the size of the tumor is not always the defining factor for invasion as there are small tumors that invade the optic nerve. The tumor may invade only the optic nerve head, and this is considered as intraocular invasion, which carries almost the same prognosis than no optic nerve invasion (Fig. 3.11) (Chantada et al. 2009; Spencer 1975; Karcioglu et al. 1997; Tosi et al. 1989; Kopelman et al. 1987). However, once in the nerve, the tumor tends to spread directly along the nerve fiber bundles toward the optic chiasm, passing through the lamina

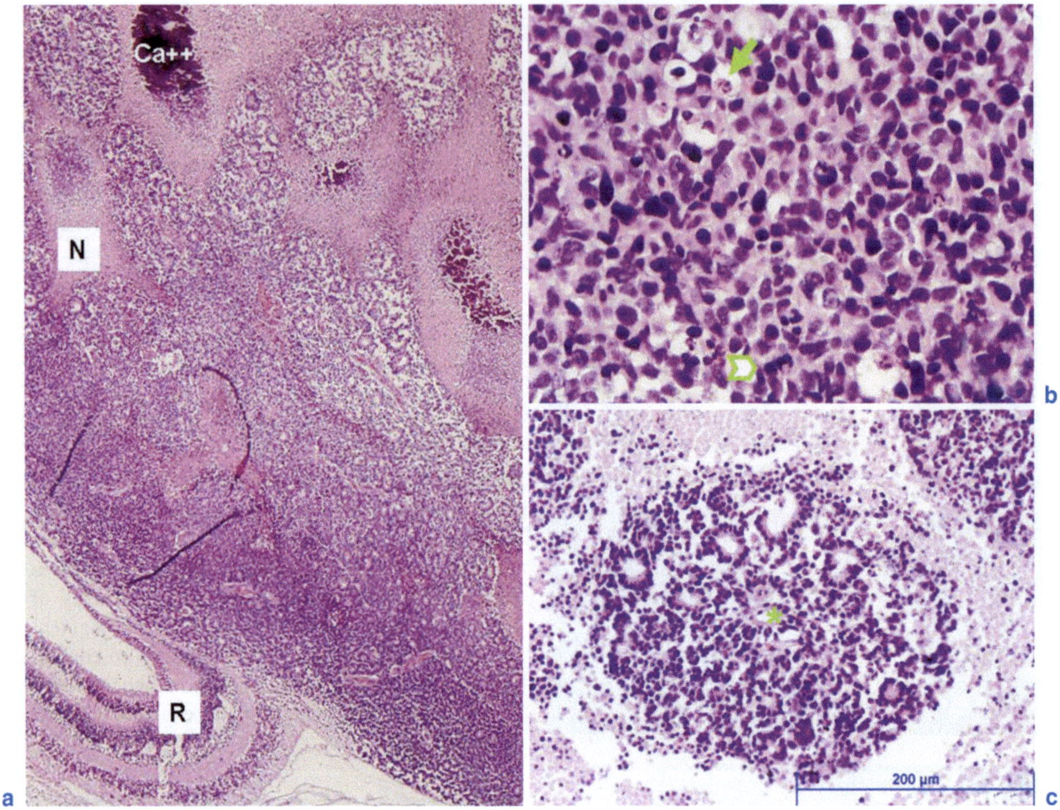

Figure 3.9 a–c

Histologic characteristics of retinoblastoma. a The tumor arises from the retina (R) and has geographic areas of necrosis (N) and dystrophic areas of calcification (Ca++). (H&E. Original magnification 10×). b The tumor is composed by medium-sized undifferentiated cells with hyperchromatic nuclei and many mitotic figures (*open arrow*) and frequent apoptosis (*solid arrow*). (H&E. Original magnification 40×). c Perivascular sleeves of tumor (pseudorosettes) seen surrounding a blood vessel (*). Away from the vessels the tumor undergoes necrosis. (H&E. Original magnification 20×)

cribrosa and into the retrolaminar area. This is now considered extraocular extension as the lamina cribrosa is the equivalent of the sclera. Patients with retrolaminar invasion carry worst prognosis for metastasis, and the prognosis is worse as the tumor infiltrates farther toward the chiasm and nearer the surgical margin. The tumor may also infiltrate through the pia into the subarachnoid space and from there into the brain and the spine (McLean et al. 1994; Hurwitz et al. 2002; Chévez-Barrios et al. 2007; Chantada et al. 2009; Spencer 1975; Karcioglu et al. 1997; Tosi et al. 1989; Kopelman et al. 1987) .

Uveal invasion: The second major route of spread is through massive involvement of the choroid into the orbit via either scleral canals or by direct extension through the sclera (McLean et al. 1994; Hurwitz et al. 2002; Chévez-Barrios et al. 2007; Chantada et al. 2009; Spencer 1975; Karcioglu et al. 1997; Tosi et al. 1989; Kopelman et al. 1987). Extraocular extension generally

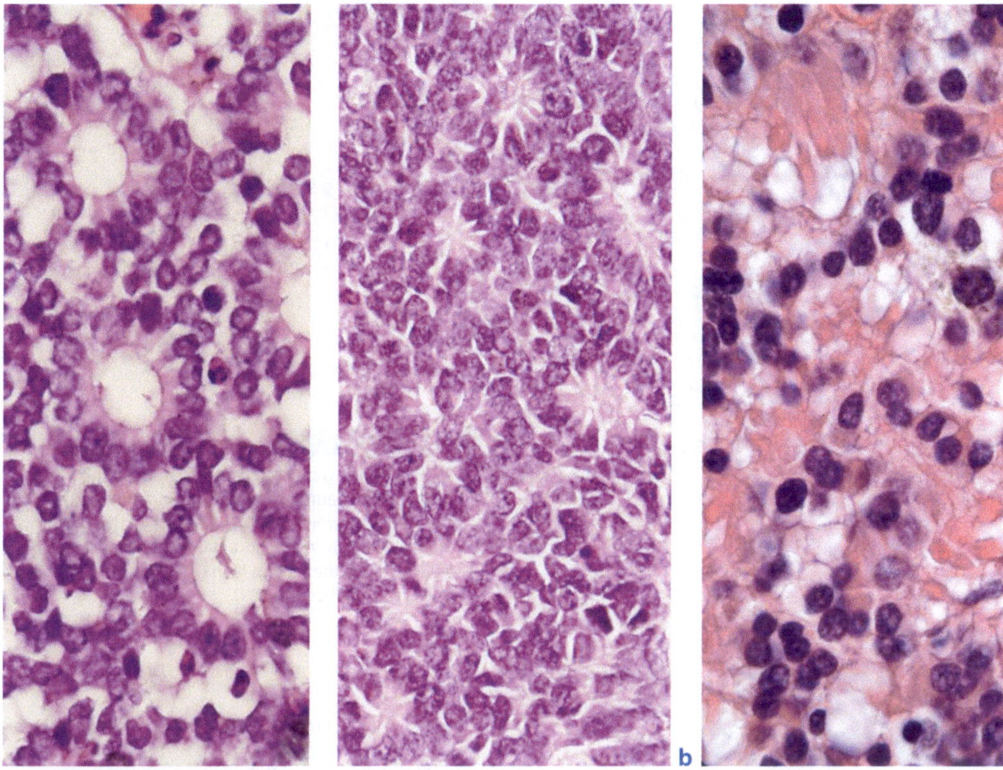

Figure 3.10 a–c

Characteristic formation of tumor cells into rosettes and fleurettes. a Flexner-Wintersteiner rosettes show an empty center and a membrane similar to that of the outer limiting membrane in the normal retina. b Homer Wright rosettes display a center that is filled by cellular prolongations of the cytoplasm. c Fleurettes are very well-differentiated structures that closely resemble groups of photoreceptors. Mitoses or apoptosis are rarely seen in these cells

occurs within six months if intraocular tumors are left untreated. The definition of focal versus massive choroidal invasion and the decision to treat have been controversial (Chantada et al. 2009; Spencer 1975; Karcioglu et al. 1997; Tosi et al. 1989; Kopelman et al. 1987). Recently, the Children's Oncology Group (COG) and the International Retinoblastoma Staging Working Group have proposed an objective classification based on specific anatomic location and size of the tumor. Focal choroidal invasion is then defined as any focus that is less than 3 mm in maximum diameter and does not reach the sclera (Fig. 3.12). Massive choroidal invasion is any focus of tumor measuring 3 mm or more in maximum diameter and reaches the sclera. However, if the tumor is more than 3 mm but does not reach the sclera, it is considered massive invasion. Currently, there are ongoing clinical prospective trials testing these definitions and their prognostic value through COG (ARET0332).

Extraocular extension dramatically increases the chances of hematogenous and lymphatic spread. Tumor may reach metastatic sites through four routes (Table 3.5) (McLean et al. 1994; Hurwitz et al. 2002; Chévez-Barriose ta l. 2007).

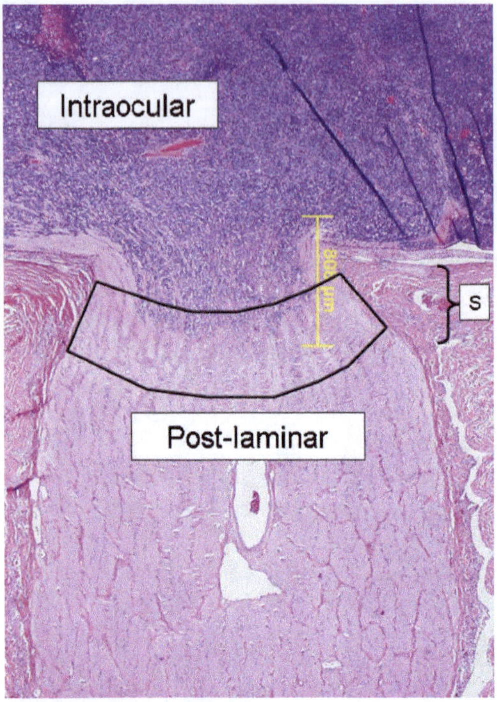

Figure 3.11

Optic nerve invasion by retinoblastoma tumor. The tumor in this photograph is invading mostly the prelaminar (*intraocular*) portion of the optic nerve. However, the tumor invades the superficial layers of the lamina cribrosa (depicted by the black line). The depth of invasion is approximately 0.8 mm. The lamina cribrosa is the area of the optic nerve corresponding to the sclera(s). The postlaminar optic nerve is free of tumor in this example. (H&E. Original magnification 2×)

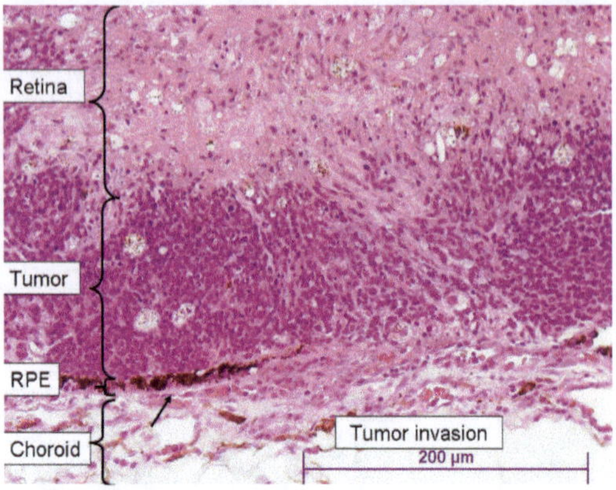

Figure 3.12

Choroidal invasion by retinoblastoma. The tumor arising and invading the retina has penetrated Bruch's membrane (*arrow*) and invaded the choroid. This example is of a focal choroidal invasion as the focus measures less than 3 mm in maximum diameter. (H&E. Original magnification 10×)

Table 3.5. Routes of retinoblastoma tumor to distant metastasis

1. Direct infiltration of tumor:
   (a) Optic nerve into the brain
   (b) Choroid into the orbit soft tissues and bones
2. Dispersion of the tumor cells through the subarachnoid space of the optic nerve to:
   (a) Opposite optic nerve
   (b) CSF into the brain and spine
3. Hematogenous dissemination to lung, bone, and brain secondary to:
   (a) Orbital and bone invasion
   (b) Lymphatic invasion reaching the lymph nodes
4. Lymphatic dissemination:
   (a) Tumors with anterior spread into conjunctiva and eyelids
   (b) Conjunctiva and skin lymphatic channels drain into regional lymph nodes.

3.12 Metastasis

Histologically, metastases of retinoblastoma are less differentiated than intraocular tumors. Rosettes are rarely encountered and fleurettes have never been described. When very well-differentiated extraocular tumors appear outside of the orbit, a differential diagnosis of a primary primitive neuroectodermal tumor (PNET) must be considered (McLean et al. 1994; Hurwitz et al. 2002; Chévez-Barrios et al. 2007).

3.13 Prognostic Factors for Metastasis

Metastatic disease is still associated with a poor prognosis. Most clinical findings are not useful in predicting the occurrence of metastasis in children with retinoblastoma. However, histopathologic features may provide a good evaluation. Multivariate statistical analysis has suggested the correlation of certain histopathologic findings and prognostic risk factors (Chantada et al. 2009; Spencer 1975; Karcioglu et al. 1997; Tosi et al. 1989; Kopelman et al. 1987). The two most important prognostic indicators for the development of metastasis are the presence of tumor in the optic nerve posterior to the lamina cribrosa at the site of surgical transection and extrascleral extension of tumor into the orbit (McLean et al. 1994; Hurwitz et al. 2002; Chévez-Barrios et al. 2007; Chantada et al. 2009; Spencer 1975; Karcioglu et al. 1997; Tosi et al. 1989; Kopelman et al. 1987). The extent of tumor invasion in the optic nerve correlates with prognosis. Superficial invasion of the optic disc is associated with a mortality rate of 10%, a rate similar to that seen when the optic nerve is not involved. The presence of tumor up to the lamina cribrosa is associated with a mortality rate of 29%. Invasion of tumor posterior to the lamina cribrosa is associated with a mortality rate of 42%, while the presence of tumor at the transected surgical margin is associated with a mortality of 80% (Chantada et al. 2009; Spencer 1975; Karcioglu et al. 1997; Tosi et al. 1989; Kopelman et al. 1987).

Choroidal invasion: Massive, but not focal, invasion of the choroid by tumor increases the possibility for hematogenous spread, either through vascular permeation of choroidal vessels or more frequently by extension through the sclera into the orbital tissues (Tosi et al. 1989; Kopelman et al. 1987) (Fig. 3.12).

Other factors: Extensive ocular tissue and tumor necrosis (more than 95% of tumor) has been associated with histologic high-risk prognostic factors for tumor metastasis and mortality (Chong et al. 2006). Vascularization of tumor is also a proposed risk factor for metastasis that is currently under study (Jia et al. 2007; Jockovich et al. 2007; Apte and Harbour 2007; Marback et al. 2003). Other factors that had been proposed are invasion into the iris and neovascularization of the iris with secondary glaucoma (Baez et al. 1994).

3.14 Trilateral Retinoblastoma and Other Tumors

Trilateral retinoblastoma is a well-recognized, although rare, syndrome. Primary retinoblastomas of the pineal and parasellar sites have been called trilateral retinoblastoma and usually present as single tumors. Tumors of the suprasellar region tend to present earlier than tumors of the pineal region after the diagnosis of intraocular tumors. Most of the cases involved patients with a family history of retinoblastoma, and the disease is usually fatal. The prognosis of children who develop trilateral retinoblastoma is dismal with current treatment strategies. Because patients who were asymptomatic at the time of diagnosis of intracranial disease had a better overall survival than those who were symptomatic, screening for intracranial tumors may be a valuable strategy in the management of patients with bilateral and/or hereditary retinoblastoma (Antoneli et al. 2007; Shields et al. 2001b; Kivelä 1999; Paulino 1999). In recent years, coinciding with the use of systemic chemotherapy for the treatment of bilateral retinoblastoma, there has been a decrease in the number of patients with trilateral presentation. The reason may be the adjuvant treatment of small incipient tumors in the pineal and parasellar sites with the chemotherapy used for the ocular tumors (Shields et al. 2001b). These tumors may appear several years after successful treatment of intraocular retinoblastoma. They may be far more differentiated than the primary tumor and may contain numerous rosettes, fleurettes, and individual cells showing photoreceptor differentiation. Trilateral retinoblastoma is different from metastatic retinoblastoma; in that metastatic retinoblastoma presents as multiple, undifferentiated tumors within the first two years of initial treatment.

3.15 Processing of Eyes with Retinoblastoma for Histopathologic Examination

It is important to adequately process the eye with retinoblastoma after enucleation because the histopathologic features may guide adjuvant treatment and prognosis. It is also recommended that in unilateral retinoblastoma, genetic studies of the tumor be performed. To this end, the eye needs to be opened immediately after enucleation to obtain fresh tumor. In general, the first step is to orient the eye to decide where to perform the incision. The orientation of the eye is performed by the localization of the inferior oblique that inserts directly in the sclera under the macular area (temporal to the optic nerve). After orientation, cross-section of the optic nerve margin should be obtained to avoid contamination with fresh tumor. The optic nerve section is submitted for histologic examination in a separate cassette. The eye is then open creating a controlled opening at the level of the equator, carefully avoiding forceful manipulation or involving structures of the optic nerve. Samples of the tumor (3–4 mm in maximum diameter) may be obtained from the cup of sclera created by the section, especially avoiding traction of the retina or other intraocular structures. The tumor is immediately frozen for future studies. The eye can then be placed in adequate amount of formalin to allow fixation for at least 48 h. After adequate fixation, the eye can be further sectioned to obtain a central section that includes the pupil of the iris and the optic nerve – the PO section. The two caps of the eye resulting from this cut are referred as calottes and

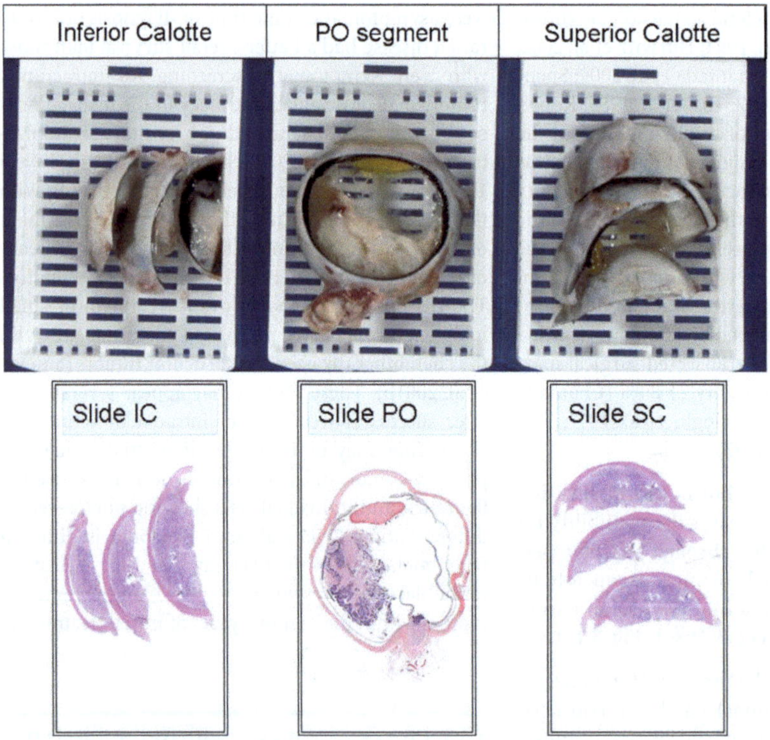

Figure 3.13

Processing of eyes with retinoblastoma. The top row shows the eye after sectioning. The central portion of the eye that contains the pupil and the optic nerve (PO segment) is submitted in one cassette. The inferior and superior calottes are further sectioned into anterior–posterior segments and submitted in one cassette per calotte. The bottom row represents the sections on the slides from each cassette to demonstrate the representation of the structures in each slide

should be also submitted for examination. It is preferable to further section these calottes in an anterior-posterior direction to obtain 3–4 segments to evaluate as much choroidal surface as possible. The calottes segments can be submitted in one cassette per calotte (Fig. 3.13). The resulting slides to be examined should include levels of the PO section, the 2 calottes and the cross-section of the optic nerve (Fig. 3.13).

References

Ajaiyeoba AI, Olusanya BA, Komolafe OO, Akang EE (2007) Clinical presentation of retinoblastoma: a tertiary hospital experience. Afr J Med Med Sci 36(3):289–290

Amoaku WM, Willshaw HE, Parkes SE, Shah KJ, Mann JR (1996) Trilateral retinoblastoma. A report of five patients. Cancer 78(4):858–863

Antoneli CB, Ribeiro Kde C, Sakamoto LH, Chojniak MM, Novaes PE, Arias VE (2007) Trilateral retinoblastoma. Pediatr Blood Cancer 48(3):306–310

Apte RS, Harbour JW (2007) Inhibiting angiogenesis in retinoblastoma. Ophthalmic Res 39(4):188–190

Apushkin MA, Apushkin MA, Shapiro MJ, Mafee MF (2005) Retinoblastoma and simulating lesions: role of imaging. Neuroimaging Clin N Am 15(1):49–67

Azar D, Donaldson C, Dalla-Pozza L (2003) Questioning the need for routine bone marrow aspiration and lumbar puncture in patients with retinoblastoma. Clin Experiment Ophthalmol 31(1):57–60

Badhu B, Sah SP, Thakur SK, Dulal S, Kumar S, Sood A, Das H, Sah RP (2005) Clinical presentation of retinoblastoma in Eastern Nepal. Clin Experiment Ophthalmol 33(4):386–389

Baez KA, Ulbig MW, Cater J, Shields CL, Shields JA (1994) Iris neovascularization, increased intraocular pressure and vitreous hemorrhage as risk factors for invasion of the optic nerve and choroid in children with retinoblastoma. Ophthalmologe 91(6):796–800

Bagley LJ, Hurst RW, Zimmerman RA, Shields JA, Shields CL, De Potter P (1996) Imaging in the trilateral retinoblastoma syndrome. Neuroradiology 38(2):166–170

Balasubramanya R, Pushker N, Bajaj MS, Ghose S, Kashyap S, Rani A (2004) Atypical presentations of retinoblastoma. J Pediatr Ophthalmol Strabismus 41(1):18–24

Balmer A, Munier F (1999) Leukokoria in a child: emergency and challenge. Klin Monatsbl Augenheilkd 214(5): 332–335

Bowman RJ, Mafwiri M, Luthert P, Luande J, Wood M (2008) Outcome of retinoblastoma in east Africa. Pediatr Blood Cancer5 o(1):160–162

Brisse HJ, Guesmi M, Aerts I, Sastre-Garau X, Savignoni A, Lumbroso-Le Rouic L, Desjardins L, Doz F, Asselain B, Bours D, Neuenschwander S (2007) Relevance of CT and MRI in retinoblastoma for the diagnosis of postlaminar invasion with normal-size optic nerve: a retrospective study of 150 patients with histological comparison. Pediatr Radiol 37(7):649–656

Chantada G, Doz F, Antoneli CB, Grundy R, Clare Stannard FF, Dunkel IJ, Grabowski E, Leal-Leal C, Rodríguez-Galindo C, Schvartzman E, Popovic MB, Kremens B, Meadows AT, Zucker JM (2006) A proposal for an international retinoblastoma staging system. Pediatr Blood Cancer 47(6):801–805

Chantada GL, Guitter MR, Fandiño AC, Raslawski EC, de Davila MT, Vaiani E, Scopinaro MJ (2009) Treatment results in patients with retinoblastoma and invasion to the cut end of the optic nerve. Pediatr Blood Cancer 52(2):218–222

Chévez-Barrios P, Eagle RC, Marbach P (2007) Histological features and risks for metastatic spread of retinoblastoma. In: Singh AD, Damato B, Pe'er J, Murphree AL, Perry JD (eds) Clinical ocular oncology, 1st edn. Elsevier, Saunders, London Section 6–77

Chong EM, Coffee RE, Chintagumpala M, Hurwitz RL, Hurwitz MY, Chevez-Barrios P (2006) Extensively necrotic retinoblastoma is associated with high-risk prognostic factors. Arch Pathol Lab Med 130(11):1669–1672

Croxatto JO, Fernandez Meijide R, Malbran ES (1983) Retinoblastoma masquerading as ocular inflammation. Ophthalmologica 186:48–53

Dimaras H, Khetan V, Halliday W, Orlic M, Prigoda NL, Piovesan B, Marrano P, Corson TW, Eagle RC Jr, Squire JA, Gallie BL (2008) Loss of RB1 induces non-proliferative retinoma: increasing genomic instability correlates with progression to retinoblastoma. Hum Mol Genet 17(10):1363–1372

Duncan JL, Scott IU, Murray TG, Gombos DS, van Quill K, O'Brien JM (2001) Routine neuroimaging in retinoblastoma for the detection of intracranial tumors. Arch Ophthalmol 119(3):450–452

Fernandes BF, Odashiro AN, Maloney S, Zajdenweber ME, Lopes AG, Burnier MN Jr (2006) Clinical-histopathological correlation in a case of Coats' disease. Diagn Pathol 1:24

Field M, Shanley S, Kirk J (2007) Inherited cancer susceptibility syndromes in paediatric practice. J Paediatr Child Health 43(4):219–229

Gündüz K, Müftüoglu O, Günalp I, Unal E, Taçyildiz N (2006) Metastatic retinoblastoma clinical features, treatment, and prognosis. Ophthalmology 113(9):1558–1566 Epub 2006 Jul 7

Hurwitz RL, Chévez-Barrios P, Chintagumpala M, Shields C, Shields J (2002) Retinoblastoma. In: Pizzo PA, Poplack D (eds) Principles and practice of pediatric oncology, 4th edn. Lippincott-Raven, Philadelphia, pp 825–846 (4th 2002 and 5th edn 2006)

Imhof SM, Moll AC, Schouten-van Meeteren AY (2006) Stage of presentation and visual outcome of patients screened for familial retinoblastoma: nationwide registration

in the Netherlands. Br J Ophthalmol 90(7):875–878 Epub 2006 Apr 13
Jia RB, Zhang P, Zhou YX, Song X, Liu HY, Wang LZ, Luo M, Lu J, Ge SF, Fan XQ (2007) VEGF-targeted RNA interference suppresses angiogenesis and tumor growth of retinoblastoma. Ophthalmic Res 39(2):108–115
Jockovich ME, Suarez F, Alegret A, Piña Y, Hayden B, Cebulla C, Feuer W, Murray TG (2007) Mechanism of retinoblastoma tumor cell death after focal chemotherapy, radiation, and vascular targeting therapy in a mouse model. Invest Ophthalmol Vis Sci 48(12):5371–5376
Karcioglu ZA (2002) Fine needle aspiration biopsy (FNAB) for retinoblastoma. Retina 22(6):707–710
Karcioglu ZA, Al Mesfer SA, Abboud E et al (1997) Workup for metastatic retinoblastoma. A review of 261 patients. Ophthalmology1 04:307–312
Kiss S, Leiderman YI, Mukai S (2008) Diagnosis, classification, and treatment of retinoblastoma. Int Ophthalmol Clin4 8(2):135–147
Kivelä T (1999) Trilateral retinoblastoma: a meta-analysis of hereditary retinoblastoma associated with primary ectopic intracranial retinoblastoma. J Clin Oncol 17(6):1829–1837
Kopelman JE, McLean IW, Rosenby SH (1987) Multivariate analysis of risk factors for metastasis in retinoblastoma treated by enucleation. Ophthalmology 94:371–377
Maat-Kievit JA, Oepkes D, Hartwig NG, Vermeij-Keers C, van Kamp IL, van de Kamp JJ (1993) A large retinoblastoma detected in a fetus at 21 weeks of gestation. Prenat Diagn1 3(5):377–384
Marback EF, Arias VE, Paranhos A Jr, Soares FA, Murphree AL, Erwenne CM (2003) Tumour angiogenesis as a prognostic factor for disease dissemination in retinoblastoma. Br J Ophthalmol 87(10):1224–1228
Margo C, Hidayat A, Kopelman J, Zimmerman LE (1983) Retinocytoma. A benign variant of retinoblastoma. Arch Ophthalmol1 01(10):1519–1531
McLean IW, Burnier M, Zimmerman L, Jakobiec F (1994) Tumors of the retina. In: McLean IW, Burnier MN, Zimmerman LE, Jakobiec FA (eds) Atlas of tumor pathology. Tumors of the eye and ocular adnexa. Armed Forced Institute of Pathology, Washington, DC, pp 100–135
Nork TM, Schwartz TL, Doshi HM et al (1995) Retinoblastoma. Cell of origin. Arch Ophthalmol 113:791–802
O'Brien JM (2001) Retinoblastoma: clinical presentation and the role of neuroimaging. AJNR Am J Neuroradiol 22(3):426–428
Paulino AC (1999) Trilateral retinoblastoma: is the location of the intracranial tumor important? Cancer 86(1):135–141
Pierro L, Brancato R, Capoferri C (1993) Prenatal detection and early diagnosis of hereditary retinoblastoma in a family. Ophthalmologica 207(2):106–111
Rao A, Rothman J, Nichols KE (2008) Genetic testing and tumor surveillance for children with cancer predisposition syndromes. Curr Opin Pediatr 20(1):1–7
Robertson DM (1997) Fine-needle biopsy and retinoblastoma. Ophthalmology 104(4):567–568
Shanmugam MP, Biswas J (1997) Fine needle aspiration biopsy in the diagnosis of intraocular mass lesions. Indian J Ophthalmol 45(2):105–108
Shields JA, Shields CL, Eagle RC et al (1988) Spontaneous pseudohypopyon secondary to diffuse infiltrating retinoblastoma. Arch Ophthalmol 106:1301–1302
Shields CL, Shields JA, Shah P (1991) Retinoblastoma in older children. Ophthalmology 98(3):395–399
Shields JA, Shields CL, Honavar SG, Demirci H (2001a) Clinical variations and complications of Coats disease in 150 cases: the 2000 Sanford Gifford Memorial Lecture. Am J Ophthalmol 131(5):561–571
Shields CL, Meadows AT, Shields JA, Carvalho C, Smith AF (2001b) Chemoreduction for retinoblastoma may prevent intracranial neuroblastic malignancy (trilateral retinoblastoma). Arch Ophthalmol 119(9):1269–1272
Singh AD, Santos CM, Shields CL, Shields JA, Eagle RC Jr (2000) Observations on 17 patients with retinocytoma. Arch Ophthalmol 118(2):199–205
Smith JH, Murray TG, Fulton L, O'Brien JM (2000) Siblings of retinoblastoma patients: are we underestimating their risk? Am J Ophthalmol 129(3):396–398
Spencer WH (1975) Optic nerve extension of intraocular neoplasms. Am J Ophthalmol 80:465–471
Sun MH, Kao LY, Kuo YH (2003) Persistent hyperplastic primary vitreous: magnetic resonance imaging and clinical findings. Chang Gung Med J 26(4):269–276
Tosi P, Cintorino M, Toti P et al (1989) Histopathological evaluation for the prognosis of retinoblastoma. Ophthalmic Paediatr Genet 10:173–177
Ts'o MO, Fine BS, Zimmerman LE (1970a) The nature of retinoblastoma. II. Photoreceptor differentiation: an electron microscopic study. Am J Ophthalmol 69: 350–359
Ts'o MO, Zimmerman LE, Fine BS (1970b) The nature of retinoblastoma. I. Photoreceptor differentiation: a clinical and histopathologic study. Am J Ophthalmol 69:339–349
Wallach M, Balmer A, Munier F, Houghton S, Pampallona S, von der Weid N, Beck-Popovic M, Swiss Pediatric Oncology Group, Swiss Childhood Cancer Registry (2006) Swiss patients with retinoblastoma treated from 1963 to 2004. Pediatrics 118(5):e1493–e1498
Wolach B, Sinnreich Z, Uziel Y, Gotesman G, Pomerantz A (1995) Toxocariasis: a diagnostic dilemma. Isr J Med Sci 31(11):689–692

Genetics of Retinoblastoma and Genetic Counseling

H. Dimaras · B.L. Gallie

Contents

4.1 Introduction 41
4.2 Molecular Genetic Progression of Retinoblastoma 41
4.2.1 The *RB1* Gene, Protein, and Function 42
4.2.2 Cell of Origin 42
4.2.3 Transient Arrest: Senescence Halts Retinoma 43
4.2.4 Post-*RB1* Progressive Events 43
4.2.4.1 Genomic Gain of 1q: *KIF14* 43
4.2.4.2 Genomic Gain of 6p: *DEK* and *E2F3* 44
4.2.4.3 Genomic Gain of 2p: *NMYC4* 44
4.2.4.4 Genomic Loss of 16q: *CDH11* . . . 44
4.2.4.5 Deregulation of Apoptosis: Loss of Expression of p75^NTR^ 45
4.2.5 Murine Models of Retinoblastoma 45
4.2.5.1 *RB1* Knockout Mouse Models . . . 45
4.2.5.2 Viral Oncoprotein-induced Murine Retinoblastoma 45
4.2.5.3 Conditional *RB1* Knockout Murine Retinoblastoma Models 46
4.2.5.4 Limitations of Mouse Models . . . 46
4.2.6 Summary: A Model of Retinoblastoma Development 46
4.3 Genetic Counseling 46
4.3.1 Heritability of Retinoblastoma 46
4.3.2 Role of Environmental Factors 48
4.3.3 Molecular Genetic Testing 48
4.3.4 *RB1* Test Strategies 48
4.3.4.1 Sporadic Bilateral or Familial Retinoblastoma 48
4.3.4.2 Sporadic Unilateral Retinoblastoma 49
4.3.4.3 Prenatal Testing 49
4.3.4.4 *RB1* Mutation Identification 49
4.3.4.5 Missense Mutations 49
4.3.4.6 Frameshift and Nonsense Mutations 50
4.3.4.7 Aberrant Splicing 50
4.3.4.8 Epigenetic Mutations 50
4.3.4.9 Translocations and Gross Deletions 50
4.3.4.10 Penetrance of Retinoblastoma 51
4.3.4.11 Mosaicism 51
4.3.4.12 Parent of Origin Effect 51
4.4 Conclusions and Significance 51
4.5 Glossary 52
References 52

4.1 Introduction

Retinoblastoma was the first cancer to be described as a genetic disease. The progression of a normal retinal cell to the eventual malignant tumor involves a stepwise accumulation of molecular genetic alterations, which correlate with clinical stage and pathology of the tumor. This chapter gives an overview of the current state of knowledge of retinoblastoma genetics and its implications for genetic counseling.

4.2 Molecular Genetic Progression of Retinoblastoma

The journey of a developing retinal cell to retinoblastoma begins with mutation or loss of expression of the retinoblastoma tumor suppressor gene (*RB1*). Alfred Knudson's classic hypothesis predicted that "two hits" are rate-limiting for the disease (Knudson 1971), and indeed, it was later shown that loss of both alleles (M1 and M2) of *RB1* is necessary, but not sufficient, for retinoblastoma development (Fig. 4.1). Why the loss of *RB1* specifically initiates childhood tumors of

C. Rodriguez-Galindo and M.W. Wilson (eds.), *Retinoblastoma*, Pediatric Oncology,
DOI 10.1007/978-0-387-89072-2_4, © Springer Science+Business Media, LLC 2010

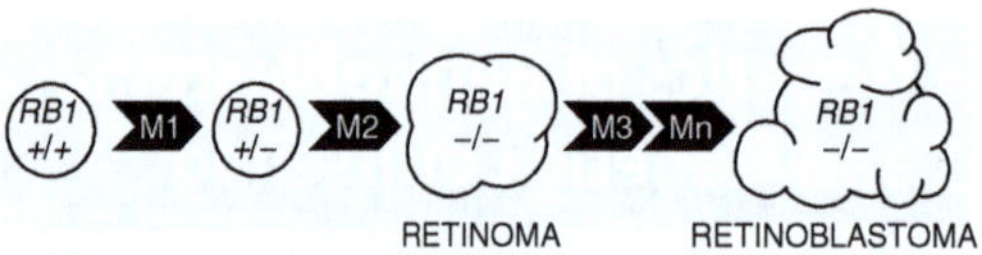

Figure 4.1

Retinoblastoma is initiated by the loss of *RB1*. Loss of both alleles of *RB1* (M1 and M2 mutational events) are necessary, but not sufficient, for retinoblastoma development. The M1 event can either be inherited or arise sporadically in a susceptible retinal cell, while M2 is always sporadic. Loss of *RB1* in a susceptible retinal cell predisposes to the benign tumor retinoma, while a number of subsequent mutational events (M3–Mn) usually eventually lead to retinoblastoma.

the retina and a few specific second primary tumors, remains unclear. Let us explore the key features of *RB1* and its protein product, pRB, to begin to learn about how retinoblastoma arises in its absence.

4.2.1 The *RB1* Gene, Protein, and Function

The *RB1* gene is located within a 183 kB region on human chromosome 13q14. Its promoter lacks any of the usual consensus TATA- or CAAT-binding elements, but instead contains binding sites for transcription factors Sp1 and ATF. The 5′ region of the gene harbors a CpG island, which is normally unmethylated. The gene is made up of 27 exons, which produce a 4.7 kB mRNA that is translated into a 928 amino acid protein called pRB.

Two highly conserved domains of pRB, termed domain A and domain B, create a pocket that serves to bind proteins with the consensus amino acid sequence LxCxE (where "x" is any amino acid). Proteins with this motif include the E2F family of transcription factors as well as viral oncoproteins, such as Simian Virus 40 Large T-antigen and adenovirus E1A. Pocket domains are also found in p107 and p130, which together with pRB constitute the retinoblastoma family of proteins.

pRB is posttranslationally modified by phosphorylation. Phosphorylation of pRB is cell cycle regulated and carried out by cyclin-dependent kinases (cdks), which are bound to and activated by cyclins. The C-terminal domain of pRB contains the binding site for the cyclin–cdk complex. pRB is phosphorylated at the G_1 to S phase transition by complexes cdk4/6, cyclin D or cdk2, and cyclin E. The protein is increasingly phosphorylated at different sites as the cell cycle proceeds, first by cdk2-cyclin A from S phase to G_2, followed by cdc2-cyclin B in M phase. Dephosphorylation of pRB is mediated by phosphoprotein phosphatase 1 (PP1), producing a hypophosphorylated pRB that is present during G_0 and G_1p hases.

The phosphorylation status affects the physical interaction between pRB and the E2F proteins. E2F family members activate genes involved in the G_1–S phase transition; thus, they promote cell cycle progression. Hypophosphorylated pRB can bind to E2Fs and thereby inhibit this function to halt the cell cycle. As pRB is phosphorylated, it loses its ability to bind E2Fs, allowing them to activate genes that promote the cell cycle. Similarly, in retinoblastoma, mutation of *RB1* leading to nonfunctional or absent pRB would result in constant activation of E2Fs and steady stimulation of the cell cycle, a feature beneficial to tumor development.

Additional functions of pRB include apoptosis and differentiation and are often mediated through interactions of pRB with its numerous and varied binding partners. Deregulation of cell death or differentiation pathways normally controlled by *RB1* could also be important to retinoblastoma tumorigenesis.

4.2.2 Cell of Origin

The identity of the retinal cell that is uniquely susceptible to developing retinoblastoma continues to evade researchers. Early studies pinpointed the cells of the outer nuclear layer as the origin based on the fact that structures called Flexner-Wintersteiner rosettes, characteristic of retinoblastoma, resemble an attempt at photoreceptor differentiation (Flexner 1891; Tso 1980). However, more recent studies suggest that the cell of origin lies in the inner nuclear layer, based on the topology of emerging tumors in the human retina (Gallie et al. 1999).

It is logical to assume that the cell of origin must be a retinal cell that normally requires expression of *RB1* during development; interestingly, this also implicates specific cells of the inner nuclear layer, namely the Müller glia, bipolar, and horizontal cells (Spencer et al. 2005). Observation of *Rb1*-deficient murine retina revealed that bipolar and horizontal cells die by apoptosis, while Müller glia and amacrine cells survive *Rb1* loss (Chen et al. 2004). Many mouse models of retinoblastoma also report tumors arising from the inner nuclear layer (Chen et al. 2004; Windle et al. 1990; MacPherson et al. 2004) likely indicating that these cells are most prone to tumorigenesis after loss of *RB1*, whereas other retinal cells may suffer different fates.

It is likely that stem cells, which are primitive, inherently self-renewing cells, are the origin of retinoblastoma, as is clear for hematopoietic malignancies. Retinoblastoma emerges during the time in retinal development when stem cell-like progenitor (uncommitted; can give rise to any cell type) and precursor (restricted to certain cell types) cells make up a large part of the retina, and after a few years of age as retina becomes nonproliferative, even a person with a germline *RB1* mutation develops no new retinoblastomas. Within the tumors, only a specific subset of cells may maintain stem cell characteristics, and continuously generate cells that attempt differentiation, forming tumor with abortive differentiation to form photoreceptor-like structures.

4.2.3 Transient Arrest: Senescence Halts Retinoma

Retinoma is a clinically benign retinal tumor originally described as an elevated, gray, translucent lesion with areas of 'cottage cheese'-like calcification (Gallie et al. 1982). It has a distinct pathology, marked by the presence of benign appearing cells and fleurettes (Margo et al. 1983), features not shared by retinoblastoma, though the two distinct lesions can be found in the same eye. It was hypothesized that retinoma represented an intermediate stage between normal retina and retinoblastoma (Gallie et al. 1999).

Due to its rarity, retinoma has only recently begun to be studied at the molecular level, mainly from eyes enucleated for retinoblastoma found also to contain retinoma (Dimaras et al. 2005; Dimaras 2007). Consistent with the initial hypothesis, retinoma was found to contain the same two *RB1* mutations as its adjacent retinoblastoma (Dimaras et al. 2005; Dimaras 2007). The loss of *RB1* potentially triggers a limited number of cell divisions and aberrant proliferation, resulting in the development of retinoma (Dimaras 2007).

The question remains, however, as to what keeps retinoma from progressing to retinoblastoma in cases where it remains clinically benign for the lifetime of the patient. The answer may lie in the fact that retinoma is associated with expression of p16^{INK4a}, not detected in retina or retinoblastoma (Dimaras et al. 2005; Dimaras 2007). Senescence that is induced after oncogenic stimulation is thought to be mediated by p16^{INK4a}, a cell cycle inhibitor (Collado et al. 2005; Braig et al. 2005; Braig and Schmitt 2006); expression of p16^{INK4a} in benign tumors and deregulated expression in malignant tumors have been observed in gastrointestinal cancer (Sabah et al. 2004) and melanoma (Radhi 1999). Thus, the transition from benign to malignant retinal cancer could occur after a reversal of the senescent state as is observed in the development of other cancers, and the rare cases of retinoma that do not progress to retinoblastoma could be an example of stable arrest. At this time, we are unable to study these specimens beyond the clinic, since eyes affected only with retinoma do not require treatment or enucleation, only clinical surveillance.

4.2.4 Post-*RB1* Progressive Events

Since most retinoblastoma tumors display genomic imbalances, it was hypothesized that chromosomes that are frequently gained or lost in retinoblastoma may harbor candidate oncogenes or tumor suppressors, respectively. Numerous studies on retinoblastoma using comparative genomic hybridization (CGH) revealed most frequent gains of chromosomes 1q, 2p, and 6p and loss of chromosome 16q. These were subsequently narrowed down to the smaller, most commonly gained or lost regions within the chromosomes, pinpointing candidate oncogenes and tumor suppressor genes harbored by those regions (Corson and Gallie 2007).

4.2.4.1 Genomic Gain of 1q: *KIF14*

Over 50% of retinoblastoma tumors show gain at chromosomal arm 1q by CGH (reviewed in (Corson et al. 2007)). The minimal region of gain was narrowed to 1q31-32, gained in about half of tumors with 1q gain. Using quantitative multiplex (QM) PCR, the region was further narrowed to 1q32.1. From this region containing 12 genes, the mitotic kinesin *KIF14* was identified as a potential retinoblastoma oncogene, since it was amplified in one case of retinoblastoma and overexpressed in all retinoblastoma tumors compared to normal retina by quantitative RT-PCR.

KIF14 is a mitotic kinesin that functions during cytokinesis. Therefore, in tumors, *KIF14* overexpression may facilitate the proliferation that leads to tumor growth. In addition to its potential role as an oncogene in retinoblastoma, *KIF14* overexpression has been correlated with higher tumor grade and worse outcome in lung and breast cancers.

It has also been suggested that *MDM4* might be the candidate oncogene at 1q, since it inhibits the transcriptional activity of p53 and stabilizes MDM2, which targets p53 for degradation. A study using array CGH and Fluorescence *In Situ* Hybridization (FISH) found that *MDM4* was gained in a subset of retinoblastoma tumors (Laurie et al. 2006). Hence, could there be two oncogenes essential for tumorigenesis at a single minimal region of gain? Or does perhaps only one gene have functional importance in tumorigenesis, while the other gene is simply 'along for the ride'? Clearly, further investigation is warranted.

4.2.4.2 Genomic Gain of 6p: *DEK* and *E2F3*

The most common region of gain on chromosome 6 was first identified as an isochromosome and later narrowed down to 6p22 (gained in 44% of retinoblastoma tumors) (Chen et al. 2001). Initially, the potential oncogene in this region was thought to be the kinesin *KIF13A*, later coined *RBKIN* for its hypothesized role as an oncogenic kinesin in retinoblastoma. Subsequent expression analysis eliminated *RBKIN* as the candidate 6p oncogene, but identified two others: *E2F3* and *DEK*. *E2F3* plays a role in initiation of the cell cycle, and was recently found to regulate *DEK*. *DEK* is a known oncogene in many cancers and is translocated in leukemia. It has been implicated in a number of different functions, including chromatin remodeling, mRNA splicing, and transcriptional regulation.

The roles of DEK and E2F3 in the retina and how they might function either alone or in combination when overexpressed in retinoblastoma are unclear. Knockdown of either candidate in retinoblastoma cell lines with 6p22 gain causes massive cell death (DEK) and decreases cellular growth rates (DEK and E2F3); therefore, it is possible that both genes could play a cooperative role in retinoblastoma development(Orlic 2007).

4.2.4.3 Genomic Gain of 2p: *NMYC*

Another chromosomal region frequently gained in retinoblastoma occurs on chromosome 2p. The minimal region of gain at 2p24 contains the gene *NMYC*, known to be amplified in neuroblastoma. Since the retinoblastoma cell line Y79 also showed *NMYC* amplification, this gene was assumed to be the retinoblastoma oncogene at this region. Since then, *NMYC* amplification has been observed in various frequencies of retinoblastoma tumors tested. The function of overexpression of *NMYC* or other 2p genes in retinoblastoma remains to be elucidated.

4.2.4.4 Genomic Loss of 16q: *CDH11*

Approximately 31% of retinoblastoma tumors show loss at chromosome 16q22 (Marchong et al. 2004), a region that contains two cadherin genes, *CDH11* and *CDH13*. Expression studies pinpointed *CDH11* as the potential tumor suppressor gene, which unlike *CDH13*, was expressed in retina but decreased or lacking in the majority of retinoblastoma tumors studied.

Although the precise mode of function of CDH11 is not well known, it belongs to the cadherin family of proteins, which are involved in cellular adhesion. The ability of the tumor to surpass cellular adhesion might be important for metastasis or vitreous seeding. This does not exclude other roles for *CDH11;* however, as studies from a murine model of retinoblastoma indicate, *Cdh11* loss causes an increase in the rate of cellular proliferation in developing tumors (Marchong 2007).

The techniques used to narrow the regions harboring potential retinoblastoma oncogenes and tumor suppressors detect gross chromosomal deletions or aberrations, but are likely to miss point mutations or small deletions, as well as epigenetic modifications, that might play a role in tumor progression. For example, CGH studies did not identify frequent loss of chromosome 13q, the location of *RB1*, likely because most *RB1* mutations are not large deletions. A candidate gene approach can be used to discover potential retinoblastoma tumor suppressor genes and oncogenes not suggested by genomic studies. This approach was used to identify $p75^{NTR}$ as a potential retinoblastoma tumor suppressor gene, as discussed in the following section.

4.2.4.5 Deregulation of Apoptosis: Loss of Expression of $p75^{NTR}$

Loss of *RB1* in many tissues leads to apoptosis; yet for reasons unknown, in the retina, $RB1^{-/-}$ cells can survive and form tumors. This led to the hypothesis that perhaps a mutational event downstream of *RB1* loss targeted a gene responsible for initiating cell death in response to tumorigenic insult. The p53 gene, a well-known tumor suppressor gene involved in the regulation of apoptosis, was studied for potential deregulation in retinoblastoma. However, retinoblastomas commonly show a few cells expressing p53, and radiation of retinoblastoma cell lines results in normal upregulation of p53. In addition, no mutations of p53 have been found in retinoblastoma cell lines or primary tumors. *MDM4* overexpression, observed in a subset of retinoblastoma, could potentially cause deregulation of p53, as it directly inhibits the transcriptional activity of the tumor suppressor.

Another candidate for a pro-apoptotic tumor suppressor in the retina is *NGFR*, which encodes $p75^{NTR}$, a modulator of developmental cell death in the retina. Expression analysis revealed t hat retinoblastoma tumors show reduced or lost $p75^{NTR}$ mRNA expression and complete absence of the protein, while retina and retinoma express normal levels of the protein (Dimaras et al. 2006). Functional evidence in mice and retinoblastoma cell lines indicate a pro-apoptotic role of $p75^{NTR}$ and support the idea that $p75^{NTR}$ is a tumor suppressor in retinoblastoma (Dimaras 2007).

4.2.5 Murine Models of Retinoblastoma

The functional study of retinoblastoma and its stepwise accumulation of genetic events depend on study of a murine retinoblastoma model that precisely mimics human retinoblastoma progression, since only late stage human retinoblastomas are available for molecular studies when eyes are removed for therapy. The existing murine retinoblastoma mouse models are reviewed in the following sections.

4.2.5.1 *RB1* Knockout Mouse Models

Heterozygote $RB1^{+/-}$ mice developed pituitary and thyroid tumors after somatic inactivation of the second *RB1* allele in the appropriate tissue; however, retinoblastoma was not observed (Hu et al. 1994; Lee et al. 1992). The first transgenic *RB1* knockout proved to be embryonic lethal (Lee et al. 1992; Jacks et al. 1992; Clarke et al. 1992), later attributed to a placental defect (de Bruin et al. 2003). However, even with a replacement normal placenta, $RB1^{-/-}$ mice did not survive past birth (de Bruin et al. 2003). Multiple $RB1^{+/-}$ transgenics in combination with knockout of *E2F1* (Tsai et al. 1998), *p107* (Lee et al. 1996), and *p53* (Morgenbesser et al. 1994) were made, yet none resulted in murine retinoblastoma; the latter two, however, developed retinal dysplasia.

4.2.5.2 Viral Oncoprotein-induced Murine Retinoblastoma

Using papillomavirus E7 and E6 to inhibit pRB and related proteins, retinal tumors were induced in mice (Griep et al. 1998; Howes et al. 1994). In an attempt to create a murine model for pituitary tumors using Simian Virus 40 Large T-antigen (TAg), one mouse lineage serendipitously developed tumors specifically in the retina that very closely mimicked the human condition. The TAg-induced retinoblastoma (TAg-RB) transgene is 100% penetrant and the tumors display characteristic Flexner-Wintersteiner and Homer Wright rosettes (Windle et al. 1990). These mice have been used in several clinical studies to test potential treatments for retinoblastoma (Escalona-Benz et al. 2005; Jockovich et al. 2006; Murray et al. 1997). Furthermore, the TAg-RB murine tumors mice show M3–Mn events like human retinoblastoma: loss of $p75^{NTR}$, *CDH11* (Marchong et al. 2004), gain of *DEK, E2F3* (Orlic et al. 2006; Grasemann et al. 2005), and *KIF14*.

4.2.5.3 Conditional *RB1* Knockout Murine Retinoblastoma Models

Most recent mouse models have attempted to mimic human retinoblastoma by knocking out *RB1* specifically in the retina using the Cre-lox system, either on a p107 null (Chen et al. 2004) or p130 null genetic background (MacPherson et al. 2004), or by Cre-mediated inactivation of *pRB* and p107 on a p53 null background (Zhang et al. 2004). A retinal-specific promoter is used to drive Cre expression, resulting in *RB1* knockout at different stages in retinal development in each mouse. The tumors develop Homer Wright rosettes; however, Flexner-Wintersteiner rosettes or M3–Mn events have not been reported.

4.2.5.4 Limitations of Mouse Models

Although mouse models can yield functional information that cannot be attained by the use of human clinical samples, we must be critical of the information garnered from these models and how it relates to the human disease. For example, the conditional models mentioned above develop retinal tumors in a completely mutant retina, which is not the case in humans, where the tumor most often initiates in one mutant cell in an otherwise normal retina. Morphological and molecular features are important when translating knowledge from murine models to human. The TAg-RB mouse model that most closely mimics the clonal nature of human retinoblastoma presents with similar histological features and acquires the same M3–Mn events as human retinoblastoma.

4.2.6 Summary: A Model of Retinoblastoma Development

Although the number and combination of events required for retinoblastoma initiation and progression is inconclusive, it is tempting to design a model of retinoblastoma progression, the precise order of events, as well as is proposed the number and combination of events required for malignancy, remains inconclusive. In general, a susceptible retinal cell loses both copies of *RB1* and undergoes a limited bout of proliferation, forming a benign retinoma lesion. Absence of *RB1* permits low-level genomic instability that is halted by $p16^{INK4a}$-mediated senescence forming a benign retinoma. A rare cell escapes this arrest by downregulation of $p16^{INK4a}$, perhaps also escaping apoptosis by early loss of $p75^{NTR}$. Cell proliferation resumes, followed and provoked by the accumulation of further genomic imbalances, perhaps some of which were initiated at a low level at the retinoma stage to begin with. A combinatory gain of oncogenes *NMYC, KIF14, E2F3,* and/or *DEK* ensues, along with loss of *CDH11*, resulting in full-blown malignant retinoblastoma.

4.3 Genetic Counseling

Genetic counseling provides valuable information to retinoblastoma patients and their families about the nature of the disease, inheritance patterns, risks to family members, and implications for family planning. This section covers the features of retinoblastoma that impact genetic counseling such as hereditability and transmission of the disease, risk for second primary cancers, and implications of molecular genetic testing.

4.3.1 Heritability of Retinoblastoma

Both *RB1* alleles have to be deregulated in order for retinoblastoma to develop in a developing retinal cell. However, the mutant *RB1* allele behaves as an autosomal dominant trait, since heterozygous carriers of an *RB1* mutation will almost always lose the second allele and develop retinoblastoma.

The majority of retinoblastoma cases (90%) arise *sporadically* in the tissues of the affected *proband* or the parental germline; they are also referred to as *isolated* cases because there is no family history of the disease. If the initial *RB1* mutation arises in a germ cell before conception, or in the early embryo, the risk for retinoblastoma will be *heritable* (Table 4.1). If two somatic *RB1* mutations occur in a susceptible retinal cell leading to retinoblastoma, but the germline is not affected, the tendency to retinoblastoma will not be heritable. Sporadic retinoblastoma more commonly arises in only one eye (*unilateral*); however, it can also affect both eyes (*bilateral*). Sporadic tumors are likely to be *unifocal*; however, *mutifocal* tumors have also been observed. Care must be taken to ensure that tumors described as "multifocal" are actually "new", and not actually a result of recurrent or disseminated tumors, as this affects the probability of the proband carrying a germline mutation (Table 4.2). For this reason, multifocal tumors cannot be clearly identified in eyes displaying vitreous or subretinal seeding, or tumors with poor prognosis features (International Intraocular Retinoblastoma Classification C, D, E (Murphree 2005)).

The minority of retinoblastoma cases (10%) are *familial*, in other words, *inherited* from an affected parent or unaffected carrier parent. Familial cases are always heritable, since the first *RB1* mutation is present in all cells of the body including the germline. As a result, familial cases are commonly bilateral and multifocal, though some unilateral cases have been observed.

Table 4.1. Heritability of retinoblastoma

Clinical presentation in proband	% of RB patients	Genetic mechanism		Inherited?	Heritable?
Familial (mostly bilateral; sometimes unilateral)	10%	Inherited mutant *RB1* allele		Yes	Yes
Sporadic bilateral	30%	88%	New mutation arising in germline of father (>90%) or mother (<10%)	No	Yes
		12%	Mutational mosaicism	No	(Yes)[a]
Sporadic unilateral	60%	85%	Somatic mutations of both *RB1* alleles	No	No
		15%	New mutation arising in germline (often mosaic)	No	Yes

[a]Germline mosaicism can only be measured in males (Sippel et al. 1998)

Table 4.2. Probability that proband has germline mutation

Family History	Clinical presentation: Unilateral – Unifocal	Clinical presentation: Unilateral – Multifocal	Clinical presentation: Bilateral	Probability
Positive[a]		+		100%
	+			100%
			+	100%
Negative[b]			+	100%
	+			15%
		+[c]		15-?%

[a]Positive = more than one affected family member
[b]Negative = only one affected individual in the family (the proband)
[c]True multifocal tumors, not disseminated tumors

In addition to retinoblastoma, *RB1* mutation predisposes to other primary cancers, including osteosarcoma, malignant melanoma, and soft tissue sarcoma (Eng et al. 1993; Fletcher et al. 2004). These second primary neoplasms present later in life, but earlier than the same tumors in persons with no *RB1* mutation. No particular *RB1* mutation has been shown to predispose to second tumors in retinoblastoma patients (Lohmann 1999); however, unknown modifier genes can potentially increase the risk as shown for lipoma (Genuardi et al. 2001). Also, treatment of retinoblastoma with external beam radiation has been shown to increase the risk for second primary tumors to as high as 50% by 50 years of age (Wong et al. 1997).

In the absence of molecular diagnosis, it is important to screen all first-degree relatives of retinoblastoma patients when it is the first identified case in the family. Eye examinations may identify underlying retinal lesions (retinoma, retinal scarring) even if they do not develop retinoblastoma.

4.3.2 Role of Environmental Factors

No environmental factors have been shown to contribution to the development to retinoblastoma (Buckley 1992). However, certain paternal occupations (metal manufacturing, welder-machinist) can predispose their future offspring to retinoblastoma, perhaps because of an increased risk of germline mutagenesis (Bunin et al. 1990).

4.3.3 Molecular Genetic Testing

The heritable nature of retinoblastoma and risk for other cancers necessitates genetic testing in the proband and their family, since the relative risk to family members and future offspring depends on whether or not the proband has germline *RB1* mutation (Tables 4.1 and 4.2). Technological advances have made genetic testing of the proband rapid and highly sensitive, identifying the heritable *RB1* mutation in 92.2% of cases (Retinoblastoma Solutions Test Sensitivity 2007), further enabling testing of other family members for the presence or absence of the mutation. Genetic counseling for family members found to have increased risk of developing retinoblastoma and/or transmitting the mutation to their offspring improves the quality of clinical care for retinoblastoma patients and their at-risk relatives. Furthermore, identifying noncarriers of the *RB1* mutation eliminates the requirement for obtrusive and costly clinical surveillance, as only family members found to carry the mutation need to be monitored for the potential development of tumors. Molecular testing has improved the standard of care for retinoblastoma, and has yet to be emulated in the treatment and management of other cancers, where the initiating molecular events are not as clearlyd efined.

4.3.4 *RB1* Test Strategies

4.3.4.1 Sporadic Bilateral or Familial Retinoblastoma

Genetic testing of constitutional DNA (usually from a sample of peripheral blood) in hereditary cases of retinoblastoma identifies over 90% of causative mutations (Retinoblastoma Solutions Test Sensitivity 2007). The second *RB1* mutation can be detected only from tumor DNA; however, for bilateral or familial cases, this is usually not required (Lohmann et al. 2007).

For sporadic bilateral retinoblastoma, analysis of peripheral blood may not always lead to the detection of the causative *RB1* mutation. In such cases, testing of tumor DNA may reveal either two *RB1* mutations or one *RB1* mutation together with evidence of LOH. The constitutional blood can then be retested specifically for the presence of the mutation(s); if neither is detected, it is assumed that the patient is mosaic. (Note: the lowest level of mosaic mutation detectable is dependent on the methodology used and currently varies from 2% to 20% (Lohmann et al. 2007)).

If a causative mutation is detected as heterozygous in the proband's blood, then the proband's parents should be tested for the mutation. Most cases of sporadic bilateral retinoblastoma are *de novo*, in other words, caused by a new mutation. In a small number of cases, the parent may be low-level mosaic, undetectable by current methodologies. For this reason, all siblings of the proband should also be tested for the proband's mutation. Children of the proband are at 50% risk of inheriting the mutation.

4.3.4.2 Sporadic Unilateral Retinoblastoma

For sporadic unilateral cases, the peripheral blood DNA is usually normal (85% of patients), and DNA from the tumor must be analyzed to identify both *RB1* mutations. The peripheral blood DNA should then be tested for the identified mutations, as 15% of patients are likely to be heterozygous carriers (germline) or mosaic.

If neither *RB1* mutation is identified in the blood (only in the tumor DNA), then this is most likely a non-germline, sporadic case of retinoblastoma, and parents and siblings are not at risk. There exists, however, the rare possibility that one of the tumor mutations is low-level mosaic, so future offspring of the proband should be tested for the presence of the mutation.

In some cases where no tumor or tumor DNA is available, blood from unilateral isolated patients can be screened using comprehensive molecular techniques (discussed below) to identify a germline mutation. The finding of no mutation lowers the risk of a germline mutation from 15% to 1.7% if the laboratory test sensitivity is 90%.

4.3.4.3 Prenatal Testing

Transmission of an *RB1* mutation from an affected parent to their offspring can be detected prenatally in DNA from amniotic fluid. If the familial mutation is detected, premature labor can be induced at 8 months gestation in order to start immediate treatment on the tumor. This can potentially save the child's vision before the tumor reaches a stage necessitating enucleation.

4.3.4.4 *RB1* Mutation Identification

Over a thousand distinct *RB1* mutations leading to retinoblastoma have been identified (Richter et al. 2003) suggesting that there are virtually an infinite number of ways to break the gene and initiate retinoblastoma. Mutations range from exonic or whole gene deletions causing frameshifts or loss of the entire gene, respectively, to point mutations causing splicing defects, missense or nonsense mutations. The range of mutation types can be found as either the first (M1) or second (M2) *RB1* mutations; however, the second mutation, in the tumor cells, is usually (65% of cases) mitotic recombination resulting in the same *RB1* mutation on both chromosomes, recognized first as loss of heterozygosity (Cavenee et al. 1983; Hagstrom and Dryja 1999; Zhu et al. 1992).

A variety of molecular genetic techniques are employed to find the identity of an unknown *RB1* mutation (Table 4.3). Methylation-specific PCR or Southern Blot with methylation-specific restriction endonucleases can be used to detect *RB1* hypermethylation (Zeschnigk et al. 1999). Cytogenetic aberrations, such as translocations or gross deletions of 13q, can be detected by FISH using lymphocytes from peripheral blood.

Gross deletions and duplications can also be identified by multiplex ligation-dependent probe amplification (MLPA), or quantitative multiplex-PCR with high-resolution fragment length analysis. The latter additionally detects length variations resulting from small insertions or deletions in the coding sequence.

Point mutations (leading to frameshifts, missense, nonsense, or splice mutations, as above) can be identified by standard sequence analysis and/or mutation scanning. Also, RNA from blood can be tested to detect splicing defects or rearrangements of *RB1* (Lohmann et al. 2007).

4.3.4.5 Missense Mutations

Missense mutations result in the alteration of the normal sequence of amino acids in the translated protein. Most *RB1* missense mutations leading to retinoblastoma create a protein with complete or partial loss of function of the pocket domain. Many missense mutations result in incomplete penetrance of retinoblastoma (discussed below) (Lohmann 1999).

Table 4.3. Clinical tests

Molecular test	Mutations detected	Rate of detection[a]
FISH	Submicroscopic deletions and translocations	>8%
QM-PCR	Submicroscopic deletions, insertions and rearrangements	37%
MLPA	Deletions, insertions	16%
Mutation scanning Sequence analysis	Single base substitutions, small length mutations	70–75%
Targeted mutation analysis (Allele-specific PCR)	Specific recurrent point mutations	30%
Methylation analysis	Promoter hypermethylation	10–12%[b]
Analysis of RNA from blood	(Deep intronic) splice mutations, gross rearrangements	<5%[c]

[a] From (Lohmann et al. 2002)
[b] In tissue from retinoblastoma tumor
[c] In individuals where mutation could not be identified in DNA

4.3.4.6 Frameshift and Nonsense Mutations

Frameshift and nonsense *RB1* mutations in retinoblastoma have been identified throughout the gene, resulting from point mutations or deletions or duplications within the gene. Mutations resulting in a premature termination codon can sometimes produce a partially functional mutant protein; however, this is not usually observed in retinoblastoma. This has been suggested to be a result of nonsense-mediated decay, a natural cellular surveillance mechanism that recognizes and initiates the destruction of transcripts containing premature stop codons.

4.3.4.7 Aberrant Splicing

Point mutations within introns or exons of *RB1* can affect the normal splicing of the gene. Often, splicing errors will result in frameshift mutations leading to a premature termination codon, the consequences of which are described above. However, if the mutation affects intronic splicing signals, which are less conserved, then its effect is variable and may sometimes both normal and splice normally, while at other times it may produce a mutant transcripts, may be produced. Mutations affecting the highly conserved, invariant +1, +2, −1, −2 intronic nucleotides tend to be highly penetrant, while those in other intronic positions that variably affect splicing have more variable effects and are more likely to lead to reduced penetrance (see below for discussion of penetrance) (Zhang et al. 2008).

4.3.4.8 Epigenetic Mutations

In addition to these genetic mutations, epigenetic mutations can also lead to retinoblastoma by inhibiting the expression of the gene. For example, hypermethylation of the CpG island of the *RB1* promoter results in transcriptional inhibition of the *RB1* gene. Current knowledge suggests that methylation of the *RB1* promoter only occurs in the somatic retinal cells, present in about 10–12% of retinoblastoma tumors, one or both *RB1* alleles are inactivated by hypermethylation as the causative events tested (Richter et al. 2003; Klutz et al. 1999; Ohtani-Fujita et al. 1997).

4.3.4.9 Translocations and Gross Deletions

Some cases of retinoblastoma are caused by translocations and/or large deletions of 13q14, the chromosomal region where *RB1* is located (Ejima et al. 1988; Bunin et al. 1989). About 5% of children have deletion of a large region of 13q (also referred to as 13q deletion syndrome) and in addition to retinoblastoma, present with other signs of genetic disease. However, even large deletions can show a reduced penetrance if the deletion is in frame, resulting in a truncated stable protein (Chen et al. 2004).

4.3.4.10 Penetrance of Retinoblastoma

RB1 mutations, such as frameshift or nonsense mutations that lead to null alleles and no functional protein, almost invariably lead to bilateral retinoblastoma (99% of cases). Full *penetrance* of an *RB1* mutation means that the majority of family members develop retinoblastoma. Since the distribution of tumors between the two eyes is random, highly penetrant *RB1* mutant alleles usually cause bilateral retinoblastoma (affecting both eyes).

As mentioned previously, there exist rare cases (<10%) of reduced penetrance mutations, evident in families with fewer affected children and more unaffected carriers. Reduced penetrance retinoblastoma is caused by distinct *RB1* mutations (specific splicing defects, promoter mutations, missense mutations) that leave some residual, partial function of the pRB protein (Lohmann et al. 2007). In addition, large deletions that span DNA beyond the *RB1* gene also show reduced penetrance, presumably because an unknown adjacent gene(s) is also deleted that is essential for cell survival, so that loss of heterozygosity results in cell death before a tumor can form. In these cases, tumors have a different intragenic *RB1* second mutant allele. In general, reduced penetrance of an *RB1* mutation is also reflected in reduced *expressivity*, so those who are affected develop fewer tumors, commonly unilateral. *Trilateral* retinoblastoma can also arise where one or both eyes and an intracranial primitive neuroectodermal tumor, usually in the pineal gland, develops.

4.3.4.11 Mosaicism

If a sporadic *RB1* mutation occurs as a postzygotic event early in the development of the fetus, only a subset of constitutional cells will harbor the mutation and the individual will be *mosaic* for the mutant allele (Sippel et al. 1998). The distribution of cells mutant for *RB1* varies depending on the timing and location of the mutation in the embryo. The mosaic individual may or may not develop retinoblastoma, and the mutation will be heritable only if the germline is affected. Individuals with mosaicism for *RB1* mutations usually present with fewer tumors that are likely to be unilateral.

4.3.4.12 Parent of Origin Effect

One specific *RB1* mutation (base substitution in intron 6 leading to missplicing of exon 6) (IVS6+1G-->T) in several unrelated families has been shown to result in earlier and more tumors in children who inherited the mutant allele from their father, and far fewer and later onset tumors if they inherited the mutant allele from their mother (Klutz et al. 2002). RNA analysis revealed lower mutant mRNA compared to normal RNA in patients with the paternally inherited allele, showing the usual effect of nonsense-mediated decay associated with premature termination of translation. Individuals with exactly the same, but maternally inherited, mutant allele had equal levels of normal and mutant transcript.

In more than 90% of bilateral isolated cases, prezygotic *RB1* mutation has arisen that does not show the mutation in the parent's blood cells. Most commonly, LOH on the child's tumor shows that the new germline *RB1* mutation originates on a paternal allele rather than the maternal (Zhu et al. 1989). This may reflect a difference between male and female gametogenesis that makes mutations more likely to occur in the male.

4.4 Conclusions and Significance

In conclusion, the definition of retinoblastoma as a genetic disease and the careful study of its molecular genetic development have contributed significant knowledge that has positively impacted clinical outcomes. Knowledge of the initiating molecular events in retinoblastoma progression, namely the loss of both alleles of the *RB1* gene (M1 and M2), has been developed into clinical tests that can achieve high sensitivity to discover the family's unique *RB1* mutant allele(s) and use that knowledge to improve outcomes for affected children and remove from surveillance those who do not carry the mutation. The delineation of post-*RB1* loss events (M3-Mn) has also led to the development of further molecular tools with clinical and diagnostic potential. Finally, the recognition that retinoma is an intermediate lesion between normal retina and retinoblastoma suggests a model of molecular progression to cancer that holds promise toi mpact onf uture treatmenta ndo utcomes.

4.5 Glossary

Bilateral retinoblastoma	retinoblastomat hat affects both eyes.
de novo germline mutation	new mutation, arising sporadically in a germ cell of the proband's parent or in early stages of embryogenesis of the proband.
Expressivity	the phenotypich eterogeneity in the presentation of the disease.
Familial retinoblastoma	the *RB1* allele that resulted in retinoblastoma was transmitted from a parent; children with familial retinoblastoma are constitutionally heterozygous for *RB1* mutant alleles.
Heritable retinoblastoma	offspring of probands with heritable retinoblastoma are at 50% risk to inherit the mutant allele.
Isolated or sporadic retinoblastoma	no family history of retinoblastoma; may or may not have a constitutional *RB1* mutanta llele.
Mosaic	the *RB1*m utation occurred early in development, affecting only a subset of constitutional cells.
Multifocal retinoblastoma	twoo rm orer etinoblastoma tumors affecting one eye.
Penetrance	thef requencya tw hicha genotype (mutation) is expressed at the phenotypic level.
Proband	the first patient in a family to be diagnosed with retinoblastoma.
Trilateral retinoblastoma	retinoblastoma develops in both eyes (or only one eye) in addition to pinealoblastoma or a primitive neuroectodermal brain tumor.
Unifocal retinoblastoma	a singler etinoblastoma tumor in one eye.
Unilateral retinoblastoma	retinoblastomat hat affectso nee ye.

References

Braig M, Schmitt CA (2006) Oncogene-induced senescence: putting the brakes on tumor development. Cancer Res 66(6):2881–2884

Braig M et al (2005) Oncogene-induced senescence as an initial barrier in lymphoma development. Nature 436(7051):660–665

Buckley JD (1992) The aetiology of cancer in the very young. Br J Cancer Suppl 18:S8–S12

Bunin GR et al (1989) Frequency of 13q abnormalities among 203 patients with retinoblastoma. J Natl Cancer Inst 81(5):370–374

Bunin GR et al (1990) Occupations of parents of children with retinoblastoma: a report from the Children's Cancer Study Group. Cancer Res 50(22):7129–7133

Cavenee WK et al (1983) Expression of recessive alleles by chromosomal mechanisms in retinoblastoma. Nature 305(5937):779–784

Chen D, Gallie BL, Squire JA (2001) Minimal regions of chromosomal imbalance in retinoblastoma detected

by comparative genomic hybridization. Cancer Genet Cytogeneti 29(1):57–63
Chen D et al (2004) Cell-specific effects of RB or RB/p107 loss on retinal development implicate an intrinsically death-resistant cell-of-origin in retinoblastoma. Cancer Cell5(6):539–551
Clarke AR et al (1992) Requirement for a functional Rb-1 gene in murine development. Nature 359(6393):328–330
Collado M et al (2005) Tumour biology: senescence in premalignant tumours. Nature 436(7051):642
Corson TW, Gallie BL (2007) One hit, two hits, three hits, more? Genomic changes in the development of retinoblastoma. Genes Chromosomes Cancer 46(7):617–634
Corson TW et al (2007) KIF14 messenger RNA expression is independently prognostic for outcome in lung cancer. Clin Cancer Res 13(11):3229–3234
de Bruin A et al (2003) Rb function in extraembryonic lineages suppresses apoptosis in the CNS of Rb-deficient mice. Proc Natl Acad Sci U S A 100(11):6546–6551
Dimaras H (2007) The molecular progression from retina through retinoma to retinoblastoma and the role of the p75NTR neurotrophin receptor, Department of Molecular and Medical Genetics. University of Toronto, Toronto, p 158
Dimaras H et al (2006) The loss of p75 neurotrophin receptor expression accompanies malignant progression to human and murine retinoblastoma. Mol Carcinog 45(5):333–343
Dimaras H et al (2008) Loss of RB1 induces non-proliferative retinoma: increasing genomic instability correlates with progression to retinoblastoma. Hom Mol Genet 17(10):1363–1372
Ejima Y et al (1988) Types, rates, origin and expressivity of chromosome mutations involving 13q14 in retinoblastoma patients. Hum Genet 79(2):118–123
Eng C et al (1993) Mortality from second tumors among long-term survivors of retinoblastoma. J Natl Cancer Inst8 5(14):1121–1128
Escalona-Benz E et al (2005) Combretastatin A-4 prodrug in the treatment of a murine model of retinoblastoma. Invest Ophthalmol Vis Sci 46(1):8–11
Fletcher O et al (2004) Lifetime risks of common cancers among retinoblastoma survivors. J Natl Cancer Inst 96(5):357–363
Flexner S (1891) A peculiar glioma (neuroepithelioma?) of the retina. Johns Hopkins Hosp Bull 2:115
Gallie BL et al (1982) Retinoma: spontaneous regression of retinoblastoma or benign manifestation of the mutation? Br J Cancer 45(4):513–521
Gallie BL et al (1999) Developmental basis of retinal-specific induction of cancer by RB mutation. Cancer Res 59(7S uppl):1731s–1735s
Genuardi M et al (2001) Multiple lipomas linked to an RB1 gene mutation in a large pedigree with low penetrance retinoblastoma. Eur J Hum Genet 9(9):690–694
Grasemann C et al (2005) Gains and overexpression identify DEK and E2F3 as targets of chromosome 6p gains in retinoblastoma. Oncogene 24(42):6441–6449
Griep AE et al (1998) Multiple genetic loci modify risk for retinoblastoma in transgenic mice. Invest Ophthalmol Vis Sci 39(13):2723–2732
Hagstrom SA, Dryja TP (1999) Mitotic recombination map of 13cen-13q14 derived from an investigation of loss of heterozygosity in retinoblastomas. Proc Natl Acad Sci U S A 96(6):2952–2957
Howes KA et al (1994) Apoptosis or retinoblastoma: alternative fates of photoreceptors expressing the HPV-16 E7 gene in the presence or absence of p53. Genes Dev 8(11):1300–1310
Hu N et al (1994) Heterozygous Rb-1 delta 20/+mice are predisposed to tumors of the pituitary gland with a nearly complete penetrance. Oncogene 9(4):1021–1027
Jacks T et al (1992) Effects of an Rb mutation in the mouse. Nature 359(6393):295–300
Jockovich ME et al (2006) Anecortave acetate as single and adjuvant therapy in the treatment of retinal tumors of LH(BETA)T(AG) mice. Invest Ophthalmol Vis Sci 47(4):1264–1268
Klutz M, Horsthemke B, Lohmann DR (1999) RB1 gene mutations in peripheral blood DNA of patients with isolated unilateral retinoblastoma. Am J Hum Genet 64(2):667–668
Klutz M, Brockmann D, Lohmann DR (2002) A parent-of-origin effect in two families with retinoblastoma is associated with a distinct splice mutation in the RB1 gene. Am J Hum Genet 71(1):174–179
Knudson AG Jr (1971) Mutation and cancer: statistical study of retinoblastoma. Proc Natl Acad Sci U S A 68(4):820–823
Laurie NA et al (2006) Inactivation of the p53 pathway in retinoblastoma. Nature 444(7115):61–66
Lee EY et al (1992) Mice deficient for Rb are nonviable and show defects in neurogenesis and haematopoiesis. Nature 359(6393):288–294
Lee MH et al (1996) Targeted disruption of p107: functional overlap between p107 and Rb. Genes Dev 10(13): 1621–1632
Lohmann DR (1999) RB1 gene mutations in retinoblastoma. Hum Mutat 14(4):283–288
Lohmann DR, Gallie BL (2007) GENE reviews: retinoblastoma http://www.ncbi.nlm.nih.gov/bookshelf/br.fcgi?book=gene&part=retinoblastoma
Lohmann D, Scheffer H, Gallie BL (2002) Best practice guidelines for molecular analysis of retinoblastoma. European Molecular Genetics Quality Network (EMQN)
MacPherson D et al (2004) Cell type-specific effects of Rb deletion in the murine retina. Genes Dev 18(14):1681–1694
Marchong MN (2007) Identification of CDH11 as a candidate tumor suppressor in retinoblastoma and characterization of its role in retina and retinoblastoma, Department of Medical Biophysics. University of Toronto, Toronto

Marchong MN et al (2004) Minimal 16q genomic loss implicates cadherin-11 in retinoblastoma. Mol Cancer Res 2(9): 495–503
Margo C et al (1983) *Retinocytoma.* A benign variant of retinoblastoma. Arch Ophthalmol 101(10):1519–1531
Morgenbesser SD et al (1994) p53-dependent apoptosis produced by Rb-deficiency in the developing mouse lens. Nature 371(6492):72–74
Murphree AL (2005) Intraocular retinoblastoma: the case for a new group classification. Ophthalmol Clin North Am1 8:41–53
Murray TG et al (1997) Subconjunctival carboplatin therapy and cryotherapy in the treatment of transgenic murine retinoblastoma. Arch Ophthalmol 115(10):1286–1290
Ohtani-Fujita N et al (1997) Hypermethylation in the retinoblastoma gene is associated with unilateral, sporadic retinoblastoma. Cancer Genet Cytogenet 98(1): 43–49
Orlic M (2007) Identification of the 6p22 Oncogene in Retinoblastoma, in Molecular and Medical Genetics. University of Toronto, Toronto
Orlic M et al (2006) Expression analysis of 6p22 genomic gain in retinoblastoma. Genes Chromosomes Cancer 45(1):72–82
Radhi JM (1999) Malignant melanoma arising from nevi, p53, p16, and Bcl-2: expression in benign versus malignant components. J Cutan Med Surg 3(6):293–297
Retinoblastoma Solutions Test Sensitivity (2007) Available at: http://www.retinoblastomasolutions.org/testsent.html. Accessed 24 Oct 2007
Richter S et al (2003) Sensitive and efficient detection of RB1 gene mutations enhances care for families with retinoblastoma. Am J Hum Genet 72(2):253–269
Sabah M et al (2004) Loss of heterozygosity of chromosome 9p and loss of p16INK4A expression are associated with malignant gastrointestinal stromal tumors. Mod Pathol 17(11):1364–1371
Sippel KC et al (1998) Frequency of somatic and germ-line mosaicism in retinoblastoma: implications for genetic counseling. Am J Hum Genet 62(3):610–619
Spencer C et al (2005) Distinct patterns of expression of the RB gene family in mouse and human retina. Gene Expr Patterns 5(5):687–694
Tsai KY et al (1998) Mutation of E2f-1 suppresses apoptosis and inappropriate S phase entry and extends survival of Rb-deficient mouse embryos. Mol Cell 2(3):293–304
Tso MO (1980) Clues to the cells of origin in retinoblastoma. Int Ophthalmol Clin 20(2):191–210
Windle JJ et al (1990) Retinoblastoma in transgenic mice. Nature 343(6259):665–669
Wong FL et al (1997) Cancer incidence after retinoblastoma. Radiation dose and sarcoma risk. JAMA 278(15):1262–1267
Zeschnigk M, Lohmann D, Horsthemke B (1999) A PCR test for the detection of hypermethylated alleles at the retinoblastoma locus. J Med Genet 36(10):793–794
Zhang J, Schweers B, Dyer MA (2004) The first knockout mouse model of retinoblastoma. Cell Cycle 3(7):952–959
Zhang K et al. (2008) Patterns of missplicing caused by RB1 gene mutations in patients with retinoblastoma and association with phenotypic expression. Hum Mutat. 29(4):475–484
Zhu XP et al (1989) Preferential germline mutation of the paternal allele in retinoblastoma. Nature 340(6231): 312–313
Zhu X et al (1992) Mechanisms of loss of heterozygosity in retinoblastoma. Cytogenet Cell Genet 59(4):248–252

Radiation Therapy in the Management of Retinoblastoma

T. E. Merchant

Contents

5.1 Introduction 55
5.2 Treatment Methods 56
5.3 Extraocular and High-Risk Retinoblastoma . . . 60
5.4 Secondary Malignant Tumors 61
5.5 Nonmalignant Side Effects from Radiation Therapy 63
5.6 Controversies in the Management of Retinoblastoma 63
5.7 Recommendations 64
References 64

5.1 Introduction

Radiation therapy is a primary treatment for retinoblastoma resulting in high rates of disease control and functional organ preservation. Late effects from treatment, including secondary tumor formation in patients with genetic predisposition have, during the past 15 years, led investigators to pursue treatment approaches that delay or omit radiation therapy. Currently, the role of radiation therapy in the management of retinoblastoma remains in a state of uncertainty, and the number of patients irradiated using external beam methods is on the decline even as cure rates continue to increase (Broaddus et al. 2009). Investigators and caregivers await firm evidence that visual outcomes and eye preservation are equivalent with newer approaches that include episcleral plaque brachytherapy as a component of local therapy in the current front-line management for selected patients (Antoneli et al. 2006).

In the treatment of retinoblastoma, radiation therapy provides the benchmark for the evaluation of tumor control, for eye preservation, and for side effects. Its role has been diminished by its known contribution to secondary tumors in a high-risk population and the move toward chemotherapy combined with local ophthalmic therapy (Wilson et al. 2001). Radiation therapy is the most effective nonsurgical treatment for retinoblastoma. It is the only treatment for which long-term data identify attribution of late effects in vulnerable young patients and those with genetic susceptibility to malignancy induction. Radiation therapy has an excellent track record in preservation of the eye. In patients with Reese–Ellsworth group I–II disease, tumor control rates measured at

C. Rodriguez-Galindo and M.W. Wilson (eds.), *Retinoblastoma*, Pediatric Oncology, DOI 10.1007/978-0-387-89072-2_5, © Springer Science+Business Media, LLC 2010

5 years are in excess of 95%. In patients with more advanced disease (Reese–Ellsworth groups III and IV), 5-year control rates reduce to approximately 50%, partly owing to the greater tumor burden and intraocular extent of disease (Blach et al. 1996). Patients with Reese–Ellsworth group VB disease have 5-year eye-preservation rates of approximately 53% (Abramson et al. 2004a). Poor tumor control in advanced cases is often attributed to vitreous seeding. Although data on visual acuity are relatively limited, most patients are reported to have good visual acuity (20/20–20/40) after radiation therapy; the rest have at least some prospect for functional vision (20/50–20/400) (Egbert et al. 1978; Hall et al. 1999). Visual acuity and field after therapy are affected by tumor location, tumor size, and treatment (Abramson et al. 2004b), which often depend on the patient's age at the time of diagnosis; younger patients are more likely to have tumors about the macula (Brinkert et al. 1998).

5.2 Treatment Methods

The promise of more advanced external beam radiation therapy methods has yet to be realized. The advent of newer treatments coincided with the movement away from the use of front-line radiation therapy. With the advent of conformal radiation therapy methods, investigators eager to focally irradiate localized disease also realized that the price of increased conformity and a potentially lower integral patient dose was an increase in the volume receiving lower doses.

Treatment methods used for fractionated irradiation of localized retinoblastoma have been extensively reviewed (Munier et al. 2008). The governing hypothesis surrounding the use of newer methods is that increased conformity of treatment will reduce dose to normal tissues and subsequently the side effects of radiation therapy. At stake is a broad spectrum of side effects ranging from the treatable endocrinopathies to lifelong and apparent deformity to the development of an incurable secondary tumor. More recently, external beam irradiation is utilized as a second-line therapy for patients with tumors not amenable to local therapies, including episcleral plaque brachytherapy. These cases often have vitreous seeding for which lens-sparing treatment might compromise the volume at risk for tumor progression, whole-globe irradiation is required, and the advantage of some focal methods may be reduced.

Most clinicians are familiar with the D-shaped fields used to treat unilateral or bilateral disease, with the isocenter placed 2–3 mm behind the lens at the level of the surgical limbus (Fig. 5.1). With the advent of three-dimensional radiation therapy, a variety of methods have been used to treat retinoblastoma, including intensity-modulated radiation therapy. The various methods may be compared on a dosimetry basis by comparing dose–volume histograms for normal tissue, assuming adequate coverage of the targeted volume. Although each method may be used to achieve conformity (i.e., shaping the radiation field so that the highest doses are centrally focused on the targeted

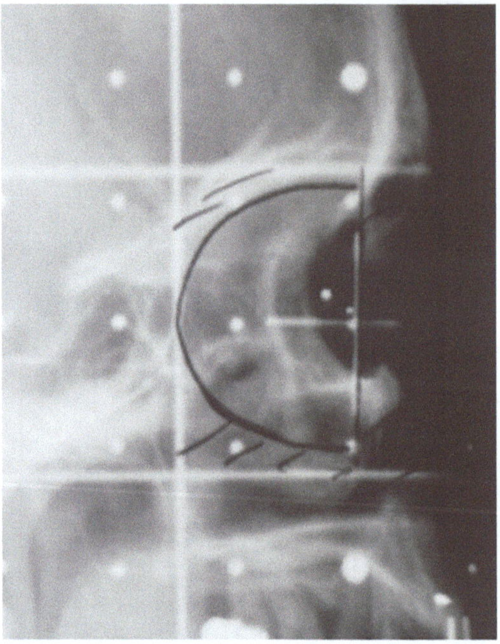

Figure 5.1

Typical D-shaped field used to treat unilateral or bilateral retinoblastoma volume), each method has different characteristics in terms of normal tissue irradiation. A recent report demonstrated the advantages of intensity-modulated radiation therapy over three-dimensional conformal radiation therapy and conventional two-dimensional irradiation in terms of the dose delivered to normal tissue structures (Krasin et al. 2004). Although, for most techniques, increasing the conformity of the highest doses results in a relatively sharp decline of the dose–volume curve at the higher doses, this gain comes at the expense of increasing the volume of normal tissue that receives the lowest doses. Consider the dose to the bony orbit, a common site of secondary malignancies: even optimally applied intensity-modulated radiation therapy will result in 50% of the orbit receiving 50% of the prescribed dose. Higgins et al. (2006) used fractionated stereotactic radiation therapy to treat the orbit in children under anesthesia. They found a maximum average deviation to be ± 2 mm. In their estimate, the normal tissue complication probability for growth inhibition of the orbit was reduced from 95–100% using standard techniques to less than 16% using their methods. Sahgal et al. (2006) used similar techniques in a small group of patients and found no acute or late side-effects in patients treated to a focal portion of the retina. The lone patient who required treatment of the entire globe developed cataract and corneal ulceration.

Proton beam radiation therapy has been available for decades. Only recently have protons become the modality of choice to deliver a precise dose to the target yet minimize the dose to normal tissues. A proton beam has exquisite stopping power in tissue and produces essentially no lateral scatter, whereas photon beams traversing the tissue slowly lose energy and deposit decreasing doses of radiation along the path through the tissue. Where the photon beam enters the tissue, it deposits most of its dose superficially, then continues to deposit dose gradually until it exits the patient. The proton beam, with its sharp Bragg peak, can penetrate deeply and deposit dose in the targeted volume, leaving no exit trail (Fig. 5.2). The proton beam can be modulated to achieve a more widely spread Bragg peak and used to uniformly irradiate the tumor or target at a particular depth. Comparing photons or X-rays with protons,

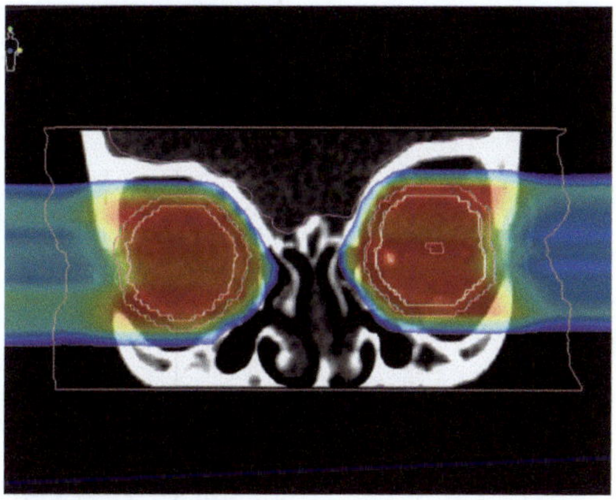

Figure 5.2

Coronal digital reconstruction of a CT image demonstrating the unique stopping ability of protons in a case of bilateral retinoblastoma

it is easy to see that proton beam irradiation can be used to control tumors at any depth without the entrance and exit doses associated with photon beam irradiation that are largely responsible for the complications we see in patients given radiation therapy for retinoblastoma. The advantage of protons over photons in reducing doses to normal tissue (lens, lacrimal gland, bony orbit, and soft tissues) has been demonstrated for of tumors in various sites in the retina (Lee et al. 2005). One study showed that for tumors located in the nasal retina, central retina, or temporal retina, irradiation of normal tissue can be avoided by using beam positioning and eye positioning techniques. Krengli et al. (2005) used tumor volumes from three patients with retinoblastoma were compared on the basis of treatment planning using conformal, electron and intensity-modulated radiation therapy. Protons beam therapy had the best orbital bone sparing dose distribution. Only 10% of the bone exceeded 5 Gy using protons compared to 25% for 3D-CRT electrons, 69% for IMRT, 41% for a single 3D lateral beam, 51% for a 3D anterolateral beam with a lens block, and 65% for a 3D anterolateral beam without a lens block. This finding opens up the possibility of selective retinal

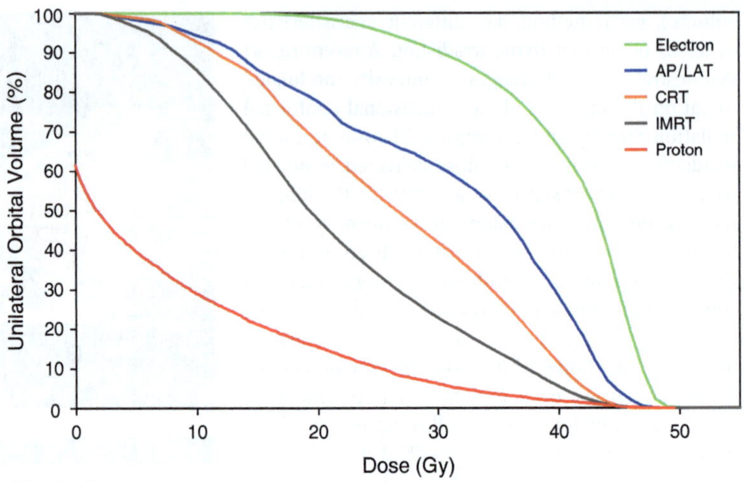

Figure 5.3

Dose–volume curves comparing different treatment techniques

irradiation by using an external beam. Enhancements that allow fine-beam (pencil-beam) scanning and new methods of achieving stereotaxy (including image guidance and robotics) will enable very precise proton-beam treatment of the retina in patients with retinoblastoma. Given plans to increase the availability of proton beam radiation therapy in the US, the relatively small number of cases (based on current trends) that will require radiation therapy, and the obvious dosimetric advantages in these high-risk patients, proton beam radiation therapy will become the standard modality for external beam irradiation of retinoblastoma. Fig. 5.3 shows the differences in orbital bone irradiation for a patient with unilateral retinoblastoma treated with conventional radiation therapy using *en face* electrons or paired photons beams, conformal or intensity-modulated radiation therapy methods, and proton beam radiation therapy. The differences in normal tissue irradiation likely correlate with risk for late effects including secondary tumors and abnormalities in growth and development although long-term data are lacking in this patient population treated with newer methods including proton beam radiation therapy.

Newer methods of irradiation combine advanced methods of patient immobilization and verification with three-dimensional treatment planning and delivery methods. The goal is to limit the highest doses to the targeted volume and minimize dose to normal tissues. In the setting that the tumor is confined to the retina, lens sparing treatment should be a primary consideration to reduce cataract formation. This may be achieved simply by irradiating the posterior aspect of the globe. When more focused methods are employed or the target is prone to motion, fixation of the globe is required. Such immobilization is available at highly specialized centers of ocular oncology(Fi g. 5.4).

Episcleral plaque brachytherapy has enjoyed resurgence and is employed primarily as a consolidative therapy after induction chemotherapy for tumors that have not completely responded yet meet the criteria for plaque treatment (see chapter 7). It has been used successfully to salvage progression of local failures after chemotherapy and radiation therapy in numerous reports. Indeed, episcleral plaque brachytherapy is the only radiation therapy option in the current portfolio of localized retinoblastoma protocols in the

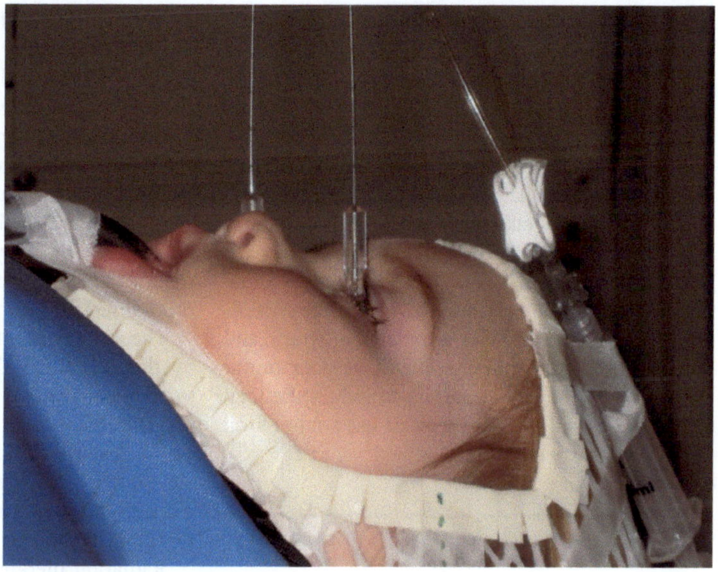

Figure 5.4
Unique immobilization of the globe for the treatment of retinoblastoma using proton therapy

Children's Oncology Group (COG). The current COG trial of systemic neoadjuvant chemotherapy for group B intraocular retinoblastoma,[1] which generally enrolls patients with tumors >3 mm in dimension with or without subretinal fluid and no evidence of vitreous seeding, includes episcleral plaque brachytherapy as a local therapy along with cryotherapy, thermotherapy, and laser photocoagulation. Local therapies are allowed during cycles 2–6 of chemotherapy. Patients who require external beam radiation therapy are considered treatment failures. Similarly, the COG is conducting a single arm trial of vincristine, etoposide and systemic and subtenon carboplatin chemotherapy for groups C and D intraocular retinoblastoma.[2] Episcleral plaque brachytherapy is included as one of the local therapies, which are withheld until the third course of chemotherapy and assessment of response. In this latter study, which includes patients with vitreous seeding, plaque therapy can be viewed only as a supportive therapy and does not replace the role of external beam treatment when progressive vitreous disease is present.

Episcleral plaque brachytherapy has the advantages that it is highly focal, it allows irradiation of normal tissue to be limited, and it has a high rate of lesion control. Its disadvantages include its lack of availability or applicability as a treatment technique. It requires extensive operator experience and in some instances produces significant adverse effects in the retina. A standard dose is 40 Gy to the apex at 40–50 cGy per hour and may require inpatient admission. Common sources include iodine 125 (^{125}I), but other sources have been investigated. In the largest reported series from Philadelphia, tumor control rates in excess of 86% were achieved in 102 cases (Shields

[1] Trial of Systemic Neoadjuvant Chemotherapy for Group B Intraocular retinoblastoma (ARET0331)
[2] A Single Arm Trial of Systemic and Subtenon Chemotherapy for Groups C and D Intraocular Retinoblastoma (ARET0231)

et al. 2001). The St. Jude series included a relatively small number of cases and a lesion control rate of 96% (Merchant et al. 2004). Responses to episcleral plaque brachytherapy are seen rapidly and in some cases during the brief course of application (Fig. 5.4). Discussion of all the radiation techniques reported for treatment of unilateral and bilateral tumors and of all the measures taken to spare the lens and minimize irradiation of normal tissue are beyond the scope of this chapter. Indeed, given that a substantial number of patients are diagnosed with vitreous seeding (Reese–Ellsworth IVB) after chemotherapy and require whole eye irradiation and have poor tumor control, it may be less important to reduce the total dose of radiation, spare the lens, or use a more focal radiation delivery technique.

5.3 Extraocular and High-Risk Retinoblastoma

Patients with extraocular and high-risk retinoblastoma include a group of children who are not commonly seen in clinical practice in the US. Radiation therapy is indicated for extraocular retinoblastoma and after enucleation when high-risk features are present including scleral involvement and involvement of the margins of the optic nerve based on anatomic pathologic examination (see chapter 8) (Stannard et al. 1979). Based on orbital or regional involvement, patients should receive radiation therapy to initially involved sites after induction chemotherapy. Delaying radiation therapy is meant to allow for response evaluation to chemotherapy, the possibility of cytoreduction, and reduced treatment volume. The fundamental target volume is the orbit for most cases of pathologically defined extraocular tumor and extends to include regional sites and lymph nodes based on clinical and imaging evidence of tumor extension. In the rare instance that regional sites or lymph node involvement are documented in the absence of local pathologic evidence of extraocular tumor, the orbit may be omitted from the primary treatment volume. The dose used for treatment of the orbit or regional extraocular sites is typically 45 Gy.

The aforementioned approach has been adopted by the Children's Oncology Group in their trial for extraocular and high-risk retinoblastoma.[3] The target volumes and doses for patients with orbit-confined and regional disease are included in Table 5.1. An example case demonstrating the definitions of clinical and planning target volume is included in Fig. 5.5.

Radiation therapy may be indicated for patients with metastatic retinoblastoma based on response to chemotherapy. In most treatment protocols, patients with hematogenous metastases or CNS involvement who achieve a complete response to induction chemotherapy are not irradiated; however, incompletely responding patients are most often irradiated at the completion of chemotherapy that includes consolidation using high-dose therapy and stem-cell rescue. This sequence is mandated for patients who require craniospinal irradiation. Typical doses include 36 Gy to non-CNS metastatic sites in patients who appear to respond to chemotherapy. Based on age, older patients who require craniospinal irradiation should receive

Table 5.1. Target volumes and doses for patients with orbit-confined and regional retinoblastoma

Stage/Site	GTV	CTV	PTV	PTV doses
Orbital involvement	Residual tumor	Orbit[a] including GTV	CTV+5 mm	45 Gy
Orbital and regional extraorbital involvement	Residual tumor and regional lymph nodes	Orbit including GTV and extraorbital and regional lymph nodes	CTV+5 mm	45 Gy

Orbit = internal bony orbit, optic foramen and optic nerve to chiasm
GTV gross tumor volume, *CTV* clinical target volume, *PTV* planning target volume
[a]Orbit may be omitted from the treatment volume when local pathologic evidence of extraocular tumor is not present

[3] A trial of intensive multimodality therapy for extraocular retinoblastoma. (ARET0321).

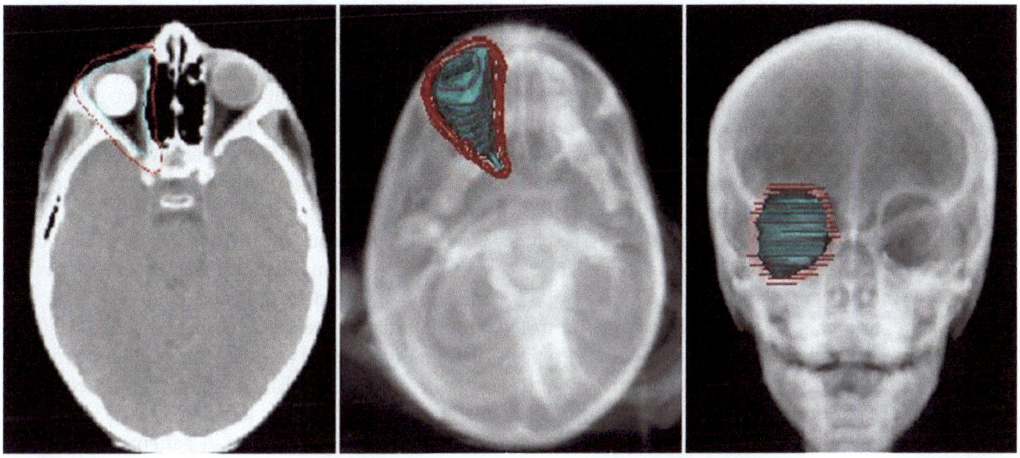

Figure 5.5

Three-dimensional radiation therapy targeting of the orbit. Clinical (*inner contour*) and planning (*outer contour*) target volume contours are shown (*left image*) along with superior (*center image*) and anterior (*right image*) projection of the volumetric orbital target volume

36 Gy to the neuraxis and 45 Gy to residual disease. Younger patients should receive at least 23.4 Gy to the neuraxis. There is evidence to suggest that clinically defined disease has limited microscopic tumor infiltration so that the clinical target volume surrounds the clinically identifiable residual tumor (gross tumor volume), may be as small as 5 mm. These patients have a poor prognosis (Leal-Leal et al. 2006).

5.4 Secondary Malignant Tumors

The risk of second malignant neoplasms is highest among patients with the germline mutation of the *RB1* gene (for more information on second malignancies in retinoblastoma survivors, see chapter 9). They may occur without the use of radiation therapy (Mahajan et al. 2008) and in patients treated with chemotherapy (Gombos et al. 2007). Chemotherapy is known to enhance the development of second malignant neoplasms in irradiated patients (Marees et al. 2008). Radiation-induced tumors are the most frequent and bone and soft-tissue sarcomas are the most common (Kleinerman et al. 2005). It appears that more patients die from radiation-induced sarcomas than from retinoblastoma itself (Kleinerman et al. 2007).

The report by Wong et al. (1997) had a major impact on the use of radiation therapy. The report covered a 70-year experience and included 604 patients with bilateral retinoblastoma. It estimated that the 50-year cumulative incidence of second malignant neoplasms in irradiated patients was 51% for patients with bilateral disease, but only 5% for patients with unilateral disease. The data also showed that radiation-induced tumors were the leading cause of death among long-term survivors.

More recent data show that the incidence is lower. Marees et al. (2008) reported on 668 retinoblastoma survivors treated from 1945 to 2005 who were in the Dutch registry. With a median follow-up of 21.9 years, they showed that the standardized incidence ratio for the development of a secondary tumor was 20.4 among irradiated patients with hereditary retinoblastoma versus 1.86 among those who were not irradiated. The cumulative incidence of a secondary tumor at 40 years was estimated to be 28% (95% CI 21–35). Kleinerman et al. reported on 1601 previously studied retinoblastoma survivors through the year 2000 (Kleinerman et al. 2005). The analysis included nearly 1,000 patients with irradiated or unirradiated hereditary tumors. The standardized incidence ratio (ratio of observed to expected cancers) was 22 in the irradiated group and 7 in the unirradiated group, a threefold difference. The cumulative incidence of new cancers at 50 years was 36% (95% CI 31–41) among those irradiated.

While these reports are more refined and control groups more acceptable than in the past, these type of data will continue to be challenged for their potential bias with regard to treatment era and techniques, the statistical handling of trilateral retinoblastoma, the attribution of low-dose therapeutic exposures and diagnostic imaging, the fundamental lack of long-term data for patients treated only with chemotherapy, and the suspicion that patients treated decades ago with "radiotherapy alone" may have had poorly documented chemotherapy exposure. Radiation oncologists acknowledge the attribution of radiation therapy but remain concerned that functional outcomes and vision in this patient group have lost ground in the current era hoping that an improved assessment of the risks for malignancy induction, including a refined evaluation of genetic predisposition, will identify a role for their modality.

The risk of secondary cancer overrides most decisions about treatment. Abramson et al. (Abramson and Frank 1998) determined that the risk of a second malignancy was reduced in patients older than 12 months compared to those younger than 12 months when irradiated. Statistically, the risk of secondary malignancies in patients irradiated when older than 12 months was equal to that in patients who did not receive radiation therapy. They concluded that delaying radiation therapy until the patient was older than 1 year appeared to reduce the risk of a second malignancy. Similar findings were observed by Moll et al., who reviewed the Dutch Registry and patients with hereditary retinoblastoma (Moll et al. 2001) (Fig. 5.6).

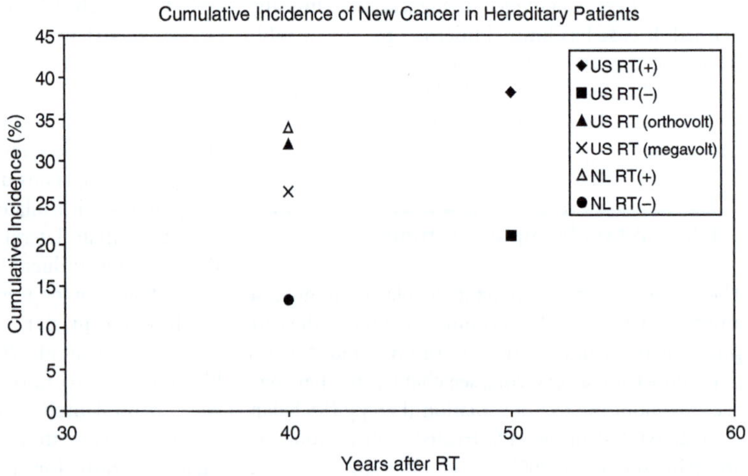

Figure 5.6

Plot of dose versus incidence of radiation-induced secondary tumors based on published data. US = United States, NL = The Netherlands, RT(+) = Radiation Therapy, RT(-) = No Radiation Therapy

5.5 Nonmalignant Side Effects from Radiation Therapy

There are a variety of potential side effects from radiation therapy that impact the goals of organ preservation, preservation of vision, and maintaining length and quality of life. The side effects of radiation therapy have framed current clinical trial designs to include avoidance of radiation therapy for patients with retinoblastoma. These side effects include (Tawansy et al. 2006; Pomarede et al. 1984; Srithavaj and Thaweboon 2006; Miller et al. 2005; Kase et al. 2008;G uyuron 1990;O 'Dohertye ta l. 2005).

Ophthalmic and nonophthalmic complications include:

- Retinald etachment
- Vitreoush emorrhage
- Cataractf ormation
- Glaucoma
- Endocrinopathy
- Xerophthalmia
- Altered oral ecology
- Orbitalh ypoplasia.

Destruction of any portion of the eye, including phthisis bulbi, is an uncommon but potential complication along with ocular glaucoma, which negates all potential benefits of radiation therapy and leaves the patient with the burden of radiation exposure since enucleation is usually required. Less severe but equally problematic is retinal detachment. Xerophthalmia is an expected complication of radiation therapy when the sebaceous meibomian glands or lacrimal glands are included in the irradiated volume. Cataract formation is a frequent side effect from radiation therapy. The true incidence of cataract formation is unclear; however, Miller et al. (2005) reported on a series of patients where the median interval from diagnosis to cataract surgery was 42 months (range, 28–95 months). Even with directed irradiation of the anterior chamber, cataract formation is not guaranteed suggesting that predisposing factors are contributory. Kase et al. (2008) showed that growth factors produced by retinoblastoma cells may lead to cataract formation. TGF-beta is known to potentiate radiation effects. There are no clinical data evaluating TGF-beta levels in cataracts induced by irradiation. Hopefully with newer techniques of irradiation, hourglass deformity is a thing of the past (Guyuron 1990).

5.6 Controversies in the Management of Retinoblastoma

Radiation therapy may be indicated when the globe is penetrated traumatically or surgically in advance of the diagnosis of retinoblastoma (Gass 1963). Investigators at the Will's Eye Institute (Shields et al. 2000) reported on the management of retinoblastoma in patients after vitrectomy. Their series included 900 patients from which 11 (1%) cases treated with vitrectomy prior to the diagnosis of retinoblastoma were identified. In no case was retinoblastoma suspected prior to vitrectomy performed to treat vitreous hemorrhage, toxocariasis, toxoplasmosis, or endophthalmitis. All cases were sporadic and the median age was 6 years. Retinoblastoma was diagnosed after cytologic evaluation of the vitrectomy specimen in most cases and less often at the time of the procedure. With a median follow-up of 7 years, none of the patients treated with adjuvant therapy experience tumor recurrence. Treatment included enucleation in all, but one patient and orbital irradiation was administered in 9 patients and a similar were treated with chemotherapy. Others have reported on the treatment of retinoblastoma following ocular surgery (Stevenson et al. 1989). Extraocular retinoblastoma was the initial presentation for three patients previously treated with ocular surgery that included biopsy, vitrectomy, or lensectomy. The time from surgery to presentation ranged from 3 to 18 months and all were successfully treated with combined modality therapy that included orbital irradiation to 44 Gy. There are also case reports citing dissemination of unsuspected retinoblastoma in patients following hyphema drainage (Murthy et al. 2007). One such case reported conjunctival presentation, cervical lymphadenopathy 7 months after surgery. The 6-year-old patient died of metastatic disease.

One wonders if controlled surgery on the eye is an indication for adjuvant therapy including radiation therapy. Twelve high-volume ocular oncology clinics were queried with regard to their patients diagnosed with retinoblastoma following controlled fine needle aspiration (Karcioglu 2002). Among 3,651 patients, eight were biopsied and six were diagnosed with retinoblastoma following fine needle aspiration biopsy with the clinical diagnosis of uveitis/endophthalmitis using 25–27 g needles through the limbus and pars plana. Most were older than 4 years of age at the time of diagnosis. Five were treated with enucleation and one with cryotherapy and I-125 brachytherapy. With follow-up of 10.8 years, there have been no cases of recurrent disease.

5.7 Recommendations

A number of measures may be taken to reduce the likelihood of second malignant neoplasms and treatment effects if radiation therapy is required including delaying radiation therapy until the patient is 12 months old, reducing the total dose, using episcleral plaque brachytherapy as a local therapy after chemotherapy, new external beam treatment methods and modalities, including conformal or intensity-modulated radiation therapy and proton beam radiation therapy.

Our recommendations for patients with newly diagnosed retinoblastoma include 36 Gy for Reese-Ellsworth group I or II disease and standard-dose irradiation (45 Gy) for more advanced (Reese–Ellsworth group III-V) disease. For patients whose disease progresses after chemotherapy, our preference is to irradiate with standard doses (outside a protocol) and to use episcleral plaque brachytherapy when possible. We recommend defining the clinical target volume as the optic globe and the treatment planning target volume as the optic globe with a 3–5 mm margin. Lens sparing can be accomplished on an individual basis when no evidence of retinal seeding is apparent. Additional individualized techniques include using a conventional split beam to spare the lens and using electrons, conformal irradiation, intensity-modulated radiation therapy, and, soon to be more widely available, proton beam radiation therapy.

References

Abramson DH, Frank CM (1998) Second nonocular tumors in survivors of bilateral retinoblastoma: a possible age effect on radiation-related risk. Ophthalmology 105:573–9

Abramson DH, Beaverson KL, Chang ST et al (2004a) Outcome following initial external beam radiotherapy in patients with Reese-Ellsworth group Vb retinoblastoma. Arch Ophthalmol 122:1316–23

Abramson DH, Melson MR, Servodidio C (2004b) Visual fields in retinoblastoma survivors. Arch Ophthalmol 122(9):1324–30

Antoneli CB, Ribeiro KC, Steinhorst F, Novaes PE, Chojniak MM, Malogolowkin M (2006) Treatment of retinoblastoma patients with chemoreduction plus local therapy: experience of the AC Camargo Hospital, Brazil. J Pediatr Hematol Oncol 28(6):342–5

Blach LE, McCormick B, Abramson DH (1996) External beam radiation therapy and retinoblastoma: long-term results in the comparison of two techniques. Int J Radiat Oncol Biol Phys 35:45–51

Brinkert AW, Moll AC, Jager MJ et al (1998) Distribution of tumors in the retina in hereditary retinoblastoma patients. Ophthalmic Genet 19:63–7

Broaddus E, Topham A, Singh AD (2009) Survival with retinoblastoma in the USA: 1975–2004. Br J Ophthalmol 93(1):24–7 Epub 2008 Aug 21

Egbert PR, Donaldson SS, Moazed K, Rosenthal AR (1978) Visual results and ocular complications following radiotherapy for retinoblastoma. Arch Ophthalmol 96:1826–30

Gass DM (1963) Retinoblastoma obscured by recent trauma. Arch Ophthalmol 69(5):583–584

Gombos DS, Hungerford J, Abramson DH, Kingston J, Chantada G, Dunkel IJ, Antoneli CB, Greenwald M, Haik BG, Leal CA, Medina-Sanson A, Schefler AC, Veerakul G, Wieland R, Bornfeld N, Wilson MW, Yu CB (2007) Secondary acute myelogenous leukemia in patients with retinoblastoma: is chemotherapy a factor? Ophthalmology 114(7):1378–83

Guyuron B (1990) The hourglass facial deformity. J Craniomaxillofac Surg 18(5):187–91

Hall LS, Ceisler E, Abramson DH (1999) Visual outcomes in children with bilateral retinoblastoma. J AAPOS 3:138–42

Higgins PD, Gerbi BJ, Macedon M, Dusenbery KE (2006) Fractionated stereotactic radiotherapy for pediatric patients with retinoblastoma. J Appl Clin Med Phys 7(2):9–17

Karcioglu ZA (2002) Fine needle aspiration biopsy (FNAB) for retinoblastoma. Retina 22(6):707–10

Kase S, Parikh JG, Youssef PN, Murphree AL, Rao NA (2008) Transforming growth factor beta in retinoblastoma-related cataract. Arch Ophthalmol 126(11):1539–42

Kleinerman RA, Tucker MA, Tarone RE, Abramson DH, Seddon JM, Stovall M, Li FP, Fraumeni JF Jr (2005) Risk of new cancers after radiotherapy in long-term survivors of retinoblastoma: an extended follow-up. J Clin Oncol2 3(10):2272–9

Kleinerman RA, Tucker MA, Abramson DH, Seddon JM, Tarone RE, Fraumeni JF Jr (2007) Risk of soft tissue sarcomas by individual subtype in survivors of hereditary retinoblastoma. J Natl Cancer Inst 99(1):24–31

Krasin MJ, Crawford BT, Zhu Y et al (2004) Intensity-modulated radiation therapy for children with intraocular retinoblastoma: potential sparing of the bony orbit. Clin Oncol (R Coll Radiol) 16:215–22

Krengli M, Hug EB, Adams JA et al (2005) Proton radiation therapy for retinoblastoma: comparison of various intraocular tumor locations and beam arrangements. Int J Radiat Oncol Biol Phys 61:583–93

Leal-Leal CA, Rivera-Luna R, Flores-Rojo M, Juárez-Echenique JC, Ordaz JC, Amador-Zarco J (2006) Survival in extra-orbital metastatic retinoblastoma:treatment results. Clin Transl Oncol 8(1):39–44

Lee CT, Bilton SD, Famiglietti RM, Riley BA, Mahajan A, Chang EL, Maor MH, Woo SY, Cox JD, Smith AR (2005) Treatment planning with protons for pediatric retinoblastoma, medulloblastoma, and pelvic sarcoma: how do protons compare with other conformal techniques? Int J Radiat Oncol Biol Phys 63(2):362–72

Mahajan S, Juneja M, George T (2008) Osteosarcoma as a second neoplasm after chemotherapeutic treatment of hereditary retinoblastoma: a case report. 1. Quintessence Int 39(5):439–452

Marees T, Moll AC, Imhof SM, de Boer MR, Ringens PJ, van Leeuwen FE (2008) Risk of second malignancies in survivors of retinoblastoma: more than 40 years of follow-up. J Natl Cancer Inst 100(24):1771–9 Epub 2008 Dec 9

Merchant TE, Gould CJ, Wilson MW et al (2004) Episcleral plaque brachytherapy for retinoblastoma. Pediatr Blood Cancer4 3:134–9

Miller DM, Murray TG, Cicciarelli NL, Capo H, Markoe AM (2005) Pars plana lensectomy and intraocular lens implantation in pediatric radiation-induced cataracts in retinoblastoma. Ophthalmology 112(9):1620–1624

Moll AC, Imhof SM, Schouten-Van Meeteren AY et al (2001) Second primary tumors in hereditary retinoblastoma: a register-based study, 1945–1997: is there an age effect on radiation-related risk? Ophthalmology 108:1109–14

Munier FL, Verwey J, Pica A, Balmer A, Zografos L, Abouzeid H, Timmerman B, Goitein G, Moeckli R (2008) New developments in external beam radiotherapy for retinoblastoma: from lens to normal tissue-sparing techniques. Clin Experiment Ophthalmol 36(1):78–89

Murthy R, Honavar SG, Vemuganti GK, Naik MN, Reddy VP (2007) Systemic metastasis following hyphema drainage in an unsuspected retinoblastoma. J Pediatr Ophthalmol Strabismus 44(2):120–3

O'Doherty M, Lanigan B, Breathnach F, O'Meara A, Gallie B, Chan H, O'Keefe M (2005) A retrospective review of visual outcome and complications in the treatment of retinoblastoma. Ir Med J 98(1):17–20

Pomarede R, Czernichow P, Zucker JM, Schlienger P, Haye C, Rosenwald JC, Labib A, Rappaport R (1984) Incidence of anterior pituitary deficiency after radiotherapy at an early age: study in retinoblastoma. Acta Paediatr Scand 73(1):115–9

Sahgal A, Millar BA, Michaels H, Jaywant S, Chan HS, Heon E, Gallie B, Laperriere N (2006) Focal stereotactic external beam radiotherapy as a vision-sparing method for the treatment of peripapillary and perimacular retinoblastoma: preliminary results. Clin Oncol (R Coll Radiol) 18(8):628–34

Shields CL, Honavar S, Shields JA, Demirci H, Meadows AT (2000) Vitrectomy in eyes with unsuspected retinoblastoma. Ophthalmology 107(12):2250–5

Shields CL, Shields JA, Cater J et al (2001) Plaque radiotherapy for retinoblastoma: long-term tumor control and treatment complications in 208 tumors. Ophthalmology 108:2116–21

Srithavaj T, Thaweboon S (2006) Determination of oral microflora in irradiated ocular deformed children. Southeast Asian J Trop Med Public Health 37(5):991–5

Stannard C, Lipper S, Sealy R, Sevel D (1979) Retinoblastoma: correlation of invasion of the optic nerve and choroid with prognosis and metastasis. Br J Ophthalmol 63:560–570

Stevenson KE, Hungerford J, Garner A (1989) Local extraocular extension of retinoblastoma following intraocular surgery. Br J Ophthalmol 73(9):739–42

Tawansy KA, Samuel MA, Shammas M, Murphree AL (2006) Vitreoretinal complications of retinoblastoma treatment. Retina 26(7 Suppl):S47–52

Wilson MW, Rodriguez-Galindo C, Haik BG et al (2001) Multiagent chemotherapy as neoadjuvant treatment for multifocal intraocular retinoblastoma. Ophthalmology 108:2106–14 discussion 2114–5

Wong FL, Boice JD Jr, Abramson DH et al (1997) Cancer incidence after retinoblastoma. Radiation dose and sarcoma risk. JAMA 278:1262–7

Chemotherapy in the Management of Retinoblastoma

C. Rodriguez-Galindo

Contents

6.1 **Introduction** . . . 67
6.2 **Ocular Pharmacokinetics** . . . 68
6.2.1 Ocular Drug Transporters . . . 69
6.3 **Chemotherapy in the Treatment of Intraocular Retinoblastoma** . . . 69
6.3.1 Unilateral Retinoblastoma . . . 69
6.3.2 Bilateral Retinoblastoma . . . 70
6.3.3 New Tumor Formation on Chemotherapy . . . 72
6.3.4 Therapy-Related Leukemia . . . 73
6.4 **Periocular Administration of Chemotherapy** . . . 73
6.4.1 Mechanisms for Transscleral Drug Delivery . . . 73
6.4.2 Periocular Chemotherapy in Retinoblastoma . . . 75
6.5 **Intravitreal and Intrarterial Chemotherapy for Intraocular Retinoblastoma** . . . 77
6.6 **Treatment of Extraocular Retinoblastoma** . . . 77
6.6.1 Orbital and Locoregional Retinoblastoma . . . 77
6.6.2 Metastatic Retinoblastoma . . . 78
6.7 **Translational Research and Emergent Therapies in Retinoblastoma** . . . 79
6.8 **Specific Agents** . . . 81
6.8.1 Vincristine . . . 81
6.8.2 Carboplatin . . . 81
6.8.3 Etoposide (VP-16) . . . 82
6.8.4 Doxorubicin . . . 82
6.8.5 Cyclophosphamide . . . 83
6.8.6 Cisplatin . . . 84
6.8.7 Topotecan . . . 85
6.8.8 Thiotepa . . . 85
References . . . 86

6.1 Introduction

Treatment of retinoblastoma aims to save life and preserve useful vision, and thus needs to be individualized. Factors that need to be considered include unilaterality or bilaterality of the disease, potential for vision, and intraocular and extraocular staging. A multidisciplinary approach is pivotal, and it is in this context that the role of chemotherapy must be discussed.

The first clinical experience with chemotherapy in the treatment of retinoblastoma using nitrogen mustard was reported in 1953 (Kupfer 1953). Institutional experiences in the management of extraocular retinoblastoma were reported subsequently, usually applying regimens modeled after the treatment regimens for metastatic neuroblastoma (Lonsdale et al. 1968; Pratt et al. 1985). Since then, the role of chemotherapy has been expanding, and now it is a main component in the management of intraocular disease.

Retinoblastoma is a very chemosensitive disease; in general, chemotherapy is indicated in patients with extraocular disease, in the subgroup of patients with intraocular disease with high-risk histologic features, and in patients with bilateral disease in conjunction with aggressive focal therapies. Agents with documented efficacy include microtubule inhibitors (vincristine and paclitaxel), platinum compounds (cisplatin and carboplatin), topoisomerase II inhibitors (teniposide and etoposide), alkylating agents (cyclophosphamide and ifosfamide), anthracyclines (doxorubicin and idarubicin), and topoisomerase I inhibitors (topotecan) (Schouten-van Meeteren et al. 2002;R odriguez-Galindoe ta l. 2007).

C. Rodriguez-Galindo and M.W. Wilson (eds.), *Retinoblastoma*, Pediatric Oncology,
DOI 10.1007/978-0-387-89072-2_6,

6.2 Ocular Pharmacokinetics

Application of new therapeutic possibilities for cancer treatment involves drug delivery in many forms, but ocular drug delivery is hampered by the barriers protecting the eye (Fig. 6.1). The eye is protected from the xenobiotics of the blood stream by blood-ocular barriers. The anterior blood-eye barrier (*blood-aqueous barrier*) is constituted by the endothelial cells in the uvea. This barrier limits the access of hydrophilic drugs from plasma into the aqueous humor; however, inflammation may disrupt the integrity of this barrier causing unlimited drug distribution to the anterior chamber. The posterior blood-eye barrier (*blood-retina barrier*) is formed by the neural retina and the retinal pigment epithelium (RPE), and the tight walls of retinal capillaries. The inner border of the neural retina faces the vitreous, and the outer border

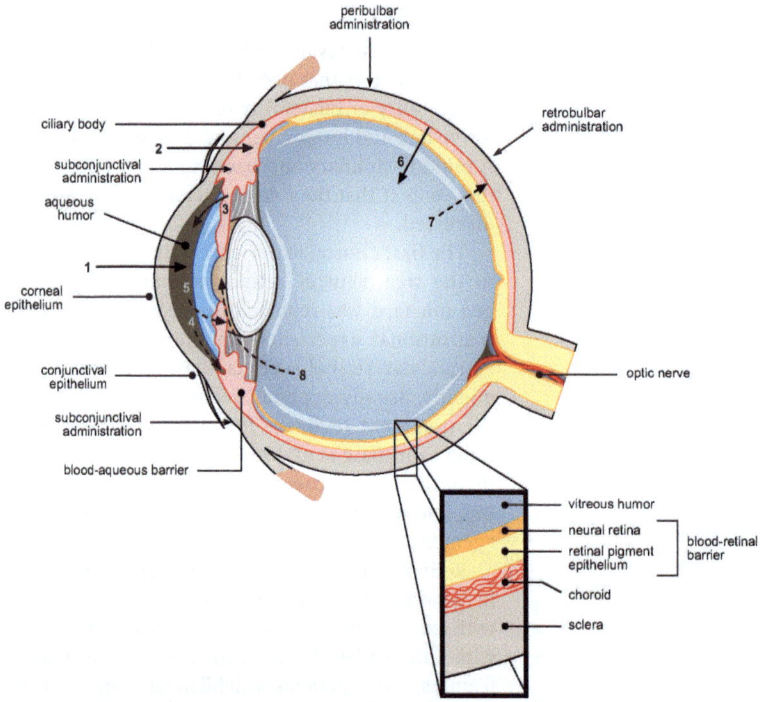

Figure 6.1

Schematic representation of the eye with routes of periocular drug administration and ocular kinetics (modified from Urtti A.(Urtti 2006)) (1) Transcorneal permeation into the anterior chamber; (2) non-corneal drug permeation across the conjunctiva and sclera into the uvea; (3) Drug distribution from the blood into the anterior chamber through the blood-aquesous barrier; (4) Clearance of drug from the anterior chamber through the trabecular meshwork and Schlemm's canal; (5) Drug clearance from the aqueous humor into the systemic circularion across the blood-aqueous barrier; (6) drug distribution from the blood into the posterior eye across the blood-retinal barrier; (7) Drug elimination from the vitreous via posterior route across the blood-retinal barrier; and (8) Drug clearance from the vitreous via anterior route to the posterior chamber is next to the RPE. The neural retina is composed of nine layers, and the RPE is composed of a monolayer of polarized cells. The blood supply to the inner two-thirds of the retina is from retinal vessels; the retinal endothelial cells have basal lamina, and they are surrounded by pericytes, thus forming tight junctions. The blood supply to the outer third of the retina and the RPE comes from the choroidal circulation. Unlike the retinal capillaries, the vasculature of the choroid has extensive blood flow and leaky walls; drugs easily gain access to the choroid extravascular space, but thereafter, distribution into the retina is limited by the RPE and retinal endothelia (Mannermaa et al. 2006; Urtti 2006). Lipophilicity, molecular weight, and protein binding (it is believed that only unbound drugs can pass through the blood-retina barrier) are the main factors for penetration through the barrier. Inflammation and trauma also have important roles in breaking the blood-retina barrier by disrupting tight junctions, increasing transendothelial vesicles, and increasing pinocytosis (Ghate and Edelhauser 2006). It is possible that a similar phenomenon occurs inr etinoblastoma.

6.2.1 Ocular Drug Transporters

The blood-retina barrier restricts the movement of substances after systemic and periocular administration to the retina. The tight junctions form the penetration barrier to hydrophilic substances, thereby limiting the transfer of compounds both inward (blood to vitreous) and outward (vitreous to blood). The RPE has many important features essential for normal retinal function, such as transport of nutrients and waste products, regulation of ion, and fluid balance. RPE thus expresses many transporters and channels related to these physiological functions. Among these, the RPE and the endothelial cells also express efflux transporters, such as P-glycoprotein, MRP1, 4, 5, and BCRP. This efflux protein activity restricts the movement of certain drugs to the retina. In most cases, this is an important protective system for the retina, but it also limits drug delivery to the posterior eye segment (Mannermaa et al. 2006). Many antineoplastic agents are known substrates of efflux proteins.

6.3 Chemotherapy in the Treatment of Intraocular Retinoblastoma

6.3.1 Unilateral Retinoblastoma

In the absence of extraocular disease, enucleation alone is curative for 85–90% of children with unilateral retinoblastoma (Khelfaoui et al. 1996; Zelter et al. 1991; Schvartzman et al. 1996; Chantada et al. 2004a). However, in view of the success in treating bilateral intraocular disease with chemoreduction, early stage intraocular disease can also be treated using conservative methods (Shields and Shields 1999). Adjuvant treatment is indicated in the cases with scleral invasion and in patients with positive tumor at the transection line of the optic nerve (see below, under treatment of extraocular retinoblastoma, and chapter 9). Adjuvant treatment for the remaining patients with intraocular disease is debatable. In the absence of randomized studies, available information would suggest that the use of adjuvant chemotherapy is beneficial for the selected group of patients with higher risk of extraocular dissemination (a subset of patients with retrolaminar optic nerve invasion, patients with massive choroidal or scleral involvement, and patients with involvement of the anterior segment) (Khelfaoui et al. 1996; Chantada et al. 2004a; Uusitalo et al. 2001; Honavar et al. 2002; Chantada et al. 2007). The value of adjuvant chemotherapy in the setting of isolated retrolaminar involvement is controversial (Chantada et al. 2007). Adjuvant chemotherapy does not seem to be indicated for patients with prelaminar involvement (Uusitalo et al. 2001; Chantada et al. 1999a), or isolated focal choroidal involvement (Schvartzman et al. 1996; Chantada et al. 2004a; Uusitalo et al. 2001; Chantada et al. 1999a). Different chemotherapy regimens have been proposed. A six-month treatment with VDC (vincristine, cyclophosphamide and doxorubicin), VCE (vincristine, carboplatin and etoposide), or a hybrid with alternating courses of both regimens, appears to be effective (Zelter et al. 1991; Honavar et al. 2002) (Table 6.1). Idarubicin is also an effective agent in retinoblastoma, and can be substituted for doxorubicin (Chantada et al. 2004a; Chantada et al. 1999b).

Table 6.1. Adjuvant chemotherapy for retinoblastoma with high risk histology

Regimen	Drugs	Doses	Comments
COG-ARET0332 protocol	VCR CBP ETO	0.05 mg/kg day 1 18.6 mg/kg day 1 5 mg/kg days 1, 2	6 cycles
Chantada et al. (Chantada et al. 2004a)	VCR CYC IDA	0.05 mg/kg day 1 65 mg/kg day 1 10 mg/m² day 1	Cycles 1, 3, 5, 7
	CBP ETO	18.7 mg/kg (<10 kg) days 1, 2 560 mg/m² (≥10 kg) days 1, 2 3.3 mg/kg (<10 kg) days 1, 2, 3 100 mg/m² (≥10 kg) days 1, 2, 3	Cycles 2, 4, 6, 8
SJCRH	VCR CYC DOX	0.05 mg/kg (<12 months) day 1 1.5 mg/m² (≥12 months) day 1 40 mg/kg (<12 months) day 1 1,200 mg/m² (≥12 months) day 1 1.5 mg/kg (<12 months) day 1 45 mg/m² (≥12 months) day 1	Cycles 1, 3, 5
	VCR CBP ETO	0.05 mg/kg (<12 months) day 1 1.5 mg/m² (≥12 months) day 1 AUC 6.5 mg/ml/min day 1 3.3 mg/kg (<12 months) days 1, 2, 3 100 mg/m² (≥12 months) days 1, 2, 3	Cycles 2, 4, 6

VCR vincristine, *CBP* carboplatin, *ETO* etoposide, *CYC* cyclphosphamide, *IDA* idarubicin, *DOX* doxorubicin, *SJCRH* St. Jude Children's Research Hospital

6.3.2 Bilateral Retinoblastoma

Patients with germline mutation of the *RB1* gene develop multiple, bilateral retinoblastomas at an earlier age, and they are at risk of developing new tumors until the completion of retinal differentiation (Mohney et al. 1998). Treatment of patients with bilateral retinoblastoma incorporates up-front chemotherapy, which intends to achieve maximum chemoreduction of the intraocular tumor burden early in the treatment, followed by aggressive focal therapies. Intraocular retinoblastoma is extremely chemosensitive, and disease progression during treatment is rarely seen. Noticeable responses are seen in more than 90% of the eyes; these responses are maximum after 2 cycles, and tumor regression after subsequent cycles is less pronounced (Figs. 6.2 and 6.3) (Rodriguez-Galindo et al. 2003a; Abramson et al. 2005; Dunkel et al. 2007). However, chemotherapy alone can only save less than 10% of the eyes (Rodriguez-Galindo et al. 2003a). Macular tumors are more sensitive to chemotherapy, probably because of the richer vascular supply that maximizes exposure to chemotherapy. Up to two-thirds of macular tumors can be controlled with chemotherapy alone (Shields et al. 2005), and with the addition of thermotherapy, this proportion may increase to greater than 80% (Shields et al. 2005; Schefler et al. 2007). Chemoreduction coupled with intensive use of sequential focal therapies (cryotherapy, laser photocoagulation, thermotherapy and brachytherapy) has resulted in an increase in the eye salvage rates and in the decrease (and delay) in the use of radiation therapy (see chapter 7). Different chemotherapy combinations are used although the best results are achieved with a combination of vincristine, carboplatin, and etoposide (or teniposide) (Shields et al. 2002a; Nenadov Beck et al. 2000; Murphree et al. 1996; Kingston et al. 1996; Chantada et al.

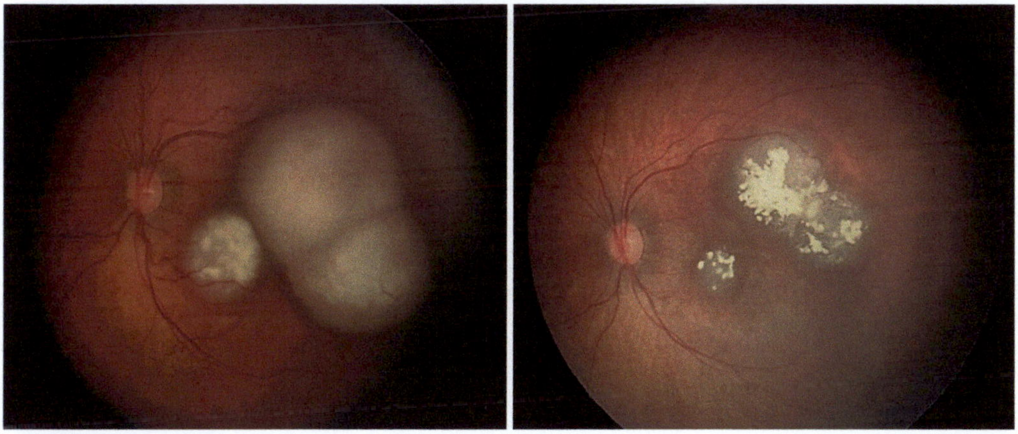

a b

Figure 6.2 a,b

Response of a group B eye a to 2 cycles of vincristine and carboplatin b

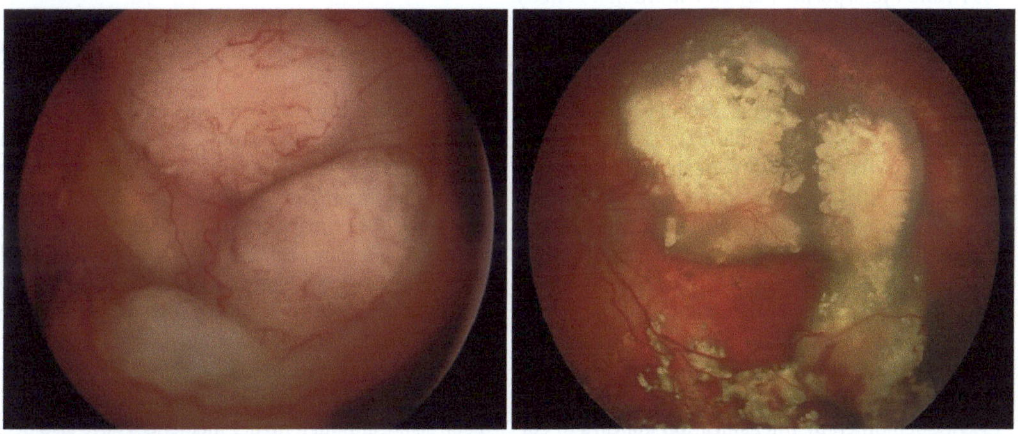

a b

Figure 6.3 a,b

Response of a group D eye a to 2 cycles of vincristine and topotecan in a patient with bilateral retinoblastoma b

2005; Menon et al. 2007; Schiavetti et al. 2005; Antonelli et al. 2006). An alternative chemotherapy regimen includes the addition of cyclosporine to the three-drug regimen (Gallie et al. 1996). The rationale for the use of cyclosporine originates from the documentation of multiple ATP-binding cassette transporters in retinoblastoma tumors (Chan et al. 1997; Wilson et al. 2006; Krishnakumar et al. 2004) and the possible correlation with treatment failure (Chan et al. 1997). The concurrent administration of cyclosporine could potentially abrogate the efflux of drugs from the cancer cell (Gallie et al. 1996; Chan et al. 1996).

Table 6.2. Recommended approach by the Children's Oncology Group to the treatment of intraocular retinoblastoma

R-E group	ABC group	Treatment		
		Focal Tx	Chemotherapy	Radiation
I–II	A	+	If PD	If PD
I–III	B	+	VCR 0.05 mg/kg d 1 CBP 18.6 mg/kg d 1 X 2–6 courses	If PD
IV–V	C–D	+ +/– subtenon carboplatin × 3	VCR 0.05 mg/kg d 1 CBP 14 mg/kg d 1, 2 ETO 6 mg/kg d 1, 2 × 6 courses + G-CSF	If PD Consider early EBRT if massive vitreous seeding at completion of chemotherapy
V b	E	Enucleation		

VCR vincristine, *CBP* carboplatin, *ETO* etoposide, *PD* progressive disease, *EBRT* external-beam radiation therapy

However, the expression of P-glycoprotein does not always seem to predict response (Krishnakumar et al. 2004), and cyclosporine may add additional toxicity. For patients with early intraocular stages (R-E I-III, International group B), a less intensive regimen with vincristine and carboplatin alone appears to be effective (Rodriguez-Galindo et al. 2003a; Chantada et al. 2005; Wilsoneta l. 2005)(Table 6.2).

Thus, the treatment of patients with advanced intraocular disease (R-E groups IV and V, International Groups C and D) remains a major challenge. Although randomized studies have not been performed, when compared to radiation and focal treatments alone, chemoreduction does not seem to improve overall ocular salvage significantly for patients with very advanced intraocular disease (Scott et al. 1999; Hungerford et al. 1995; Toma et al. 1995). Chemotherapy intensification appears to correlate with outcome, and better results are obtained with protocols that include at least 6 courses of vincristine, etoposide, and carboplatin (Shields et al. 2002a; Gündüz et al. 1998; Shields et al. 1997). Central retinal tumors usually respond better to chemotherapy than do tumors in the peripheral retina (Gombos et al. 2002), but large central tumors may be associated with subretinal seeds, which ultimately may cause treatment failure (Shields et al. 2002b). With the addition of aggressive sequential focal therapies, globe retention is no better than 50% for R-E group V eyes (Group D) and most patients eventually require radiation (Shields et al. 2002a; Nenadov Beck et al. 2000; Wilsoneta l. 2005).

6.3.3 New Tumor Formation on Chemotherapy

In the natural history of patients with germline *RB1* mutation, new tumors continue to form after diagnosis. But it is not clear whether the use of chemotherapy might alter this process . Several authors have evaluated the impact of primary systemic chemotherapy on the rate of new tumor formation in patients with hereditary retinoblastoma. For patients receiving treatment with the standard two- or three-drug regimens that include 6 to 8 cycles of chemotherapy, the cumulative incidence of new tumors following the start of chemotherapy is 10 to 24% (Wilson et al. 2007; Shields et al. 2003), although higher incidences have also been reported (Schueler et al. 2006). However, most new tumors develop after stopping chemotherapy (Rodriguez-Galindo et al. 2003a; Shields et al. 2003). The incidence of new tumors is higher if less chemotherapy or only focal treatments are given (Lee et al. 2003; Abramson et al. 1992; Abramson et al. 1994). Younger age at diagnosis, a family history of retinoblastoma, and lower Reese-Ellsworth grouping at diagnosis are factors that significantly increase the likelihood of new tumor formation (Wilson et al. 2007; Shields et al. 2003; Schueler et al. 2006). These risk factors are intrinsically tied together; patients with a family history are more likely to be screened early and diagnosed at a younger age, early in the natural history of the disease.

Importantly, the majority of the new tumors after the start of chemotherapy develop in the equatorial or peripheral retina, and less than 20% of the tumors form in the macula (Wilson et al. 2007). This tumor distribution is likely tied to retinal development rather than to the use of chemotherapy, but it is possible that small tumors in the richly vascularized central retina are effectively treated with chemotherapy before they become visible. New tumors may still retain sensitivity to the drugs used as they likely represent new somatic mutations occurring after the start of treatment.

The use of chemotherapy may alter the natural history of retinoblastoma. This could have some important implications. First, even in those cases of early diagnosis, in which the tumor(s) can be treated successfully with focal treatments, chemotherapy (probably with carboplatin alone or in combination with vincristine) may help prevent tumor development in areas in which the tumors or the focal treatments required for their control may represent a threat to vision, such as in the macula or near the optic nerve. Second, this prophylactic effect may extend to the development of pineal tumors. The incidence of trilateral retinoblastoma has decreased dramatically since systemic chemotherapy protocols have been used routinely, although the decrease in the use of radiation therapy may also have influenced this change in outcomes (Shields et al. 2001).

6.3.4 Therapy-Related Leukemia

Although patients with germline mutation of the *RB1* gene do not appear to have an increased risk of hematopoietic malignancies (Eng et al. 1993; Gombos et al. 2007), the use of etoposide adds an additional risk to this patient population (Smith et al. 1994). Epipodophyllotoxin-related leukemia shows a dose-response relation, with the highest risk associated with cumulative doses greater than 4,000 mg/m^2 (Smith et al. 1994; Pui et al. 1991). Also associated with dosage schedule, there is a higher leukemogenic potential when the medication is administered weekly than when administered every 3 or 4 weeks (Pui et al. 1991), as in the treatment of retinoblastoma. However, it should not be assumed that the risk of developing a treatment-related leukemia is only dose and schedule related. Modest exposures to these agents can induce this fatal complication (Blanco et al. 2001), so routine use of etoposide should be evaluated very carefully. Therapy-related acute myeloid leukemia after the treatment of retinoblastoma has been reported although its occurrence appears to be very low (Nishimura et al. 2001; Gombos et al. 2007).

6.4 Periocular Administration of Chemotherapy

6.4.1 Mechanisms for Transscleral Drug Delivery

Transscleral drug delivery is a potential solution to the need to achieve high intraocular concentrations of chemotherapeutic agents. Traditionally subconjunctival, subtenon and retrobulbar injections have been used to administer drugs such as steroids and local anesthetics. The high permeability of the sclera to macromolecules has revived the interest to this route of drug administration (Ranta and Urtti 2006). For transscleral drug delivery, the drug is placed into a periocular space (subconjunctival, subtenon, peribulbar, retrobulbar, or posterior juxtascleral), and it may permeate from the periocular space into the vitreous via the anterior chamber, a direct penetration pathway across the sclera, or through the systemic circulation. In the anterior chamber route, the drug reaches the aqueous humor either directly across the sclera and ciliary body or indirectly via the tear fluid and cornea, and subsequently diffuses to the posterior chamber and into the vitreous. In the direct penetration pathway, the drug permeates into the vitreous through the underlying tissues (Fig. 6.1); in the anterior eye, the drug may diffuse through the ciliary body and then to posterior chamber and vitreous, while in the posterior eye, the drug has to permeate across the choroid, retinal pigment epithelium, and neural retina in order to reach the vitreous. Finally, a small proportion of the drug enters the general circulation via conjunctival, episcleral of choroidal vessels and returns into eye with blood flow (Urtti 2006). The relative importance of each

Table 6.3. Factors affecting transscleral drug delivery (Ranta and Urtti 2006)

Tissue	Factor
Conjunctiva and Tenon's capsule	Diffusion across tissues Clearance via conjunctival blood and lymphatic flow
Sclera	Diffusion across sclera Clearance via episcleral veins
Ciliary body	Diffusion across ciliary body Clearance via circulation
Choroid, Bruch's membrane and RPE	Passive diffusion Active transport and efflux in RPE Clearance via choroidal circulation Binding to melanin
Neural retina	Diffusion across neural retina
Vitreous	Distribution and elimination in vitreous

route to vitreal drug delivery has been investigated in the animal models; the direct penetration pathway is the most important route in the vitreal delivery of most compounds with widely differing physicochemical properties (Ranta and Urtti 2006).

The pharmacokinetics of transscleral drug delivery need to consider the direct penetration of drug into the vitreous, the elimination of the drug from the vitreous, and the drug lost from the periocular space (Table 6.3). Thus, the bioavailability may be improved by either increasing the direct penetration rate or reducing the rate of loss. The loss of drug from the periocular spaces affects the efficiency of transscleral drug delivery into the posterior eye. Periocular clearance uses elimination into conjunctival lymphatics and episcleral veins, and the conjunctival lymphatic and blood flow are important mechanisms for the loss of drug from the sub-tenon space. When the drug is given as a solution into the periocular space, no sustained drug delivery is expected, and most drugs are cleared within 1 h (Li et al. 2004). In the animal model, Robinson et al. reduced the clearance via conjunctival lymphatics and blood vessels by incising a small square through the conjunctiva thus hindering lymphatic and blood flow in the area (Robinson et al. 2006). Administration of a drug in a viscous or semisolid media is an alternative method to decrease orbital clearance. As discussed below, fibrin sealants result in sustained drug delivery into the choroid, retina, and vitreous.

The drug must permeate across several tissues, and some of the barriers are different in the anterior and posterior eye. The RPE is the rate-limiting permeation barrier in the retinal delivery of hydrophilic drugs and macromolecules through the transscleral route. Permeability in RPE is determined both by physical–chemical factors (molecular weight, lipophilicity, charges) and affinity to active transporters. The transporters may decrease or increase the drug transfer across the RPE depending on the type of transporter (influx or efflux) and its location (vitreal or blood side). The permeating drug also faces active barriers such as the clearance via choriocapillaris blood flow. The choroidal blood flow is higher than in any other tissue (relative to the tissue weight) and choriocapillaris walls contain large fenestrations. Large macromolecules are able to diffuse through the fenestrations in rabbit choriocapillaris. In a rabbit model for administration of triamcinolone acetonide, elimination of the blood flow with cryotherapy did not result in improved penetration of drug after subtenon administration (Robinson et al. 2006). The orbital and conjunctival vasculature and lymphatics seem to have a larger role in drug clearance than does the choroid. The elimination of conjunctival lymphatic and blood flow by incising a small window in the conjunctiva was more effective in increasing the vitreous concentration than the elimination of the choroidal blood flow (Robinson et al. 2006). When considering the orbital clearance, the posterior subtenon location appears to be the best periocular route as it is closer to the sclera and farther from the orbital vasculature (Ghate et al. 2007). Following periocular injection, the drug must penetrate across the sclera, which is more permeable than the cornea. However, for the drug to reach the retina, it must pass across the choroid and RPE (a tighter barrier than the sclera), at which point drugs may be cleared significantly to the blood stream (Urtti 2006).

The sclera has a large surface area (16.3 cm^2) and scleral permeability shows no dependence on lipophilicity but dependence on molecular radius. The sclera is composed of collagen and proteoglycan fibers with few protein binding sites. Drugs permeate through the aqueous intercellular media of the sclera occupying the pores between the collagen fibers. Pore diameter and intercellular space are important determinants of transscleral drug delivery, particularly for drugs such as large hydrophilic peptides and oligonucleotides. The cornea is relatively impermeable to solutes with a molecular size of >1 kDa; however, dextran and albumin (69 kDa) readily penetrate the sclera. Scleral permeability is affected by an increase in intraocular pressure (Ghate and Edelhauser 2006). There are several ways to enhance scleral permeability. Treatment of many ocular diseases incorporates the use of transscleral depots, either as scleral implants (used for anti-inflammatory agents) or collagen matrix and fibrin sealants, or the use of microspheres and other nanoparticles (Ghate and Edelhauser 2006; Bu et al. 2007). Scleral permeability can also be increased through scleral thinning, increased hydration, increased temperature, or use of prostaglandins (which increase the expression of matrix metalloproteases) (Ghate and Edelhauser 2006). Additional methods for increasing scleral permeability include iontophoresis and ultrasound-induced mild hyperthermia. Iontophoresis is a noninvasive technique and employs the principle of charge repulsion for driving charged drug molecules through cellular layers (Majumdar and Mitra 2006).

6.4.2 Periocular Chemotherapy in Retinoblastoma

Control of the intraocular tumor burden requires achieving high levels of chemotherapeutic agents in all the intraocular compartments, including the vitreous, the subretinal space and the ocular coats. While effective, systemic administration of chemotherapy is limited by the blood-ocular barriers described earlier. In recent years, methods to increase the intraocular concentrations of chemotherapeutic agents have been extensively investigated, and periocular administration of carboplatin has been incorporated into most regimens for the treatment of advanced intraocular retinoblastoma.

In the transgenic murine retinoblastoma treated with intravitreous injections of carboplatin, inhibition of tumor growth occurs in a dose-dependent manner (Harbour et al. 1996), thus suggesting that higher intraocular levels of chemotherapy would be desirable. However, direct injection into the vitreous carries the risk of extraocular dissemination from the injection tract, thus limiting this option. A valid alternative to intraocular injection is periocular administration. In the transgenic mice retinoblastoma model, subconjunctival administration of carboplatin results in tumor control in a dose-dependent manner (Hayden et al. 2000), suggesting good intraocular penetration of this agent when given periocularly. Pharmacokinetic studies performed in the rabbit eye have validated this method. Hayden et al. compared the intraocular pharmacokinetics of carboplatin when given by subconjunctival injections (SC) (5 mg), by Coulomb-controlled iontophoresis (CCI) (14 mg) or intravenous (IV) administration (18.7 mg/kg) (Hayden et al. 2004). The concentrations of carboplatin in retina, choroid, optic nerve, and vitreous were higher in the SC and CCI groups than in the IV group. Furthermore, systemic levels after local administration were very low. Subconjunctival administration resulted in better intraocular penetration than CCI. Compared with intravenous administration, the subconjunctival route resulted in higher levels of carboplatin in retina, choroid, optic nerve, and vitreous. In vitreous, peak levels of 4,560 mcg/mL were achieved when compared with 1,220 mcg/mL following IV administration. The concentration vs. time curves showed statistically significant higher total levels of carboplatin in the retina, choroid, and vitreous over the 24 h period after focal delivery than with IV injection. Studies performed in the primate eye also support the use of periocular administration of carboplatin. Mendelsohn et al. compared the intraocular concentrations of agents after local or systemic administration in primates (Mendelsohn et al. 1998). Intravenous carboplatin was given at the standard dose used in humans (18.7 mg/kg), and systemic and intraocular pharmacokinetics were compared with peribulbar and episcleral injections of 10 mg of carboplatin. The intravenous administration resulted in higher levels in the aqueous humor (6.2 mcg/ml) than peribulbar (2 mcg/ml) or episcleral (1.74 mcg/ml). However, vitreous levels were significantly higher when carboplatin was administered periocularly (0.3 mcg/ml IV vs 2.38 mcg/ml PB vs. 2.95 mcg/ml EPI). Importantly, systemic absorption after periocular administration was minimal; plasma levels of carboplatin were 3% of those achieved after intravenous administration. In the same study, etoposide was administered systemically as a single dose of 5 mg/kg and, importantly, no etoposide was detected in the aqueous or vitreous humors. Etoposide is a protein-bound drug, and it likely stays in the plasma and thus has limited penetration. Studies in the mouse model have also shown little intravitreal penetration of etoposide when given intravenously. The vitreous/plasma ratios when measured as area under the curve concentrations were 0.59 for carboplatin and 0.07 for etoposide (Laurie et al. 2005). However, these models may not recapitulate the natural history of retinoblastoma as the blood-vitreous barrier is likely disrupted by tumor. In fact, intraocular carboplatin concentrations in the human retinoblastoma eye are higher after intravenous administration (18.7 mg/kg) than what the primate eye model shows; levels in the vitreous are 4.05 mcg/ml, much higher than what the animal studies would predict, and are similar to levels measured in unaffected animals when drug is given after cryotherapy (Abramson et al. 1999a). An important point of these studies, however, is the fact that pharmacokinetics in the rabbit eye are similar to the primate's, thus establishing a good model for developmental therapeutics.

Given the promising preclinical data, periocular administration of carboplatin has been progressively incorporated into the clinical practice. Patients tolerate the administration of 2 ml of the 10 mg/ml solution although orbital toxicity is significant. In the only phase II study reported, responses were seen in three of the five eyes with vitreous disease and in two of the five eyes with retinal tumors (Abramson et al. 1999b). The role of this form of administration in the management of retinoblastoma is still being evaluated prospectively. Currently, patients with advanced intraocular disease (particularly those with massive vitreous or subretinal seeding) receive up to three doses of periocular carboplatin concomitantly with systemic chemotherapy. However, great caution should be exerted if periocular carboplatin is administered; acute (periorbital edema, inflammation) and long-term (orbital fat necrosis, soft tissue and muscle fibrosis, optic neuritis) toxicities are common (Schmack et al. 2006; Mulvihill et al. 2003).

Although effective in increasing the intraocular levels, subconjunctival administration of carboplatin in aqueous media has many limitations. Most of the drug delivered is dispensed quickly throughout the subconjunctival space and surrounding orbit, thus exposing extraocular tissues to high transient concentrations of carboplatin and potential toxicities. Methods for improving periocular delivery of carboplatin while minimizing toxicity are being investigated. Using a collagen matrix vehicle, Gilbert et al. were able to provide a more controlled release of cisplatin in the rabbit eye leading to higher drug levels in several ocular tissues (Gilbert et al. 2003). Fibrin sealants have the potential to minimize not only the risk for periorbital toxicity but also for retinal toxicity associated with SC carboplatin by providing controlled, sustained drug delivery.

Human-derived fibrin protein sealant is an FDA-approved valid alternative for drug delivery. It is formulated to contain human proteins, which minimizes immunogenicity and foreign body reactions and eliminates the need for physical removal of the clot, which is naturally degraded by the body. Carboplatin appears to be a good drug candidate for this approach; studies have shown that this drug may enhance fibrin clot formation (Gorodetsky et al. 2005). One benefit of the sealant is that the anhydrous form of carboplatin can be overloaded beyond its solubility limit to provide higher levels of drug for extended periods. The scleral drug exposure is maximized, extending the duration of therapeutically significant intraocular drug penetration, and decreasing the need for repeated periocular injections. Simpson et al. compared the trans-scleral diffusion of carboplatin in the rabbit eye when administered using a fibrin sealant (FS) or a balanced salt solution (BSS) (Simpson et al. 2002). Intravitreous concentrations were higher when using an FS, and the FS was able to provide a transscleral release of carboplatin for >24 h (and carboplatin could be detected in the vitreous for up to 2 weeks). As the intraocular levels increase, so does the risk of retinal toxicity. Retinal toxicity studies in mice suggest that retinal toxicity occurs with vitreous concentrations >10 mcg/mL (Harbour et al. 1996). In the rabbit model, the peak vitreous level using FS reached 11.83 mcg/mL (Simpson et al. 2002). There was a temporary decline in retinal function as noted with transient decrease in electroretinographic amplitude at 2 days after treatment. However, at the doses used (12 mg/mL in BSS and 25 mg/mL in FS), there was no toxic effect on retinal function or structure (Pardue et al. 2004).

One of the advantages of using fibrin sealants is the ability to increase drug concentrations, thus providing the possibility of higher doses of carboplatin being delivered to the ocular structures. Van Quill et al. investigated the intraocular pharmacokinetics and ocular toxicity of high carboplatin doses administered in fibrin sealant in transgenic murine retinoblastoma (Van Quill et al. 2005). Carboplatin was delivered in concentrations of 37.5 mg/mL and 75 mg/mL in the fibrin sealants. A single injection was sufficient to induce a complete response or nearly complete response in 95% of the eyes; however, high-dose carboplatin did not prove to have superior anti-tumor effects than the lower dose, while orbital and retinal toxicity in the later group was significant. These results compare favorably to previous studies using multiple injections in the same rodent model (Hayden et al. 2004).

Given these encouraging preclinical data, many regimens now incorporate periocular carboplatin concomitantly with the intravenous administration of the standard drugs for patients with advanced intraocular disease. However, not more than three injections are currently recommended (Table 6.2).

6.5 Intravitreal and Intrarterial Chemotherapy for Intraocular Retinoblastoma

In order to achieve the maximum concentrations of chemotherapy close to the tumor and in the vitreous, investigators have attempted direct intravitreal delivery. This approach was pioneered by Swedish investigators in the 1960s (Ericson and Rosengren 1961; Ericson et al. 1964). Thiotepa was the agent selected in those initial studies, and repeated injections of 1 to 1.5 mg were administered, often in conjunction with external beam radiation therapy. Regressions were obtained, but long term control of the intraocular disease was generally not possible. This approach was recently rekindled by Seregard et al. in three cases of recurrent retinoblastoma in an only eye (Seregard et al. 1995). Patients received repeated intravitreal injections of 2 mg of thiotepa, followed by vitrectomy and weekly injections for a total cumulative dose of 10–14 mg of thiotepa; no obvious clinical responses were observed. More recently, Japanese investigators have pioneered the administration of intravitreal and intraarterial melphalan for patients with advanced or recurrent intraocular retinoblastoma (Kaneko and Suzuki 2003). Preclinical data suggests that retinoblastoma is very sensitive to melphalan, and that there is a synergistic effect with thermotherapy (Inomata and Kaneko 1987). Clinical responses in patients with progressive retinoblastoma have been obtained using intravitreal melphalan followed by hyperthermia (Kaneko and Suzuki 2003).

Chemotherapy administration directly into the tumor vasculature is a common practice in oncology. A small, localized tumor as retinoblastoma would be an excellent candidate for such approach. However, cannulation of the retinal artery is required, thus limiting the availability of this procedure. Kaneko et al. initially reported the feasibility of injecting melphalan into the ipsilateral carotid artery, with documented efficacy (Kaneko and Suzuki 2003). The technique was later perfected by Mohri using a balloon catheter that allowed for selective injection into the ophthalmic artery (Mohri 1993). More recently, Abramson et al. reported a variation of this technique that includes a direct cannulation of the ophthalmic artery using a microcatheter (Abramson et al. 2008). Using this approach, the authors reported high ocular salvage rates with minimal local and systemic toxicity after the administration of 3–5 mg of intraarterial melphalan.

6.6 Treatment of Extraocular Retinoblastoma

Four patterns of extraocular disease can be recognized: (1) Locoregional dissemination, including orbital disease, tumor extending to the cut end of the optic nerve, and lymphatic spread to the preauricular lymph nodes; (2) Central nervous system dissemination; (3) Metastatic retinoblastoma and (4) Trilateral retinoblastoma. Treatment of extraocular retinoblastoma is described in detail in chapter 8.

6.6.1 Orbital and Locoregional Retinoblastoma

Orbital retinoblastoma occurs as a result of progression of the tumor through the emissary vessels and sclera. Orbital retinoblastoma is isolated in 60–70%

of the cases; lymphatic, hematogenous, and CNS metastases occur in the remaining patients (Doz et al. 1994). Treatment should include systemic chemotherapy and radiation therapy; with this approach, 60–85% of patients can be cured. Since most recurrences occur in the CNS, regimens using drugs with well documented CNS penetration are recommended. Different chemotherapy regimens have proven to be effective, including vincristine, cyclophosphamide and doxorubicin, platinum- and epipodophyllotoxin-based regimens, or a combination of both (Zelter et al. 1991; Schvartzman et al. 1996; Doz et al. 1995; Mustafa et al. 1999; Kiratli et al. 1998; Antonelli et al. 2003; Chantada et al. 2003; Gündüz et al. 2006). For patients with macroscopic orbital disease, it is recommended that surgery is delayed until response to chemotherapy has been obtained (usually 2 or 3 courses of treatment). Enucleation should then be performed, and chemotherapy completed with an additional 4–6 courses. Local control should then be consolidated with orbital irradiation (40–45 Gy). Using this approach, orbital exenteration is not indicated (Kiratli et al. 1998; Chantada et al. 2003).

6.6.2 Metastatic Retinoblastoma

Hematogenous metastases occur to the bones, bone marrow and, less frequently, to the liver (Antonelli et al. 2003; Chantada et al. 2003; Gündüz et al. 2006; Dunkel et al. 2000; Marsubara et al. 2005). Although long term survivors have been reported with conventional chemotherapy (Gündüz et al. 2006), these cures should be considered anecdotal; metastatic retinoblastoma is not curable with conventional chemotherapy (Antonelli et al. 2003; Chantada et al. 2003). In recent years, however, small series have shown that metastatic retinoblastoma can be cured using high-dose chemotherapy and autologous stem cell rescue (Table 6.4) (Dunkel et al. 2000; Marsubara et al. 2005; Namouni et al. 1997; Kremens et al. 2003; Rodriguez-Galindo et al. 2003b; Saarinen et al. 1991). The approach is similar to metastatic neuroblastoma; patients receive short and intensive induction regimens usually containing alkylating agents, anthracyclines, etoposide and platinum compounds, and are then consolidated with autologous hematopoietic stem cell transplant. Using this approach, the outcome appears to be excellent. As for any megatherapy consolidation, the agents selected may be important. In general, recurrences are intracranial, and for this reason, agents with proven efficacy in intracranial retinoblastoma should be used. In this regard, the combination of carboplatin and etoposide has been shown to be effective against CNS disease (Doz et al. 1995), and for this reason, it should be part of the regimen. In the largest published series, seven patients received consolidation with the CARBOPEC combination (carboplatin 1,250–1,750 mg/m^2, etoposide 1,750 mg/m^2, and cyclophosphamide 6.4 g/m^2), 5 of them were cured, and two patients failed because of CNS relapse. Two other series have used a thiotepa-based consolidation (thiotepa 900 mg/m^2, etoposide 750–1,200 mg/m^2, and carboplatin 1,500 mg/m^2). There is strong rationale for using

Table 6.4. Recommended chemotherapy regimen for metastatic retinoblastoma (Dunkel et al. (2000) and COG ARTE0321)

Phase	Drugs	Doses		Days
		< 36 months	> 36 months	
Induction (4 cycles)	VCR	0.05 mg/kg	1.5 mg/m^2	1, 8, 15
	CDDP	3.5 mg/kg	105 mg/m^2	1
	CYC	65 mg/kg	1,950 mg/m^2	2, 3
	ETO	4 mg/kg	120 mg/m^2	2, 3
Consolidation	CBP	AUC 7 (max. 16.7 mg/kg)	AUC 7 (max. 500 mg/m^2)	−8, −7, −6
	TT	10 mg/kg	300 mg/m^2	−5, −4, −3
	ETO	8.3 mg/kg	250 mg/m^2	−5, −4, −3

VCR vincristine, *CDDP* cisplatin, *CYC* cyclphosphamide, *ETO* etoposide, *CBP* carboplatin, *TT* thiotepa, *AUC* area under the curve

thiotepa: retinoblastoma is responsive to alkylating agents such as thiotepa, a group of agents for which dose escalation is shown to overcome resistance. Furthermore, thiotepa has excellent CNS penetration (Dunkel et al. 2000; Heideman et al. 1989). An interesting observation is that patients with distant (outside orbit and skull) bone metastases who show good response to induction chemotherapy may not require radiation therapy when treated with autologous stem cell rescue (Namouni et al. 1997; Kremens et al. 2003). A prospective study is currently being developed by the Children's Oncology Group (ARET0321 protocol, Ira Dunkel MD, principal investigator), which includes induction with a cisplatin-based regimen and consolidation with high-dose chemotherapy (carboplatin, thiothepa and etoposide) and autologous hematopoietic stem cell rescue).

Despite the advances in the treatment of metastatic retinoblastoma, the prognosis for patients with central nervous system disease is still dismal (Chantada et al. 2004a; Kiratli et al. 1998; Antonelli et al. 2003; Chantada et al. 2003; Namouni et al. 1997; Pratt et al. 1994; Jubran et al. 2004; Gündüz et al. 2006; Marsubara et al. 2005). Treatment for these patients should include platinum-based intensive systemic chemotherapy and CNS directed therapy. Although intrathecal methotrexate (with or without cytarabine) has been traditionally used, there is no preclinical or clinical evidence to support its use (Chan et al. 1989). Other intrathecal agents with documented effect against retinoblastoma include topotecan (Blaney et al. 2003; Chantada et al. 2004b) and thiotepa (Pratt et al. 1994; Fisher et al. 2002). However, there is no evidence that their use can impact outcome. Although the use of irradiation in these patients is controversial, responses have been observed with craniospinal irradiation, using 25–35 Gy to the CNS and the spinal axis, and a boost (10 Gy) to sites of measurable disease (Antonelli et al. 2003; Chantada et al. 2003; Dunkel et al. 2000; Namouni et al. 1997; Pratt et al. 1994). Therapy intensification with high-dose chemotherapy and autologous stem cell rescue has been explored (Namouni et al. 1997), but its role is not yet clear. Despite the intensity of the treatment and the documented responses of the intracranial disease (Doz et al. 1995), patients succumb to their disease, and survivors are anecdotal (Kiratli et al. 1998; Namouni et al. 1997). Treatment of patients with extraocular disease is discussed in detail in chapter 8.

6.7 Translational Research and Emergent Therapies in Retinoblastoma

There are currently three types of rodent models of retinoblastoma. These animal models are described in more detail in chapters 1 and 4. The retinoblastoma xenograft model relies on injecting $>1\times10^6$ cultured human retinoblastoma cells into the flank of adult immunocompromised mice. For obvious reasons, this model fails to recapitulate the intraocular environment and developmental milieu that is present in children with retinoblastoma. A more accurate xenograft model can be generated with the injection of human retinoblastoma cells into the eyes of newborn rats (Laurie et al. 2005). The transgenic mouse models of retinoblastoma rely on the broad ectopic expression of the SV40 T oncogene to lead to massive hyperproliferation. The limitation of this transgenic mouse model is the lack of focal and clonal tumors; large regions of the retina are altered. Thus, one of the main limitations in understanding the pathogenesis of retinoblastoma has been the lack of a mouse model that recapitulates the developmental environment of this malignancy. Mice with hemizygous mutations of the retinoblastoma gene, generated to recapitulate the human condition, do not develop retinoblastoma (although some of them develop midbrain tumors) (Jacks et al. 1992) and "knock-out" mice die at gestational day 14 due to hematopoietic and neuronal defects (Lee et al. 1992). In the mouse retina, *p107* is upregulated in a compensatory manner when *Rb* is inactivated, thus preventing ectopic cell division. *p107* is an E2F-regulated gene, and when *Rb* repression of E2F at the *p107* promoter is relieved, *p107* expression is activated (however, this *p107* compensation does not occur in human retinal progenitor cells when *Rb* is inactivated) (Donovan et al. 2006). Both *Rb* and *p107* or *Rb* and *p130* must be inactivated in proliferating retinal progenitor cells in order for mice to develop retinoblastoma. Recently, the first knockout mouse models of retinoblastoma were generated by conditionally deleting *Rb* in retinal progenitor cells of *p107*-deficient mice (Zhang et al. 2004). When *p53* is simultaneously inactivated in *Rb; p107*-deficient retinal progenitor cells, a more aggressive form of retinoblastoma, similar to the human disease, is observed (Zhang et al. 2004).

The development of these preclinical models of retinoblastoma is the first step toward the development of new therapies (Dyer et al. 2005). Contrary to what occurs in adult cancer, where the high numbers facilitate developmental therapeutics, few children are eligible for clinical trials, thus limiting the efficiency of this process. Furthermore, development of new agents for retinoblastoma must take into consideration the uniqueness of the developmental nature of the disease and the physiology of the eye. In this regard, the information generated in the animal models is extremely relevant, and new agents with better intraocular penetration are being investigated.

Topotecan, a topoisomerase-I inhibitor with well documented efficacy against pediatric dysontogenic tumors, is a promising alternative (Rodriguez-Galindo et al. 2000). Preclinical and clinical studies have shown that topotecan penetrates the blood brain barrier, and it has good penetration into the cerebrospinal fluid (Baker et al. 1996). Since there are some structural and functional similarities between the blood brain barrier and the vitreoretinal barrier one could anticipate that topotecan could have good penetration into the vitreous. Pharmacokinetic studies performed in the rat and rabbit models show that topotecan consistently penetrates the vitreous, and that the proportion of drug that crosses the blood-vitreous barrier is similar or higher than the proportion of drug that crosses the blood-brain barrier (Laurie et al. 2005; Carcaboso et al. 2007). It must be considered, however, that because of the nature of the disease, the blood-vitreous barrier is significantly disrupted in the eye with retinoblastoma, and therefore the penetration of topotecan into the vitreous may be much higher than what the preclinical studies show. There is little information regarding the efficacy of topotecan in retinoblastoma. Anecdotal responses have been observed in previous phase I and phase II studies. One patient with recurrent retinoblastoma treated on the phase I study of 21-day continuous infusion had a response (Frangoul et al. 1999), and the only patient with recurrent retinoblastoma treated on the phase II study that used 2 mg/m^2/d for five consecutive days had a partial response that was maintained for 14 courses (Nitschke et al. 1998). Chantada et al. reported on a phase II study of topotecan in seven patients (five previously treated) with extraorbital disease. Three of these seven patients, including one patient with CNS disease, responded (Chantada et al. 2004b). Despite the paucity of information, one could anticipate that retinoblastoma is sensitive to topotecan, given the similar pattern of sensitivities between retinoblastoma and neuroblastoma. In vitro and in vivo studies show that retinoblastoma cell lines are very sensitive to topotecan. In these same studies, the combination of topotecan and carboplatin appears to be the most effective against retinoblastoma when compared with other carboplatin combinations, including the standard regimen of vincristine, carboplatin and etoposide (Laurie et al. 2005). Unfortunately, systemic administration of both agents in doses that would reach therapeutic levels in the eye results in significant systemic toxicity (Athale et al. 2001). However, we must consider that the goal is to obtain therapeutic concentrations of both agents in the eye at the same time in order to achieve the synergistic effect. The concomitant administration of periocular carboplatin with systemic topotecan may achieve this goal with limited systemic toxicity. This approach is currently under investigation at St. Jude Children's Research Hospital. An alternative is the administration of topotecan periocularly. In the animal model, periocular administration of topotecan reached potentially active levels of its active lactone moiety without significant toxicity (Carcaboso et al. 2007). However, systemic absorption was significant. A recently completed phase I study has documented the feasibility of administering 2 mg of topotecan periocularly (Chantada et al. 2009), and a phase II study is under development.

Suicide gene therapy using an adenoviral vector to locally deliver (by intraocular injection) the herpes simplex thyrosine kinase gene, followed by systemic administration of ganciclovir has been shown to be safe and to induce responses of the vitreous lesions in a recently reported phase I study (Chevez-Barrios et al. 2005). This is a promising treatment for patients with vitreous disease, and a phase II study is in progress.

Finally, the recent description of *MDMX* amplification as the mechanism of inactivation of the p53 pathway in retinoblastoma has opened the door for the use of specific targeted molecular therapies. Nutlin-3 is a small-molecule inhibitor of the MDM2-p53 interaction. MDMX and MDM2 bind p53 with similar affinities, and studies have shown that nutlin-3 prevents the MDMX-p53 interaction in retinoblastoma cells, inducing p53-mediated apoptosis in vitro and in vivo (Laurie et al. 2006; Elison et al. 2006). Importantly, subconjunctival injection of nutlin-3 to mice with intraocular retinoblastoma resulted in significant tumor responses, and the combination of nutlin-3 with a DNA damaging agent such as topotecan resulted in a synergistic effect (Laurie et al. 2006). The possibility of molecular targeted therapy using small-molecules by periocular administration may represent the most remarkable advance in the treatment of children with retinoblastoma.

6.8 Specific Agents

6.8.1 Vincristine

Standard dosage:S eeT ables 6.1, 6.2, and 6.4.

Source and Pharmacology: Vincristine is an alkaloid obtained from the periwinkle *(Vinca rosea)* plant. It reversibly binds to microtubule and spindle proteins causing metaphase arrest. Vincristine has poor penetration into the CSF. It is approximately 75% protein bound. Extensive metabolism occurs in the liver. Excretion is primarily in the bile. A dosage decrease is recommended in patients with a bilirubin >3 mg/dl.

Formulation and Stability: Vincristine is supplied in multiple-dose 1 mg/ml vials containing 1 ml, 2 ml, and 5 ml. The intact vials should be stored under refrigeration and protected from light.

Contraindications: Hypersensitivity to vincristine or any component; patients with demyelinating form of Charcot-Marie-Tooth syndrome.

Main Drug Interactions: Cytochrome P450 isoenzyme CYP3A3/4 and CYP3A5-7 substrate; isoenzyme CYP2D6 inhibitor. Concurrent administration with itraconazole may result in an increased severity of neuromuscular side effects; voriconazole may increase plasma levels of vincristine.

Toxicity: Dose limiting toxicity is neurotoxicity. This can be characterized by constipation and/or paralytic ileus, ptosis, vocal chord paralysis, weakness, jaw pain, abdominal pain, peripheral neuropathies, loss of deep tendon reflexes and "foot drop". Peripheral neuropathy is often the first sign of neurotoxicity and is initially reversible. Other toxicities reported include alopecia, mild nausea and vomiting, SIADH, myelosuppression, orthostatic hypotension, optic atrophy, transient cortical blindness, and auditory damage. Acute shortness of breath and severe bronchospasm have been reported following the administration of vinca alkaloids. Myelosuppression is rare at usual doses. Vincristine is a vesicant and may cause severe tissue damage if extravasation occurs.

6.8.2 Carboplatin

Standard Dosage:S eeT ables 6.1, 6.2, and 6.4.

Source and Pharmacology: Carboplatin is an inorganic heavy metal coordination complex that has biochemical properties similar to those of a bifunctional alkylating agent. Carboplatin must undergo activation, by aquation, to form positively charged platinum complexes that react with nucleophilic sites on DNA, producing predominantly intrastrand DNA cross-links. Carboplatin is widely distributed in body tissues and fluids with highest concentrations in the kidney, liver, skin and tumor tissue. Carboplatin does not bind significantly to plasma proteins, but the activated form does bind to tissue and plasma proteins. In adults with normal renal function, the plasma elimination half-life is ≈2–3 h. The elimination of carboplatin and its platinum-containing products is primarily dependent on glomerular filtration rate; therefore, dosages may be adjusted for renal function.

Formulation and Stability: Carboplatin is supplied in 20-ml amber vials containing 50, 150 or 450 mg of carboplatin as a white lyophilized powder. Vials should be reconstituted with sterile water for injection, D5W or 0.9% NaCl to give a concentration of 10 mg/ml and further diluted with D5W or 0.9% NaCl to concentration of 0.5 mg to 1.0 mg per ml. It is recommended that the reconstituted solution be discarded 8 hours after preparation.

Contraindications: Hypersensitivity to carboplatin, cisplatin, any component, other platinum-containing compounds, or mannitol; severe bone marrow suppression or excessive bleeding.

Main Drug Interactions: Aminoglycosides (increased ototoxicity and nephrotoxicity); nephrotoxic drugs (increased renal toxicity); decreases phenytoin serum levels.

Main Side Effects: Dose limiting toxicity is bone marrow suppression with thrombocytopenia being prominent. Nausea and vomiting of moderate severity are common. Hepatic dysfunction (after high doses), alopecia, ototoxicity, peripheral neuropathies, reversible renal toxicity, visual disturbances, and allergic reactions have all been reported less commonly. Pulmonary fibrosis is rare, but occurs most commonly in patients treated with cumulative doses >1,400 mg/m^2 or receiving bone marrow transplant dosages. Electrolyte abnormalities including hyponatremia, hypomagnesemia, hypocalcemia and hypokalemia can occur. Secondary cancers have been reported rarely. When given by subtenon administration, carboplatin may cause periorbital swelling. Direct injection close to the optic nerve may cause optic neuropathy.

6.8.3 Etoposide (VP-16)

Standard Dosage:S eeT ables 6.1, 6.2a nd 6.4.

Source and Pharmacology: Etoposide is an epipodophyllotoxin derived from *Podophyllum pelatatum*. It is thought to act mainly by inhibiting topoisomerase II, causing double and single strand DNA breaks. Etoposide is cell cycle, phase-specific, with activity in the G2 and S phases. Absorption of etoposide is approximately 30–40% and is highly variable and somewhat dose-dependent. It is extensively bound to serum proteins and is metabolized in the liver, including cytochrome P450 3A metabolism to several moieties that include a reactive oxidized species. Etoposide and its metabolites are excreted mainly in the urine with a smaller amount excreted in the feces. Dosage adjustments should be considered in patients with liver dysfunction, kidney dysfunction or hypoalbuminemia.

Formulation and Stability: Etoposide is available in multi-dose vials containing 100 mg, 150 mg, 500 mg and 1,000 mg of etoposide as a 20 mg/ml solution and 30% alcohol. Etoposide is also available as a 50 mg capsule. The intact vials of etoposide solution should be stored at room temperature. The capsules should be stored under refrigeration. Etoposide solution should be diluted in D5W or 0.9% NaCl prior to administration. Solutions with a final concentration of 0.2 and 0.4 mg/ml are stable at room temperature for 96 h and 24 h respectively.

Contraindications: Hypersensitivity to etoposide or any component; pregnancy.

Main Drug Interactions: Cytochrome P450 isoenzyme CYP3A3/4 substrate. Cyclosporine may increase the plasma levels of etoposide.

Main Side Effects: Dose limiting toxicity is myelosuppression. Nausea and vomiting (usually of low to moderate severity), diarrhea, mucositis (particularly with high doses), alopecia and anorexia are fairly common. Hypotension can occur with rapid infusions. Etoposide injection contains benzyl alcohol which may cause allergic reactions in susceptible individuals; large amounts of benzyl alcohol (≥99 mg/kg/day) have been associated with a potentially fatal toxicity ("gasping syndrome") in neonates. Other side effects reported less commonly include hepatitis, fever and chills, anaphylaxis and peripheral neuropathy. Secondary leukemia has been reported.

6.8.4 Doxorubicin

Standard Dosage: Patients <12 months of age: 1.5 mg/kg i.v.; patients ≥12 months of age: 45 mg/m^2 i.v (see Table 6.1).

Source and Pharmacology: Doxorubicin is an anthracycline antibiotic produced by *Streptomyces peucetius*. Doxorubicin exerts its anti-tumor effects in several different ways. Doxorubicin intercalates between base pairs of DNA causing steric obstruction, disruption of DNA function and inhibition of RNA synthesis. In addition, doxorubicin inhibits topoisomerase II, an enzyme responsible for allowing strands of DNA to pass through one another as they unwind. Lastly, doxorubicin undergoes enzymatic electron reduction to generate highly reactive species, including the hydroxyl free radical, which is thought to be responsible for the drug's cardiac toxicity, but may play a role in its anti-tumor activity as well. Doxorubicin is cell-cycle, phase nonspecific. Doxorubicin is widely distributed in the tissues and plasma, but does not cross the blood brain barrier to an appreciable extent. It is metabolized to doxorubicinol, which is thought to be the major active metabolite, and aglycones. Doxorubicin and its metabolites are excreted mainly in the bile and feces (≈80%). The remainder is excreted in the urine. Dosage should be reduced in patients with liver dysfunction (bilirubin > 1.2 mg/dl) or renal dysfunction (creatinine >3 mg/dl).

Formulation and Stability: Doxorubicin is available in vials containing 10, 20, 50, and 200 mg as a 2 mg/ml red-orange solution. It is also available in vials containing 10, 20, 50, 100, and 150 mg of doxorubicin as a red-orange lyophilized powder. Intact vials of doxorubicin solution should be stored under refrigeration while the lyophilized product should be stored at room temperature. Both products should be protected from light. Lyophilized doxorubicin can be reconstituted by adding 5, 10, 25, 50 or 75 ml of 0.9% NaCl respectively to the 10, 20, 50, 100, and 150 mg vials to produce a final concentration of 2 mg/ml. Bacteriostatic diluents are not recommended. After reconstitution, the resultant solution should be protected from light and is stable for 7 days at room temperature and 15 days if refrigerated.

Contraindications: Hypersensitivity to doxorubicin or any component; severe CHF, cardiomyopathy, pre-existing myelosuppression; patients who have received a total dose of 550 mg/m^2 of doxorubicin or 400 mg/m^2 in patients with previous or concomitant treatment with daunorubicin, idarubicin, mitoxantrone, cyclophosphamide, or irradiation of the cardiac region; patients who have received previous treatment with complete cumulative doses of daunorubicin, idarubicin, or other anthracycline derivatives; pregnancy.

Main Drug Interactions: Cytochrome P450 isoenzyme CYP3A3/4 substrate; isoenzyme CYP2D6 inhibitor. May potentiate the toxicity of cyclophosphamide. Ritonavir and cyclosporine decrease doxorubicin metabolism; doxorubicin decreases carbamazepine, digoxin, and phenytoin levels; paclitaxel decreases doxorubicin clearance resulting in increased toxicity if administered prior to doxorubicin; phenobarbital increases elimination of doxorubicin.

Main Side Effects: Dose-limiting toxicities include myelosuppression and cardiotoxicity. Two forms of cardiac toxicity can occur. Acute toxicity may take the form of arrhythmias, heart block or pericarditis and may be fatal. The chronic form of cardiotoxicity is related to total cumulative dose and is characterized by heart failure. Mediastinal radiotherapy and/or other cardiotoxic drugs may increase the risk of cardiotoxicity. In general, total lifetime dosages of 450–550 mg/m^2 should not be exceeded. Other toxicities include nausea and vomiting, mucositis, alopecia, diarrhea and red discoloration of the urine and other body fluids. Severe tissue damage and necrosis can occur upon extravasation. Radiation recall reactions can occur and can be severe. Rarely, allergic reactions may occur.

6.8.5 Cyclophosphamide

Standard Dosage:S eeT ables 6.1a nd 6.4.

Source and Pharmacology: Cyclophosphamide is a nitrogen mustard derivative. It acts as an alkylating agent that causes cross-linking of DNA strands by binding with nucleic acids and other intracellular structures, thus interfering with the normal function of DNA. Cyclophosphamide is cell-cycle, phase nonspecific. Cyclophosphamide is well absorbed from the GI tract with a bioavailability of >75%. Cyclophosphamide is a prodrug that requires activation. It is metabolized by mixed-function oxidases in the liver to 4-hydroxycyclophosphamide, which is in equilibrium with aldofosfamide. Aldofosfamide spontaneously splits into cyclophosphamide mustard, which is considered to be the major active metabolite, and acrolein. In addition, 4-hydroxycyclophosphamide may be enzymatically metabolized to 4-ketocyclophosphamide and aldofosfamide may be enzymatically metabolized to carboxyphosphamide which are generally considered to be inactive. Cyclophosphamide and its metabolites are excreted mainly in the urine. Dosage adjustments should be made in patients with a creatinine clearance of <50 ml/min.

Formulation and Stability: Cyclophosphamide is available in 25 and 50 mg tablets. Cyclophosphamide is also available in vials containing 100, 200, 500, 1,000, and 2,000 mg of lyophilized drug and 75 mg mannitol per 100 mg of cyclophosphamide. Both forms of the drug can be stored at room temperature. The vials are reconstituted with 5, 10, 25, 50 or 100 ml of sterile water for injection respectively to yield a final concentration of 20 mg/ml. Reconstituted solutions may be further diluted in either 5% dextrose or 0.9% NaCl containing solutions. Diluted solutions are physically stable for 24 h at room temperature and 6 days if refrigerated, but contain no preservative, so it is recommended that they be used within 24 h of preparation.

Contraindications: Hypersensitivity to cyclophosphamide or any component.

Main Drug Interactions: Cytochrome P450 isoenzyme CYP2B6, CYP2D6, and CYP3A3/4 substrate. Allopurinol (increases myelotoxicity of cyclophosphamide); phenobarbital, phenytoin, and chloral hydrate may increase conversion of cyclophosphamide to active metabolites; chloramphenicol, phenothiazines, imipramine may inhibit the metabolism of cyclophosphamide (increased bone marrow suppression); cyclophosphamide may prolong the neuromuscular blocking activity of succinylcholine.

Main Side Effects: Dose limiting toxicities of cyclophosphamide are bone marrow suppression and cardiac toxicity. Cardiac toxicity is typically manifested as congestive heart failure, cardiac necrosis or hemorrhagic myocarditis and can be fatal. Hemorrhagic cystitis may occur and necessitates withholding therapy. Other toxicities reported commonly include nausea and vomiting (may be mild to severe depending on dosage), diarrhea, anorexia, alopecia, immunosuppression and sterility. Pulmonary fibrosis, SIADH, anaphylaxis and secondary neoplasms have been reported rarely.

6.8.6 Cisplatin

Standard Dosage:S eeT able 6.4.

Source and Pharmacology: Cisplatin is an inorganic heavy metal coordination complex that has biochemical properties similar to those of a bifunctional alkylating agent. It must undergo activation, by aquation, to form positively charged platinum complexes that react with nucleophilic sites on DNA. Cisplatin is cell-cycle, phase nonspecific. Cisplatin rapidly distributes into tissues with the highest concentrations being present in the prostate, liver, and kidney and is highly protein bound (>90%). Cisplatin has an elimination half-life of 30-90 min. Platinum is bound to plasma constituents. Cisplatin is excreted predominantly via glomerular filtration, and dosage adjustments are necessary for patients with renal dysfunction.

Formulation and Stability: Cisplatin is available in an amber multi-dose vial containing 100 mg of cisplatin at a concentration of 1 mg/ml. The unopened vial should be stored at room temperature and protected from light. The undiluted solution should not be refrigerated as a precipitate will form. Once opened, the vial should be discarded after 28 days if protected from light, or 7 days if not protected from light. Cisplatin should be further diluted in NS or 1/2 NS prior to administration.

Contraindications: Hypersensitivity to cisplatin, platinum-containing agents, or any component; preexisting renal impairment, hearing impairment, and myelosuppression; pregnancy.

Main Drug Interactions: Aminoglycosides, amphotericin B, and other nephrotoxic drugs (increase risk of nephrotoxicity); loop diuretics, aminoglycosides (potentiate ototoxicity); synergistic antineoplastic activity with cytarabine, 5-fluorouracil, etoposide; reduces renal elimination of methotrexate.

Main Side Effects: Nephrotoxicity is one of the major dose-limiting side effects of cisplatin. This toxicity may be irreversible and can be minimized by providing adequate hydration before, during, and after cisplatin therapy. Other dose limiting toxicities include myelosuppression, neuropathies, and ototoxicity. Nausea and vomiting are common and can be severe. Delayed nausea and vomiting (occurring ≥24 h after drug administration) can occur. Diarrhea, anorexia, electrolyte disturbances (especially hypomagnesemia), cardiac abnormalities, allergic reactions, and transient elevations in liver enzymes can occur. Secondary cancers have been reported.

6.8.7 Topotecan

Standard Dosage: Under investigation in retinoblastoma. 2–3 mg/m^2/d for 5 days when given as single agent.

Source and Pharmacology: Topotecan is a semi-synthetic derivative of camptothecin that inhibits topoisomerase I activity. Topoisomerase I relieves torsional strain in the DNA helix during replication by inducing reversible single strand DNA breaks. Topotecan binds to the topoisomerase I-DNA complex and prevents relegation of single strand breaks. This results in double-strand DNA breaks during DNA synthesis when replication enzymes interact with the ternary complex formed by topotecan, topoisomerase I and DNA. Topotecan undergoes a rapid, pH-dependent opening of the lactone ring to yield a relatively inactive, hydroxy acid in plasma. At physiologic pH, topotecan exists mainly as the hydroxy acid. Metabolism occurs via a pH dependent hydrolysis of the lactone moiety. Metabolism to an N-demethylated metabolite represents a minor metabolic pathway. Mean elimination half-life is three hours. Approximately 30% of a dose is excreted in the urine. Dosage adjustment is recommended for patients with moderate to severe renal dysfunction).

Formulation and Stability: Topotecan is available in single-dose vials containing 4 mg of topotecan as a lyophilized light yellow to greenish powder and 48 mg of mannitol. The intact vials should be stored at room temperature and protected from light. Each vial may be reconstituted with 4 ml of sterile water for injection to yield a final concentration of 1 mg/ml. Because the reconstituted solution does not contain a preservative, it is recommended that it be used immediately after reconstitution. The reconstituted solution can be further diluted with 5% dextrose or 0.9% NaCl containing solutions. Once diluted for administration, the drug is stable for at least 24 h at room temperature and ambient lighting.

Contraindications: Hypersensitivity to topotecan.

Main Drug Interactions: Concurrent cisplatin or carboplatin with topotecan therapy results in greater myelosuppression.

Main Side Effects: The dose-limiting toxicity is myelosuppression. Other toxicities reported commonly include nausea and vomiting, diarrhea, mucositis, abdominal pain, fever, rash, alopecia, anorexia, headache, and flu-like symptoms. Toxicities reported less commonly include elevated liver function tests and paresthesia.

6.8.8 Thiotepa

Standard Dosage:S eeT able 6.4.

Source and Pharmacology: Thiotepa is a cell-cycle nonspecific polyfunctional alkylating agent. It reacts with DNA phosphate groups to produce cross-linking of DNA strands leading to inhibition of DNA, RNA and protein synthesis. Thiotepa is extensively metabolized in the liver to metabolites that retain activity, primarily triethylenephosphoramide (TEPA). The main route of elimination is via the urine, mainly as metabolites; the elimination half-life of the thiotepa is 2.5 h, and that of TEPA is 17.6 h.

Formulation and Stability: Thiotepa is supplied in single-use vials containing 15 mg of lyophilized thiotepa, 80 mg NaCl and 50 mg $NaHCO_3$. The intact vials should be stored under refrigeration and protected from light. Each vial should be reconstituted with 1.5 ml of sterile water for injection to yield a concentration of 10 mg/ml. Further dilution with sterile water for injection to a concentration of 1 mg/mL yields an isotonic solution; if larger volumes are desired for intracavitary, IV infusion, or perfusion therapy, this solution may then be diluted with 5% dextrose or 0.9% NaCl containing solutions. The 10 mg/ml reconstituted solution is chemically stable when stored in the refrigerator for up to 5 days, however, it is recommended that solutions be prepared just prior to administration since they do not contain a preservative. Reconstituted solutions should be clear to slightly opaque: the solutions may be filtered through a 0.22 micron filter to eliminate haze.

Contraindications: Hypersensitivity to thiotepa or any component.

Main Drug Interactions: Cytochrome P450 isoenzyme CYP2B6 inhibitor. Succinylcholine (thiotepa inhibits pseudocholinesterase activity; prolongs muscular paralysis); other alkylating agents such as nitrogen mustard or cyclophosphamide (intensifies toxicity).

Main Side Effects: Dose limiting toxicity is myelosuppression. The leukocyte nadir may occur at any time from 10 to >30 days. Other toxicities include pain at the injection site, nausea and vomiting, anorexia, mucositis, dizziness, headache, amenorrhea, interference with spermatogenesis, and depigmentation with topical use. Allergic reactions, including skin rash and hives, have been reported rarely. Rare cases of apnea, hemorrhagic cystitis, and renal failure have occurred. Thiotepa is mutagenic, carcinogenic, and teratogenic ina nimals.P regnancyc ategory D.

References

Abramson DH, Greenfield DS, Ellsworth RM (1992) Bilateral retinoblastoma: correlations between age at diagnosis and time course for new intraocular tumors. Ophthalmic Paediatr Genet 13:1–7

Abramson DH, Gamell LS, Ellsworth RM et al (1994) Unilateral retinoblastoma: new intraocular tumours after treatment. Br J Ophthalmol 78:698–701

Abramson DH, Frank C, Chantada G et al (1999a) Intraocular carboplatin concentrations following intravenous administration for human intraocular retinoblastoma. Ophthalmic Genet 20:31–36

Abramson D, Frank C, Dunkel I (1999b) A phase I/II study of subconjunctival carboplatin for intraocular retinoblastoma. Ophthalmology 106:1947–1950

Abramson DH, Lawrence SD, Beaverson KL, Lee TC, Rollins IS, Dunkel IJ (2005) Systemic carboplatin for retinoblastoma: change in tumour size over time. Br J Ophthalmol 89:1616–1619

Abramson DH, Dunkel IJ, Brodie SE, Kim JW, Gobin YP (2008) A phase I/II study of direct intraarterial (ophthalmic artery) chemotherapy with melphalan for intraocular retinoblastoma: initial results. Ophthalmology 115:1398–1404

Antonelli CBG, Steinhorst F, Ribeiro KCB et al (2003) Extraocular retinoblastoma: a 13-year experience. Cancer98:12 92–1298

Antonelli CBG, Ribeiro KCB, Steinhorts F, Novaes PERS, Chojniak MM, Malogolowkin M (2006) Treatment of retinoblastoma patients with chemoreduction plus local therapy: experience of the AC Camargo Hospital, Brazil. J Pediatr Hematol Oncol 28:342–345

Athale UH, Stewart C, Kuttesch JF et al (2001) Phase I study of combination topotecan and carboplatin in pediatric solid tumors. J Clin Oncol 20:88–95

Baker SD, Heideman RL, Crom WR, Kuttesch JF, Gajjar A, Stewart CF (1996) Cerebrospinal fluid pharmacokinetics and penetration of continuous infusion topotecan in children with central nervous system tumors. Cancer Chemother Pharmacol 37:195–202

Blanco J, Dervieux T, Edick M et al (2001) Molecular emergence of acute myeloid leukemia during treatment for acute lymphoblastic leukemia. Proc Natl Acad Sci USA 98:10338–10343

Blaney SM, Heideman R, Berg S et al (2003) Phase I clinical trial of intrathecal topotecan in patients with neoplastic meningitis. J Clin Oncol 21:143–147

Bu H-Z, Gukasyan HJ, Goulet L, Lou X-J, Xiang C, Koudriakova T (2007) Ocular disposition, pharmacokinetics, efficacy and safety of nanoparticle-formulated ophthalmic drugs. Curr Drug Metab 8:91–107

Carcaboso AM, Bramuglia GF, Chantada GL et al (2007) Topotecan vitreous levels after periocular or intravenous delivery in rabbits: an alternative for retinoblastoma chemotherapy. Invest Ophthalmol Vis Sci 48:3761–3767

Chan HS, Canton MD, Gallie BL (1989) Chemosensitivity and multidrug resistance to antineoplastic drugs in retinoblastoma cell lines. Anticancer Res 9:469–474

Chan H, DeBoer G, Thiessen J et al (1996) Combining cyclosporin with chemotherapy controls intraocular retinoblastoma without requiring radiation. Clin Cancer Res 2:1499–1508

Chan H, Lu Y, Grogan T et al (1997) multidrug resistance protein (MRP) expression in retinoblastoma correlates with the rare failure of chemotherapy despite cyclosporine for reversal of P-glycoprotein. Cancer Res 57:2325–2330

Chantada G, Davila MTG, Fandiño A et al (1999a) Retinoblastoma with low risk for extraocular relapse. Ophthalmic Genet 20:133–140

Chantada G, Fandiño A, Mato G, Casak S (1999b) Phase II window of idarubicin in children with extraocular retinoblastoma. J Clin Oncol 17:1847–1850

Chantada G, Fandiño A, Casak S, Manzitti J, Raslawski E, Schvartzman E (2003) Treatment of overt extraocular retinoblastoma. Med Pediatr Oncol 40:158–161

Chantada G, Fandiño A, Dávila MTG et al (2004a) Results of a prospective study for the treatment of retinoblastoma. Cancer 100:834–842

Chantada G, Fandino A, Casak S et al (2004b) Activity of topotecan in retinoblastoma. Ophthalmic Genet 25:37–43

Chantada GL, Fandiño A, Raslawski EC et al (2005) Experience with chemoreduction and focal therapy for

intraocular retinoblastoma in a developing country. Pediatr Blood Cancer 44:455–460
Chantada GL, Casco F, Fandiño AC et al (2007) Outcome of patients with retinoblastoma and postlaminar optic nerve invasion. Ophthalmology 114:2083–2089
Chantada GL, Fandino AC, Carcaboso AM et al (2009) A phase I study of periocular topotecan in children with intraocular retinoblastoma. Invest Ophthalmol Vis Sci 50:1492–1496
Chevez-Barrios P, Chintagumpala M, Mieler W et al (2005) Response of retinoblastoma with vitreous tumor seeding to adenovirus-mediated delivery of thymidine kinase followed by gancyclovir. J Clin Oncol 23:7927–7935
Donovan SL, Schweers B, Martins R, Johnson D, Dyer MA (2006) Compensation by tumor suppressor genes during retinal development in mice and humans. BMC Biol 4:14
Doz F, Khelfaoui F, Mosseri V et al (1994) The role of chemotherapy in orbital involvement of retinoblastoma. Cancer7 4:722–732
Doz F, Neuenschwander S, Plantaz D et al (1995) Etoposide and carboplatin in extraocular retinoblastoma: a study by the Société Française d'Oncologie Pédiatrique. J Clin Oncol 13:902–909
Dunkel I, Aledo A, Kernan N et al (2000) Successful treatment of metastatic retinoblastoma. Cancer 89:2117–2121
Dunkel IJ, Lee TC, Shi W et al (2007) A phase II trial of carboplatin for intraocular retinoblastoma. Pediatr Blood Cancer4 9:643–648
Dyer MA, Rodriguez-Galindo C, Wilson MW (2005) Use of preclinical models to improve treatment of retinoblastoma. PLoS Med 2:e332
Elison JR, Cobrinik D, Claros N, Abramson DH, Lee TC (2006) Small molecule inhibition of HDM2 leads to p53-mediated cell death in retinoblastoma cells. Arch Ophthalmol1 24:1269–1275
Eng G, Li FP, Abramson DH et al (1993) Mortality from second tumors among long-term survivors of retinoblastoma. J Natl Cancer Inst 85:1121–1128
Ericson LA, Rosengren BH (1961) Present therapeutic resources in retinoblastoma. Acta Ophthalmol 39:569–576
Ericson LA, Kalberg B, Rosengren BH (1964) Trials of intravitreal injections of chemotherapeutic agents in rabbits. Acta Ophthalmol 42:721–726
Fisher PG, Kadan-Lottick NS, Koroner DN (2002) Intrathecal thiotepa: reappraisal of an established therapy. J Pediatr Hematol Oncol 24:274–278
Frangoul H, Ames MM, Mosher RB et al (1999) Phase I study of topotecan administered as a 21-day continuous infusion in children with recurrent solid tumors: a report from the Children's Cancer Group. Clin Cancer Res 5:3956–3962
Gallie B, Budning A, DeBoer G et al (1996) Chemotherapy with focal therapy can cure intraocular retinoblastoma without radiotherapy. Arch Ophthalmol 114:1321–1328
Ghate D, Edelhauser HF (2006) Ocular drug delivery. Expert Opin Drug Deliv 3:275–287
Ghate D, Brook W, McCarey BE, Edelhauser HF (2007) Pharmacokinetics of intraocular drug delivery by periocular injections using ocular fluorophotometry. Invest Ophthalmol Vis Sci 48:2230–2237
Gilbert JA, Simpson AE, Rudnick DE, Geroski DH, Aaberg TM, Edelhauser HF (2003) Transscleral permeability and intraocular concentrations of cisplatin from a collagen matrix. J Control Rel 20:409–417
Gombos D, Kelly A, Coen P, Kingston J, Hungerford J (2002) Retinoblastoma treated with primary chemotherapy alone: the significance of tumor size, location, and age. Br J Ophthalmol 86:80–83
Gombos DS, Hungerford J, Abramson DH et al (2007) Secondary acute myelogenous leukemia in patients with retinoblastoma. Ophthalmology 114:1378–1383
Gorodetsky R, Peylan-Ramu N, Reshef A, Gaberman E, Levdansky L, Marx G (2005) Interactions of carboplatin with fibrin(ogen), implications for local slow release chemotherapy. J Control Release 102:235–245
Gündüz K, Shields CL, Shields JA et al (1998) The outcome of chemoreduction treatment in patients with Reese-Ellsworth group V retinoblastoma. Arch Ophthalmol 116:1613–1617
Gündüz K, Muftuoglu O, Gunalp I, Unal E, Tacyildiz N (2006) Metastatic retinoblastoma: clinical features, treatment, and prognosis. Ophthalmology 113:1558–1566
Harbour JW, Murray TG, Hamasaki D et al (1996) Local carboplatin therapy in transgenic murine retinoblastoma. Invest Ophthalmol Vis Sci 37:1892–1898
Hayden B, Murray T, Scott I et al (2000) Subconjunctival carboplatin in retinoblastoma. Impact of tumor burden and dose schedule. Arch Ophthalmol 118:1549–1554
Hayden BC, Jockovich M-E, Murray TG et al (2004) Pharmacokinetics of systemic versus focal carboplatin chemotherapy in the rabbit eye: possible implication in the treatment of retinoblastoma. Invest Ophthalmol Vis Sci 45:3644–3649
Heideman RL, Cole DE, Balis F et al (1989) Phase I and pharmacokinetic evaluation of thiotepa in the cerebrospinal fluid and plasma of pediatric patients: evidence for dose-dependent plasma clearance of thiotepa. Cancer Res 49:736–741
Honavar SG, Singh A, Shields CL et al (2002) Postenucleation adjuvant therapy in high-risk retinoblastoma. Arch Ophthalmol 120:923–931
Hungerford J, Toma N, Plowman P, Kingston J (1995) External beam radiotherapy for retinoblastoma: I Whole eye technique. Br J Ophthalmol 79:109–111
Inomata M, Kaneko A (1987) Chemosensitivity profiles of primary and cultured human retinoblastoma cells in a human tumor clonogenic assay. Jpn J Cancer Res 78:858–868
Jacks T, Fazeli A, Schmitt EM, Bronson RT, Goodell MA, Weinberg RA (1992) Effects of a Rb mutation in the mouse. Nature 359:295–300
Jubran RF, Erdreich-Epstein A, Butturini A, Murphree AL, Villablanca JG (2004) Approaches to treatment for

extraocular retinoblastoma. Children's Hospital Los Angeles experience. J Pediatr Hematol Oncol 26:31–34
Kaneko A, Suzuki S (2003) Eye-preservation treatment of retinoblastoma with vitreous seeding. Jpn J Clin Oncol 33:601–607
Khelfaoui F, Validire P, Auperin A et al (1996) Histopathologic risk factors in retinoblastoma. A retrospective study of 172 patients treated in a single institution. Cancer7 7:1206–1213
Kingston J, Hungerford J, Madreperla S, Plowman P (1996) Results of combined chemotherapy and radiotherapy for advanced intraocular retinoblastoma. Arch Ophthalmol 114:1339–1343
Kiratli H, Bilgiç S, Özerdem U (1998) Management of massive orbital involvement of intraocular retinoblastoma. Ophthalmology1 05:322–326
Kremens B, Wieland R, Reinhard H et al (2003) High-dose chemotherapy with autologous stem cell rescue in children with retinoblastoma. Bone Marrow Transplant 31:281–284
Krishnakumar S, Mallikarjuna K, Desai N et al (2004) Multidrug resistance proteins: P-glycoprotein and lung resistance protein expression in retinoblastoma. Br J Ophthalmol8 8:1521–1526
Kupfer C (1953) Retinoblastoma treated with intravenous nitrogen mustard. Am J Ophthalmol 36:1721–1723
Laurie NA, Gray JK, Zhang J et al (2005) Topotecan combination chemotherapy in two new rodent models of retinoblastoma. Clin Cancer Res 11:7569–7578
Laurie NA, Donovan SL, Shih C-S et al (2006) Inactivation of the p53 pathway in retinoblastoma. Nature 444:61–66
Lee EY, Chang CY, Hu N et al (1992) Mice deficient for Rb are nonviable and show defects in neurogenesis and haematopoiesis. Nature 359:288–294
Lee TC, Hayashi NI, Dunkel IJ, Beaverson K, Novetsky D, Abramson DH (2003) New retinoblastoma tumor formation in children initially treated with systemic carboplatin. Ophthalmology 110:1989–1995
Li SL, Molokhia SA, Jeon EK (2004) Asessment of subconjunctival delivery with model ionic permeants and magnetic resonance imaging. Pharm Res 21:2175–2184
Lonsdale D, Berry DH, Holcomb TM et al (1968) Chemotherapeutic trials in patients with metastatic retinoblastoma. Cancer Chemother Rep 52:631–634
Majumdar S, Mitra AK (2006) Chemical modification and formulation approaches to elevated drug transport accross cell membranes. Expert Opin Drug Deliv 3:511–527
Mannermaa E, Vellonen K-S, Urtti A (2006) Drug transport in corneal epithelium and blood-retina barrier: Emerging role of transporters in ocular pharmacokinetics. Adv Drug Deliv Rev 58:1136–1163
Marsubara H, Makimoto A, Higa T et al (2005) A multidisciplinary treatment strategy that includes high-dose chemotherapy for metastatic retinoblastoma without CNS involvement. Bone Marrow Transplant 35:763–766
Mendelsohn M, Abramson DH, Madden T, Tong W, Tran H, Dunkel I (1998) Intraocular concentrations of chemotherapeutic agents after systemic or local administration. Arch Ophthalmol 116:1209–1212
Menon BS, Juraida E, Alagaratnam J et al (2007) Chemoreduction for intraocular retinoblastolma in Malaysia. J Pediatr Hematol Oncol 29:2–4
Mohney B, Robertson D, Schomberg P, Hodge D (1998) Second nonocular tumors in survivors of heritable retinoblastoma and prior radiation therapy. Am J Ophthalmol 126:269–277
Mohri M (1993) The technique of selective ophthalmic arterial infusion for conservative treatment of recurrent intraocular retinoblastoma. Keio Igaku 70:679–687
Mulvihill A, Budning A, Jay V et al (2003) Ocular motility changes after subtenon carboplatin chemotherapy for retinoblastoma. Arch Ophthalmol 121:1120–1124
Murphree A, Villablanca J, Deegan W et al (1996) Chemotherapy plus local treatment in the management of intraocular retinoblastoma. Arch Ophthalmol 114:1348–1356
Mustafa M, Jamshed A, Khafaga Y et al (1999) Adjuvant chemotherapy with vincristine, doxorubicin, and cyclophosphamide in the treatment of postenucleation high risk retinoblastoma. J Pediatr Hematol Oncol 21:364–369
Namouni F, Doz F, Tanguy M et al (1997) High-dose chemotherapy with carboplatin, etoposide and cyclophosphamide followed by a haematopoietic stem cell rescue in patients with high-risk retinoblastoma: a SFOP and SFGM study. Eur J Cancer 33:2368–2375
Nenadov Beck M, Balmer A, Dessing C, Pica A, Munier F (2000) First-line chemotherapy with local treatment can prevent external-beam irradiation and enucleation in low-stage intraocular retinoblastoma. J Clin Oncol 18:2881–2887
Nishimura S, Sato T, Ueda H, Ueda K (2001) Acute myeloblastic leukemia as a second malignancy in a patient with hereditary retinoblastoma. J Clin Oncol 19:4182–4183
Nitschke R, Parkhurst J, Sullivan J, Harris MB, Bernstein M, Pratt C (1998) Topotecan in pediatric patients with recurrent and progressive solid tumors: a Pediatric Oncology Group phase II study. J Pediatr Hematol Oncol 20:315–318
Pardue MT, Hejny C, Gilbert JA, Phillips MJ, Geroski DH, Edelhauser HF (2004) Retinal function after subconjunctival injection of carboplatin in fibrin sealant. Retina 24:776–782
Pratt CB, Crom DB, Howarth C (1985) The use of chemotherapy for extraocular retinoblastoma. Med Pediatr Oncol 13:330–333
Pratt CB, Fontanesi J, Chenaille P et al (1994) Chemotherapy for extraocular retinoblastoma. Pediatr Hematol Oncol 11:301–309
Pui C-H, Ribeiro RC, Hanckok M (1991) Acute myeloid leukemia in children treated with epipodophyllotoxins for acute lymphoblastic leukemia. N Engl J Med 325:1682–1687
Ranta V-P, Urtti A (2006) Transscleral drug delivery to the posterior eye: prospects of pharmacokinetic modeling. Adv Drug Deliv Rev 58:1164–1181

Robinson MR, Lee SS, Kim H et al (2006) A rabbit model for assessing the ocular barriers to the trasscleral delivery of triamcinolone acetonide. Exp Eye Res 82:479–487
Rodriguez-Galindo C, Radomski KM, Stewart CF, Furman W, Santana VM, Houghton PJ (2000) Clinical use of topoisomerase I inhibitors in anticancer treatment. Med Pediatr Oncol 35:385–402
Rodriguez-Galindo C, Wilson MW, Haik BG et al (2003a) Treatment of intraocular retinoblastoma with vincristine and carboplatin. J Clin Oncol 21:2019–2025
Rodriguez-Galindo C, Wilson MW, Haik BG et al (2003b) Treatment of metastatic retinoblastoma. Ophthalmology1 10:1237–1240
Rodriguez-Galindo C, Chantada GL, Haik B, Wilson MW (2007) Retinoblastoma: current treatment and future perspectives. Curr Treat Options Neurol 9:294–307
Saarinen UM, Sariola H, Hovi L (1991) Recurrent disseminated retinoblastoma treated with high-dose chemotherapy, total body irradiation, and autologous bone marrow rescue. Am J Pediatr Hematol Oncol 13:315–319
Schefler AC, Cicciarelli N, Feuer W, Toledano S, Murray TG (2007) Macular retinoblastoma: Evaluation of tumor control, local complications, and visual outcomes for eyes treated with chemotherapy and repetitive foveal laser ablation. Ophthalmology 114:162–169
Schiavetti A, Hadjistilianou T, Clerico A, Bonci E, Ragni G, Castello MA (2005) Conservative therapy in intraocular retinoblastoma. response/recurrence rate. J Pediatr Hematol Oncol 27:3–6
Schmack I, Hubbard B, Kang SJ, Aaberg TM, Grossniklaus HE (2006) Ischemic necrosis and atrophy of the optic nerve after periocular carboplatin injection for intraocular retinoblastoma. Am J Ophthalmol 142:310–315
Schouten-van Meeteren A, Moll A, Imhof S, Veerman A (2002) Chemotherapy for retinoblastoma: an expanding area of clinical research. Med Pediatr Oncol 38:428–438
Schueler AO, Anastassiou G, Jurklies C, Havers W, Wieland R, Bornfeld N (2006) De novo intraocular retinoblastoma development after chemotherapy in patients with hereditary retinoblastoma. Retina 26:425–431
Schvartzman E, Chantada G, Fandiño A, de Dávila MT, Raslawski E, Manzitti J (1996) Results of a stage-based protocol for the treatment of retinoblastoma. J Clin Oncol1 4:1532–1536
Scott I, Murray T, Feuer W et al (1999) External beam radiotherapy in retinoblatoma. Tumor control and comparison of 2 techniques. Arch Ophthalmol 117:766–770
Seregard S, Kock B, TRampe E (1995) Intravitreal chemotherapy for recurrent retinoblastoma in an only eye. Br J Ophthalmol7 9:194–195
Shields CL, Shields JA (1999) Recent developments in the management of retinoblastoma. J Pediatr Ophthalmol Strabismus3 6:8–18
Shields CL, Shields JA, Needle M et al (1997) Combined chemoreduction and adjuvant treatment for intraocular retinoblastoma. Ophthalmology 104:2101–2111
Shields CL, Meadows AT, Shields JA, Carvalho C, Smith A (2001) Chemoreduction for retinoblastoma may prevent intracranial neuroblastic malignancy (trilateral retinoblastoma). Arch Ophthalmol 119:1269–1272
Shields CL, Honavar SG, Meadows AT et al (2002a) Chemoreduction plus focal therapy for retinoblastoma: Factors predictive of need for treatment with external beam radiotherapy or enucleation. Am J Ophthalmol 133:657–664
Shields CL, Honavar SG, Shields JA, Demirci H, Meadows AT, Naduvilath TJ (2002b) Factors predictive of recurrence of retinal tumors, vitreous seeds, and subretinal seeds following chemoreduction for retinoblastoma. Arch Ophthalmol 120:460–464
Shields CL, Shelil A, Cater J, Meadows AT, Shields JA (2003) Development of new retinoblastomas after 6 cycles of chemoreduction for retinoblastoma in 162 eyes of 106 consecutive patients. Arch Ophthalmol 121:1571–1576
Shields CL, Mashayekhi A, Cater J et al (2005) Macular retinoblastoma managed with chemoreduction: Analysis of tumor control with or without adjuvant thermotherapy in 68 tumors. Arch Ophthalmol 123:765–773
Simpson AE, Gilbert JA, Rudnick DE, Geroski DH, Aaberg TM, Edelhauser HF (2002) Transscleral diffusion of carboplatin. an in vitro and in vivo study. Arch Ophthalmol 120:1069–1074
Smith MA, Rubinstein L, Ungerleider RS (1994) Therapy-related acute myeloid leukemia following treatment with epipodophyllotoxins: estimating the risks. Med Pediatr Oncol 23:86–98
Toma N, Hungerford J, Plowman P, Kingston J, Doughty D (1995) External beam radiotherapy for retinoblastoma: II Lens sparing technique. Br J Ophthalmol 79:112–117
Urtti A (2006) Challenges and obstacles of ocular pharmacokinetics and drug delivery. Adv Drug Deliv Rev 58:1131–1135
Uusitalo M, Van Quill K, Scott I, Matthay KK, Murray T, O'Brien J (2001) Evaluation of chemoprophylaxis in patients with unilateral retinoblastoma with high-risk features on histopathologic examination. Arch Ophthalmol 119:41–48
Van Quill KR, Dioguardi PK, Tong CT et al (2005) Subconjunctival carboplatin in fibrin sealant in the treatment of transgenic murine retinoblastoma. Ophthalmology 112:1151–1158
Wilson MW, Haik BG, Liu T, Merchant TE, Rodriguez-Galindo C (2005) Effect on ocular survival of adding early intensive focal treatments to a two-drug chemotherapy regimen in patients with retinoblastoma. Am J Ophthalmol 140:397–406

Wilson MW, Fraga CH, Fuller CE et al (2006) Immunohistochemical detection of multidrug-resistant protein expression in retinoblastoma treated by primary enucleation. Invest Ophthalmol Vis Sci 47:1269–1273
Wilson MW, Haik BG, Billups CA, Rodriguez-Galindo C (2007) Incidence of new tumor formation in patients with hereditary retinoblastoma treated with primary systemic chemotherapy: is there a preventive effect? Ophthalmology 114:2077–2082
Zelter M, Damel A, Gonzalez G, Schwartz L (1991) A prospective study on the treatment of retinoblastoma in 72 patients. Cancer 68:1685–1690
Zhang J, Schweers B, Dyer MA (2004) The first knockout mouse model of retinoblastoma. Cell Cycle 3:952–959

Treatment of Intraocular Retinoblastoma

M. W. Wilson

Contents

7.1 Introduction 91
7.2 Primary Treatments. 91
7.3 Focal Therapies 94
7.4 Emerging Treatments 99
7.5 Conclusion 99
References. 99

7.1 Introduction

The extent of intraocular involvement, visual potential of the eye, tumor size, and status of the fellow eye are the principal considerations in devising a treatment strategy for patients with intraocular retinoblastoma. Preservation of life, the eye, and vision are what we hope to achieve. The potential risk of any treatment must be weighed against the possible benefit. The more advanced the disease, the greater the risk to the patient if there is to be any preservation of vision.

7.2 Primary Treatments

The decision making process for treatment becomes increasingly complex when we consider patients with unilateral and bilateral disease (Figs. 7.1 and 7.2). For patients with massive unilateral disease, *enucleation* remains the standard of care. In the hands of a trained ophthalmic surgeon, enucleation affords resection of the gross tumor as well as excellent cosmetic outcome. Only those ophthalmologists who are experienced in the management of the disease should perform enucleations in retinoblastoma patients.

Care must be taken to minimize the risk of inadvertent globe perforation and to ensure a maximal length of optic nerve. Traction sutures should not be placed on the eye. Rather, the medial rectus muscle should be removed, leaving 3–5 mm of tendon attached at the insertion. Using a hemostat, the medial rectus tendon can then be grasped to provide ample traction during the removal of the eye (Fig. 7.3a). The globe should

C. Rodriguez-Galindo and M.W. Wilson (eds.), *Retinoblastoma*, Pediatric Oncology,
DOI 10.1007/978-0-387-89072-2_7,

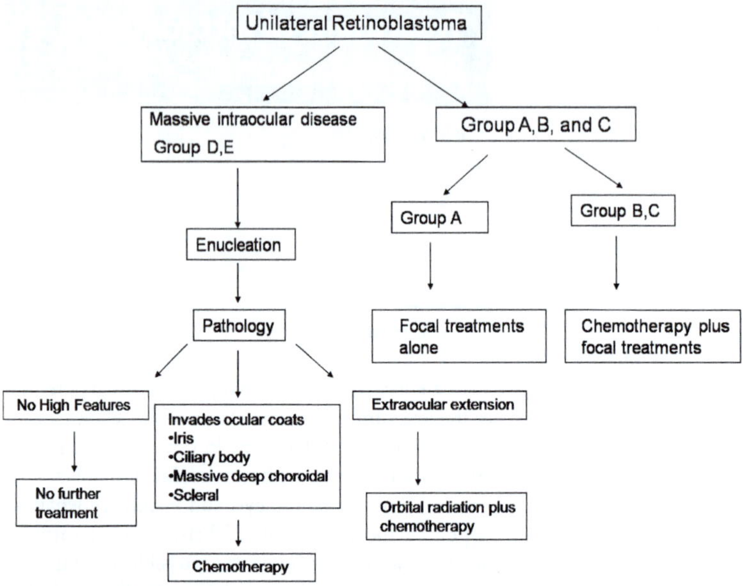

Figure 7.1

Schematic representation of consideration in treating unilateral retinoblastoma. Decisions are based on the international classification of retinoblastoma and the use of primary systemic chemotherapy

be rotated into abduction once all the muscles have been removed from the eye. Curved enucleation scissors should be avoided. Long Metzenbaum scissors should be passed posteriorly between the medial rectus muscle and the globe along the medial orbital wall until the optic nerve is identified (Fig. 7.3b). Only then should the blades of the scissors be slightly opened so as to encompass the optic nerve before transecting it. This technique affords a maximum length of optic nerve, usually in excess of 10 mm (Fig. 7.3c).

Some retinoblastoma surgeons prefer to use a snare to minimize inadvertent perforation of the globe. Technical difficulties with a snare, such as a broken wire, can necessitate the use of scissors. It is important, therefore, that the surgeon be adept at the aforementioned technique.

Once the eye is removed, it must be sent to a pathologist skilled in the handling of ophthalmic specimens as well as in the histopathology of retinoblastoma (see chapter 3). The identification of high-risk pathologic features should be followed by appropriate treatment (see chapter 8) (Chantada et al. 2007; Chong et al. 2006; Shields et al. 1993, 1994).

Patients with either bilateral disease or early unilateral disease should be considered for conservative therapy. Until the 1990s, *external beam radiotherapy* was the gold standard for the treatment of patients with bilateral retinoblastoma (Ellsworth 1969; Reese 1963). External beam radiotherapy was effective in controlling intraocular disease. However, it posed significant risk to young patients who possessed the *RB1* mutation. The risk of second cancers in patients with the *RB1* mutation appears to be significantly increased when treatment is delivered before their first birthday (Abramson and Frank 1998).

As a result of these findings, *primary systemic chemotherapy* has moved to the forefront in the conservative treatment of patients with intraocular retinoblastoma. The aim of chemotherapy is to reduce the intraocular tumor burden so that targeted focal therapies can be

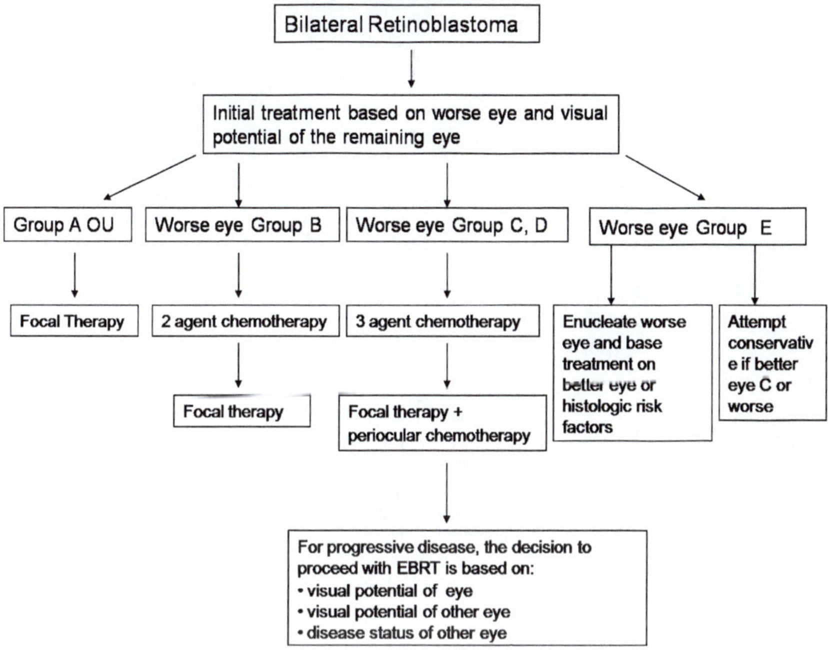

Figure 7.2

Schematic representation of consideration in treating gemline/multifocal retinoblastoma. Decisions are based on the international classification of retinoblastoma and the use of primary systemic chemotherapy

used to consolidate the tumor. The chemotherapeutic agents used and the number of cycles of chemotherapy needed have been the subject of much debate, and a consensus opinion regarding the drugs and number of cycles needed has not yet been reached (see chapter 6). Ideally, therapy should be structured to achieve maximal response with minimal toxicity. The aggressiveness of the chemotherapeutic protocol chosen should be tailored toward the severity of the intraocular disease, with particular attention directed toward the more severely affected eye. These principles should be taken into serious consideration when electing to treat unilateral disease (Beck et al. 2000; Brichard et al. 2002; Friedman et al. 2000; Gallie et al. 1996; Gombos et al. 2002; Greenwald and Strauss 1996; Kingston et al. 1996; Murphree et al. 1996; Rodriguez-Galindo et al. 2003, 2007; Shields et al. 1996, 1997, 2002a).

For Reese–Ellsworth Groups I–III and International Classification Groups A and B, it has been shown that a 2-agent regimen consisting of 6–8 cycles of carboplatin and vincristine provides equal efficacy to 6 cycles of triple-agent therapy with carboplatin, vincristine, and etoposide when coupled with aggressive focal consolidation. In cases of advanced intraocular disease, i.e., Reese–Ellsworth Groups IV and V and International Classification C–E, triple agent chemotherapy may have greater efficacy. Eyes with significant subretinal or vitreous seeding still frequently require external beam radiotherapy regardless of the chemotherapy regimen used. In these cases, chemotherapy can be used to delay radiation, hopefully allowing the child to eclipse his or her first birthday before radiation is needed (Rodriguez-Galindo et al. 2007, 2003; Wilson eta l. 2001).

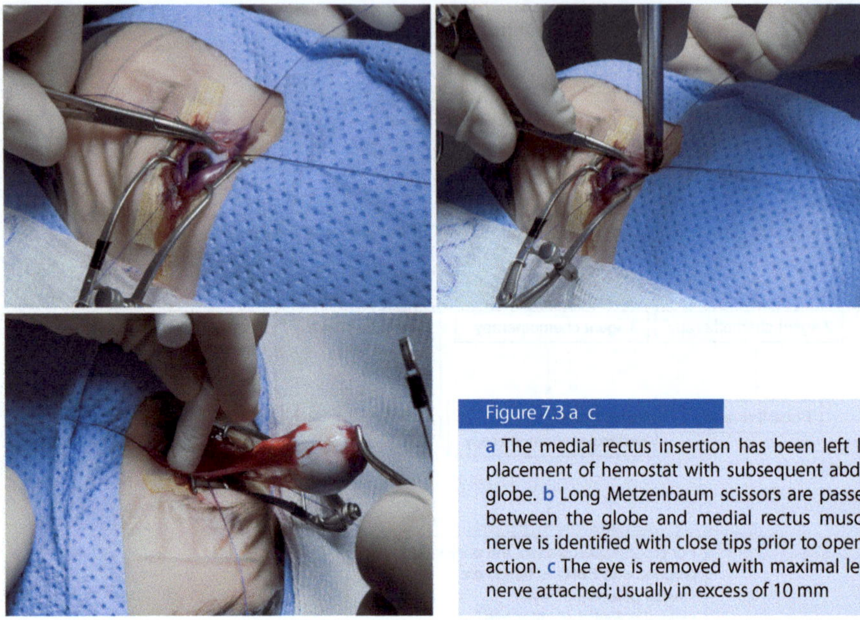

a b c

Figure 7.3 a c

a The medial rectus insertion has been left long to allow placement of hemostat with subsequent abduction of the globe. b Long Metzenbaum scissors are passed posteriorly between the globe and medial rectus muscle. The optic nerve is identified with close tips prior to opening for transaction. c The eye is removed with maximal length of optic nerve attached; usually in excess of 10 mm

7.3 Focal Therapies

Tumors will completely or partially calcify in response to chemotherapy. Reese and Ellsworth described tumor responses on the basis of their collective experience with external beam radiation. A Type I response implied complete calcification of the tumor, whereas a Type II response indicated a residual fish-flesh tumor. A Type III response indicated a combination of the two. In the era of primary systemic chemotherapy, the aforementioned patterns of tumor regression are no longer applicable, especially with regards to persistent fish-flesh tumor. Upon commencing chemotherapy, targeted focal therapies should be directed toward those tumors or parts of tumors that fail to calcify. We typically defer focal therapies until the completion of two cycles of chemotherapy to allow maximal reduction in tumor size, thereby minimizing damage to the surrounding retina, especially when visually sensitive structures, such as the fovea and optic nerve, are in close proximity to the tumor (Hamel et al. 2000).

Focal therapies can also be used in an attempt to treat a limited number of vitreous implantations in an effort to avoid external beam radiotherapy. These implants are typically seen in the inferior mid-periphery or peripheral retina in the setting of an optically clear vitreous cavity. These lesions are "assumed" to be seeds based on their multiplicity, clustering, and location. In the setting of overt vitreous seeds unresponsive to chemotherapy, focal measures alone are not adequate to control the disease. The entire vitreous cavity must be sterilized.

The current focal therapies available to treat retinoblastoma include the *argon green laser*, the *diode laser*, *cryotherapy*, *brachytherapy*, and *periocular chemotherapy*. Focal therapies are selected based on tumor location and size. Lasers are more commonly used to treat posterior tumors, while more anterior tumors are easily accessed with cryotherapy. Brachytherapy is reserved for those tumors that cannot be consolidated with laser or cryotherapy and are not in need of external beam radiotherapy, while periocular chemotherapy can be used to treat minimal vitreous seeds in an attempt to avoid external beam radiotherapy.

Two principal wavelengths of light are currently used to treat retinoblastoma. The argon green laser with a wavelength of 532 nm photocoagulates tissue by inducing a temperature in excess of 65°C. Traditionally, the argon laser has been used to treat the retina edge surrounding a tumor in an effort to deprive the tumor of its blood supply and in turn cause tumor regression. Using an indirect ophthalmoscope, a double row of subtle white burns is used to encircle the tumor; powers of 250–350 mW and burn durations of 0.3–0.5 s are used (Ellsworth 1969; Shields et al. 1990; Journée-de Korver and Keunen 2002).

Debate exists as to whether the tumor surface should be directly treated for fear of liberating tumor cells into the vitreous cavity as photocoagulation occurs. Newer generations of the 532 nm laser permit continuous delivery similar to that of the diode laser. Such modalities have led some to advocate its use in the treatment of retinoblastoma. If the tumor surface is treated, the desired endpoint remains a subtle whitening of the tumor surfaces. Laser energy should be kept at the lowest possible level necessary to achieve the desired endpoint. Powers in excess of 500 mW will result in tumor disruption and should be avoided. As with all focal therapies, treatment should be continued until the residual fish- flesh tumor regresses into a flat chorioretinal scar. Typically, lasers are administered every 3–4 weeks.

The optimal indication for direct treatment with the argon green laser is a residual fish-flesh mass overlying a largely calcified tumor (Fig. 7.4). In such situations, the uptake of the diode laser is unpredictable. Using the argon green laser, a whitening of the tumor can be seen, assuring an adequate treatment.

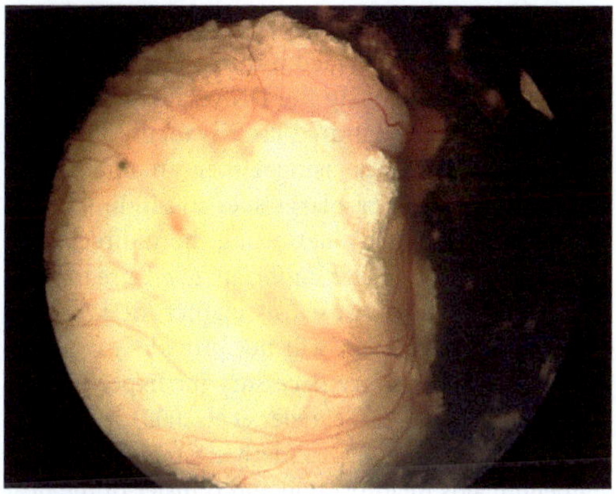

Figure 7.4

Residual fish flesh tumor overlying calcified mass. This represent an ideal scenario for newer 532 nm lasers with continuous delivery options

The argon laser has both direct and indirect cytotoxic effects. Photocoagulation directly kills tumor cells, and the thermal spread from the laser may have secondary hyperthermic effects that act synergistically with ongoing chemotherapy. Argon laser photocoagulation should not be performed if there is a retinal detachment overlying the tumor.

The diode laser (810 nm) was adapted for the treatment of retinoblastoma based on its success in the treatment of choroidal malignant melanoma. The laser energy is readily absorbed by melanin pigment and proved successful in the treatment of small melanocytic tumors. Low power settings, coupled with a large spot size (2–3 mm) and prolonged delivery, achieved hyperthermia (45–65°C) at sub-photocoagulation temperatures. The end result was a sustained penetrant burn with direct cytotoxic effects. The term *transpupillary thermotherapy*, or *TTT*, was coined to describe this technique (Journee-de Korver et al. 1992a, b; Oosterhuis et al. 1995; Shields et al. 2002b;R obertsoneta l. 1999).

The methods of TTT were subsequently adapted to treat retinoblastoma. Initially, the diode laser was used synergistically with platinum-based chemotherapy. The laser provided a direct cytotoxic effect in addition to enhancing the DNA-damaging effects of carboplatin. The infrared laser is focused directly on the tumor surface using either an ophthalmic microscope adapter or a large spot size indirect ophthalmoscope adapter. When using the indirect ophthalmoscope for TTT, it is important to ensure that the correct adapter is being used, as adapters designed for diode photocoagulation will not provide a continuous wavelength delivery necessary for hyperthermia (Lumbroso et al. 2003; Schueler et al. 2003).

For small tumors, the underlying retinal pigment epithelium aids in absorption and transfer of the heat to the tumor. The desired endpoint is a subtle whitening of the tumor free of hemorrhage. Powers are titrated based on the tumor size and pigmentation of the underlying retinal pigment epithelium. Powers should not exceed 600 mW when there is visible uptake by the surrounding/underlying retinal pigment epithelium.

Tumors with significant elevation or those residual elements that rest on adjacent calcified tumor do not readily whiten with TTT. Prolonged treatment sessions of 5–10 min using powers of 600–800 mW may be needed to achieve a therapeutic effect. Even with such prolonged treatment, a visible change in the tumor may not be seen until follow-up examination 3–4 weeks later. If available, the argon green laser may provide a more effective treatment. One of the major shortcomings in the modern treatment of retinoblastoma is our failure as a community to communicate clearly our methods of consolidation with lasers, i.e., type, duration, and power.

Tumors with significant elevation or those residual elements that rest on adjacent calcified tumor do not readily whiten with TTT. Prolonged treatment sessions of 5–10 min using powers of 600–800 mW may be needed to achieve a therapeutic effect. Even with such prolonged treatment, a visible change in the tumor may not be seen until follow-up examination 3–4 weeks later (Fig. 7.5).

Cryotherapy is ideally suited for the treatment of small anterior tumors (Ellsworth 1969; Shields et al. 1989; Tolentino and Tablante 1972). Cryotherapy is directly cytotoxic, causing cell lysis by disruption of the cell membrane that occurs after the formation of cytoplasmic ice crystals. Nitrous oxide gas is used to deliver a transcleral freeze via a cryoprobe under direct visualization. The lesion to be treated is visualized with an indirect ophthalmoscope and the scleral

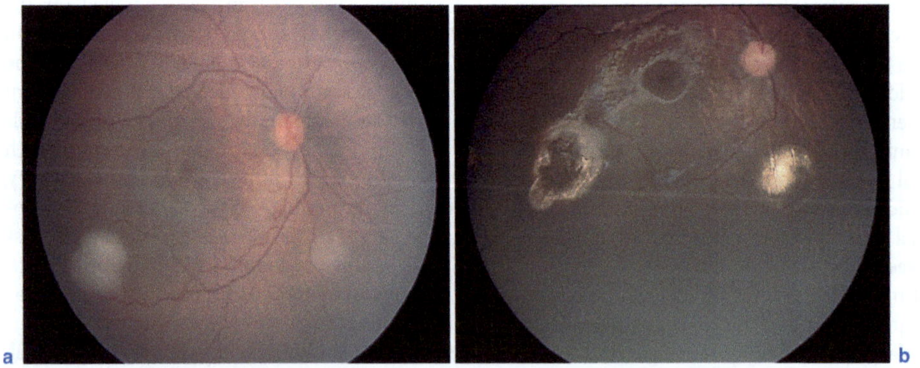

Figure 7.5 a,b

a Right eye of a patient with bilateral retinoblastoma, Group A OD and Group C OS. b Appearance of tumors after 1 treatment with diode laser. Viable tumor persists along the superior edge of the temporal most lesion

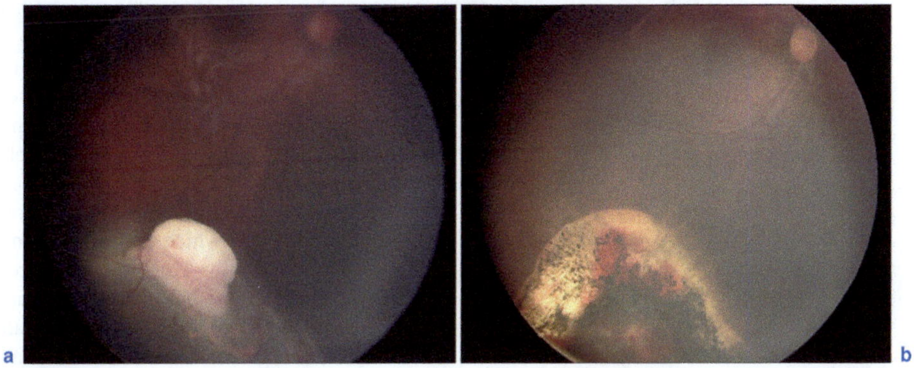

Figure 7.6 a,b

a Inferior peripheral visualized using scleral indentation with cryoprobe. b A transcleral triple-thaw freeze is administered with the "ice ball" incorporating the entire tumor as well as the adjacent retina and vitreous

underlying the tumor indented with a cryoprobe. A succession of 3 freezes with three intervening thaws is applied to the tumor. An "ice ball" should be seen to encompass the tumor and adjacent vitreous with each freeze (Fig. 7.6). Treatment should be limited to the area of the tumor to minimize damage to adjacent normal retina. Multiple tumors may be treated at one examination, but extensive treatments should be avoided. Aggressive cryotherapy may cause serious retinal detachments and iatrogenic retinal breaks. Although each cryotherapy unit may vary, we target a freezing temperature of −70°C during treatment. Treatments should be repeated at 3- to 4-week intervals until the lesion regresses to a flat chorioretinal scar.

Posterior tumors can also be treated with cryotherapy. The conjunctiva is opened in the quadrant of the tumor to be treated. The curved cryoprobe is passed along the curvature of the eye and the tumor indented. Once the tumor has been identified, the triple freeze-thaw is applied. We generally reserve "cut-down" cryotherapy for recurrent posterior tumors not amenable to laser treatment. Generally, these are tumors smaller than those for which we would consider brachytherapy.

Brachytherapy involves the implantation of a radioactive source close to the tumor. For the treatment of retinoblastoma, a carrier or "plaque" is loaded with a radioactive isotope and surgically placed on the scleral surface underlying the tumor to be treated. Traditional isotopes have included radon-222 and cobalt-60. Today, iodine-125 is the most commonly used isotope in the United States. Ruthenium-106 is more commonly used in Europe. Other, less commonly used isotopes include iridium-192, gold-198, and palladium-103. We use gold shields loaded with iodine-125. The gold shields the surrounding orbit from the emitted ionizing radiation. Brachytherapy may be used as primary therapy alone, as consolidation for tumors too large to treat with laser or cryotherapy, or as treatment for tumors that have recurred after chemotherapy and other focal therapies. The radiation damages the cellular DNA, triggering the p53 pathway and subsequent apoptosis. Target doses are 40–45 Gy to the tumor apex (see chapter 5) (Merchant et al. 2004; Shields et al. 2006).

A trained ophthalmic surgeon should perform the placement of episcleral radioactive plaques in collaboration with a designated radiation oncologist and medical physicists. The conjunctiva is opened in the quadrant in which the tumor to be treated is located. Using the technique of indirect ophthalmoscopy and scleral depression, the borders of the tumor are

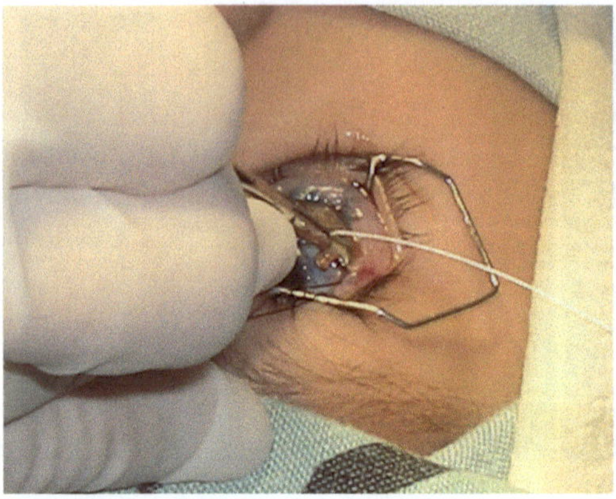

Figure 7.7

An episcleral plaque loaded with I-125 radioactive seeds is secured to the sclera overlying the tumor to be treated

demarcated and marked with methylene blue. The plaque is then sewn to the scleral surface using spatulated needles similar to those used in strabismus and scleral buckling procedures (Fig. 7.7). Extreme caution should be taken to avoid inadvertent perforation of the globe. If needed, a rectus or an oblique muscle may be transposed to allow the plaque to lie flush on the scleral surface. Treatment effects should be seen within 4 weeks. Tumors typically regress to a calcified mass with associated chorioretinal scarring.

In contrast to lasers, cryotherapy, and brachytherapy, the exact role and efficacy of *periocular chemotherapy* are less well defined (see chapter 6). The penetration of systemic chemotherapy into the vitreous cavity is highly variable. This is most likely due to the status of the blood-retina barrier at the time of treatment. Large tumors with incompetent vessels are more apt to spill chemotherapeutics into the vitreous cavity. However, as the tumor regresses and the blood-retinal barrier is restored, delivery of the chemotherapy into vitreous becomes increasingly difficult. Some investigators have advocated cryotherapy to the peripheral retina in an attempt to breakdown the blood-retinal barrier and increase diffusion of the chemotherapy into the vitreous (Murphree et al. 1996). The true efficacy of such treatment remains in doubt.

Periocular injections, specifically of carboplatin, have been used to deliver high doses of chemotherapy to the vitreous cavity in attempts to treat seeds (Abramson et al. 1999a, b; Dunkel et al. 2007). The sclera represents a porous membrane, and thus a subtenon's injection of carboplatin creates a diffusion gradient by which the carboplatin travels into the vitreous cavity. The vitreous concentrations of carboplatin exceed those that can be achieved with systemic therapy. Using a 3-cc syringe and 27" gauge needle, 20 mg of carboplatin in 2 cc of normal saline are injected into the subtenon's space. Multiple injections can be given at 3- to 4-week intervals.

A marked response to a single injection can be seen within weeks of treatment. However, sustained remissions have been difficult to achieve with periocular injections alone. Most case series report long-term treatment failures when periocular injections are used as salvage therapy. The reason for this is still uncertain. Some investigators feel it is due to a failure to treat adequately the source of the seeding; thus, there is a continued liberation of seeds into the vitreous cavity. Others postulate that the relative dormancy of the seeds makes them less susceptible to the DNA-damaging effects of carboplatin. Finally, it has been argued that when perioucular injections are used as a rescue treatment, the cells so selected are the most resistant and least likely to respond. New protocols of the Children's Oncology Group are investigating earlier incorporation of carboplatin in the treatment of International Group C and D eyes in an attempt to avoid external beam radiotherapy.

The diffusion of carboplatin into the orbit tissue can induce a profound myositis requiring temporary treatment with oral corticosteroids (Mulvihill et al. 2003). Other noted complications have been ischemic optic neuropathy and severe fibroblastic proliferation, which in turn increase the difficulty of any subsequent enucleation (Abramson et al. 1999a, b).

Newer agents and methods of transcleral delivery are being investigated. These include the use of fibrosealant glue to serve a carrier of carboplatin (Van Quill et al. 2005). Injection of the glue into the subtenon's space permits a slower diffusion of the carboplatin.

Higher sustained vitreous concentrations with diminished orbital toxicity are achieved. Other chemotherapeutics such topotecan have been shown to have good transcleral delivery in preclinical models and are currently being studied at some centers (Carcaboso eta l. 2007).

For patients with bilateral retinoblastoma who have advanced or recalcitrant vitreous disease, external beam radiotherapy remains an essential part of treatment (Shields et al. 2002c, d). External beam radiotherapy is also an important tool in the management of juxtapapillary and juxtafoveal tumors. Laser to tumors adjoining these visually sensitive areas can result in damage to adjacent healthy retina and cause visual loss. External beam radiotherapy is more likely to spare the optic nerve and retina, and preserve maximal vision. A consultation with the radiation oncologists should be made early in treatment if radiotherapy is deemed likely. Discussions should pertain to timing, the dose needed to control the intraocular disease, and potential side effects. Decisions to proceed with external beam radiotherapy should be based on the potential vision of the affected eye as well as the vision of the other eye.

Newer methods of radiation such as conformal radiotherapy and intensity-modulated radiotherapy have tightened the field of radiation thereby diminishing exposure to surrounding orbital structures. More encouraging is the potential use of proton beam radiotherapy. The tightly collimated proton beam reduces spread to adjacent tissue and its depth of penetration more strictly controlled. The long-term results and complications of these newer radiation methods have yet to be fully studied in retinoblastoma patients. A more detailed discussion of external beam radiotherapy can be found in chapter 5.

7.4 Emerging Treatments

New frontiers in the treatment of retinoblastoma include the use of both gene therapies for the treatment of vitreous seeds. Adenoviral-mediated transfection of tumor cells with thymidine kinase renders the tumor susceptible to systemically administered ganciclovir (Chevez-Barrios et al. 2005). Phase 1 clinical trials have been completed, documenting both safety and efficacy. Although currently reserved as salvage therapy for remaining eyes failing conventional modalities of treatment, there is hope that this new targeted therapy may become a mainstream treatment.

Perhaps more exciting are recent studies showing the success of targeted therapies. Laurie et al. (2006) have shown inactivation of the p53 pathway in retinoblastoma is secondary to an upregulation of *MDMX*. Using small molecular inhibitors such as nutlin, MDMX can be inactivated permitting apotosis to ensue. Molecules such as nutlin provide hope in that they can be delivered across the sclera and in turn diminish systemic toxicities.

7.5 Conclusion

The treatment of intraocular retinoblastoma requires a multidisciplinary team approach. The ophthalmologist must communicate the intraocular findings to the pediatric oncologist and radiation oncologist. The pro and cons of each treatment modality are weighed against the severity of disease and the potential for vision (Wilson et al. 2006). The team then constructs a treatment plan, which is individualized to fit the needs of the patients. Once treatment begins, the ophthalmologist monitors the response to therapy and the team modifies the treatment plan as needed. Only by working as a cohesive team of specialists can the best outcome of the retinoblastoma be obtained.

References

Abramson DH, Frank CM (1998) Second nonocular tumors in survivors of bilateral retinoblastoma: a possible age effect on radiation-related risk. Ophthalmology 105:573–579

Abramson DH, Frank CM, Chantada GL et al (1999a) Intraocular carboplatin concentrations following intravenous administration for human intraocular retinoblastoma. Ophthalmic Genet 20:31–36

Abramson DH, Frank CM, Dunkle IJ (1999b) A phase I/II study of subconjunctival carboplatin for intraocular retinoblastoma. Ophthalmology. 106:1947–1950

Beck MN, Balmer A, Dessing C et al (2000) First-line chemotherapy with local treatment can prevent external-beam irradiation and enucleation in low-stage intraocular retinoblastoma. J Clin Oncol 18:2881–2887

Brichard B, Brucycker JJ, DePotter P et al (2002) Combined chemotherapy and local treatment in the management of intraocular retinoblastoma. Med Pediatr Oncol 38:411–415

Carcaboso AM, Bramuglia GF, Chantada GL et al (2007) Topotecan vitreous levels after periocular or intravenous delivery in rabbits: an alternative for retinoblastoma chemotherapy. Invest Ophthalmol Vis Sci 48:3761–3767

Chantada GL, Dunkel IJ, Antoneli CB et al (2007) Risk factors for extraocular relapse following enucleation after failure of chemoreduction in retinoblastoma. Pediatr Blood Cancer 49:256–260

Chevez-Barrios P, Chintagumpala M, Mieler W et al (2005) Respone of retinoblastoma with vitreous tumor seeding to adenovirus-mediated delivery of thymidine kinase followed by ganciclovir. J Clin Oncol 23:7927–7935

Chong EM, Coffee RE, Chintagumpala M et al (2006) Extensively necrotic retinoblastoma is associated with high-risk prognostic factors. Arch Pathol Lab Med 130:1669–1672

Dunkel IJ, Lee TC, Shi W et al (2007) A phase II clinical trial of carboplatin for intraocular retinoblastoma. Pediatri Blood Cancer 49:643–648

Ellsworth RM (1969) Practical management of retinoblastoma. Trans Am Ophthalmol Soc 67:464–534

Friedman DL, Himelstein B, Shields CL et al (2000) Chemoreduction and local ophthalmic therapy for intraocular retinoblastoma. J Clin Oncol 18:12–17

Gallie BL, Budning A, DeBoer G et al (1996) Chemotherapy with focal therapy can cure intraocular retinoblastoma without radiotherapy. Arch Ophthalmol 114:1321–1328

Gombos DS, Kelly A, Coen PG et al (2002) Retinoblastoma treated with primary chemotherapy alone: the significance of tumor size, location and age. Br J Ophthalmol 86:80–83

Greenwald MJ, Strauss LC (1996) Treatment of intraocular retinoblastoma with carboplatin and etoposide with retinoblastoma. Ophthalmology 103:1989–1997

Hamel P, Heon E, Gallie BL, Budning AS (2000) Focal therapy in the management of retinoblastoma: when to start and when to stop. J AAPOS 4:334–337

Journée-de Korver JG, Keunen JEE (2002) Thermotherapy in the management of choroidal melanoma. Prog Retin Eye Res 21(3):303–317

Journee-de Korver JG, Oosterhuis JA, Kakebeeke-Kemme HM (1992a) Transpupillary thermotherapy (TTT) by infrared irradiation of choroidal melanoma. Doc Ophthalmol8 2:185–191

Journee-de Korver JG, Verberg-van der Marel EH, Oosterhuis JA, van Best JA, de Wolff-Rouendaal D (1992b) Tumoricidal effect of hyperthermia by near infrared irradiation on pigmented hamster melanoma. Lasers Light Ophthalmol 4:175–180

Kingston JE, Hungerford JL, Madreperla SA, Plowman PN (1996) Results of combined chemotherapy and radiotherapy for advanced intraocular retinoblastoma. Arch Ophthalmol 114:1339–1343

Laurie NA, Donovan SL, Shih CS et al (2006) Inactivation of the p53 pathway in retinoblastoma. Nature 444:61–66

Lumbroso L, Doz F, Levy C et al (2003) Diode laser thermotherapy and chemothermotherapy in the treatment of retinoblastoma. J Fr Ophtalmol 26:154–159

Merchant TE, Gould CJ, Wilson MW et al (2004) Epislceral plaque brachytherapy for retinoblastoma. Pediatr Blood Cancer 43:134–139

Mulvihill A, Budning A, Jay V et al (2003) Ocular motility changes after subtenon carboplatin chemotherapy for retinoblastoma. Arch Ophthalmol 121:1120–1124

Murphree AL, Villablanca JG, Deegan WF et al (1996) Chemotherapy plus local treatment in the management of intraocular retinoblastoma. Arch Ophthalmol 114:1348–1356

Oosterhuis JA, Journee-de Korver JG, Kakebeeke-Kemme HM, Bleeker JC (1995) Transpupillary thermotherapy in choroidal melanomas. Arch Ophthalmol 113:315–321

Reese A Retinoblastoma. In: Reese A (1963) Tumors of the eye. Harper and Row, pp 85–161

Robertson DM, Buettner H, Bennett SR (1999) Transpupillary thermotherapy as primary treatment for small choroidal melanomas. Arch Ophthalmol 117:1512–1519

Rodriguez-Galindo C, Wilson MW, Haik BG et al (2003) Treatment of intraocular retinoblastoma with vincristine and carboplatin. J Clin Oncol. 21:2019–2025

Rodriguez-Galindo C, Chantada GL, Haik BG, Wilson MW (2007) Treatment of retinoblastoma: current status and future directions. Curr Treat Options Neurol 9: 294–307

Schueler AO, Jurklies C, Heimann H et al (2003) Thermochemotherapy in retinoblastoma. Br J Ophthalmol 87:90–95

Shields JA, Parsons H, Shields CL et al (1989) The role of cryotherapy in the management of retinoblastoma. Am J Ophthalmol 108:260–264

Shields JA, Shields CL, Parsons H et al (1990) The role of photocoagulation in the management of retinoblastoma. Arch Ophthalmol 108:205–208

Shields CL, Shields JA, Baez KA et al (1993) Choroidal invasion of retinoblastoma: metastatic potential and clinical risk factors. Br J Ophthalmol 77:544–548

Shields CL, Shields JA, Baez KA et al (1994) Optic nerve invasion of retinoblastoma: metastatic potential and clinical risk factors. Cancer 73:692–698

Shields CL, De Potter P, Himelstein B et al (1996) Chemoreduction in the initial management of intraocular retinoblastoma. Arch Ophthalmol 114:1330–1338

Shields CL, Shields JL, Needle M et al (1997) Combined chemoreduction and adjuvant treatment for intraocular retinoblastoma. Ophthalmology 104:2101–2111

Shields CL, Honavar SG, Meadows AT et al (2002a) Chemoreduction for unilateral retinoblastoma. Arch Ophthalmol1 20:1653–1658

Shields CL, Shields JA, Perez N et al (2002b) Primary transpupillary thermotherapy for small choroidal melanoma in 256 consecutive cases. Ophthalmology 109:225–234

Shields CL, Honavar SG, Meadows AT et al (2002c) Chemoreduction plus focal therapy for retinoblastoma: factors predictive of need for treatment with external beam radiotherapy and enucleation. Am J Ophthalmol 133:657–664

Shields CL, Honavar SG, Shields JA et al (2002d) Factors predictive of recurrence of retinal tumors, vitreous seeds, and subretinal seeds following chemoreduction for retinoblastoma. Arch Ophthalmol 120:460–464

Shields CL, Mashayekhi A, Sun H et al (2006) Iodine-125 plaque radiotherapy as salvage treatment for retinoblastoma recurrence after chemoreduction in 84 patients. Ophthalmology 113:2087–2092

Tolentino FI, Tablante RT (1972) Cryotherapy of retinoblastoma. Arch Ophthalmol 87:52–55

Van Quill KR, Dioguardi PK, Tong CT et al (2005) Subconjunctival carboplatin in fibrin sealant in the treatment of transgenic murine retinoblastoma. Ophthalmology 112:1151–1158

Wilson MW, Rodriguez-Galindo C, Haik BG et al (2001) Multiagent chemotherapy as neoadjuvant treatment for multifocal intraocular retinoblastoma. Ophthalmology. 108:2106–2115

Wilson MW, Haik BG, Rodriguez-Galindo C (2006) Socioeconomic impact of modern multidisciplinary management of retinoblastoma. Pediatrics 118:e331–e336

Treatment of Extraocular and Metastatic Retinoblastoma

G. L. Chantada · I. J. Dunkel

Contents

8.1 **Introduction** 103
8.2 **Patients with High Risk Intraocular Disease** . . 104
8.2.1 Choroidal Invasion 105
8.2.2 Optic Nerve Invasion 105
8.3 **Patients with Microscopic Residual Disease after Enucleation** 106
8.3.1 Trans-Scleral Invasion 107
8.3.2 Future Directions 108
8.4 **Orbital and Locoregional Disease** 108
8.4.1 Orbital Relapse 109
8.4.2 Special Situations 110
8.5 **Metastatic Disease** 111
8.5.1 Stage 4a: Metastatic Disease Without CNS Involvement 111
8.5.2 Stage 4b: Distant Metastatic Disease with CNS Involvement 112
8.5.3 Future Research 112
References 113

8.1 Introduction

Retinoblastoma can extend outward through different structures of the eye. It may disseminate through the optic nerve into the CNS and through the sclera to the orbit. Retinoblastoma can also give rise to systemic metastasis after gaining access to the choroidal circulation or after locoregional dissemination to the orbit and lymph nodes. Usual metastatic sites of retinoblastoma include the CNS, bone and the bone marrow (MacKay et al. 1984). Less frequently, retinoblastoma can metastasize to other organs, such as the liver or distant lymph nodes.

The presenting signs and symptoms of metastatic retinoblastoma are quite variable and depend on the site or sites of involvement. In patients who have previously undergone enucleation, orbital recurrences often present with the parental observation that the prosthesis is no longer fitting well. More extensive orbital disease may present as a visible mass. Central nervous system disease can occur as optic nerve disease tracking posteriorly into the brain, or as diffuse leptomeningeal involvement. Again, signs and symptoms are variable, depending on the locations involved and the degree of involvement, but may include headache, irritability, emesis and/or focal neurological signs. Bone disease may present with pain, and bone marrow disease may present with abnormally low blood counts, but often, disease at those sites and liver disease may be asymptomatic and discovered only during evaluation of the extent of the disease(Table 8.1).

C. Rodriguez-Galindo and M.W. Wilson (eds.), *Retinoblastoma*, Pediatric Oncology,
DOI 10.1007/978-0-387-89072-2_8,

Table 8.1. Extent of disease evaluation for suspected metastatic disease

- Brain and orbit MRI with and without contrast
- Lumbar puncture for CSF cytology
- Spine MRI with and without contrast (if CNS disease is present or appropriate focal neurological signs are present)
- Abdominal CT with IV contrast
- Bone scan
- Bone marrow aspirate and biopsy

The treatment of high risk intraocular and extraocular retinoblastoma can be divided into four different scenarios that will be discussed below:

- Patients with high risk intraocular disease
- Patients with microscopic extraocular residue aftere nucleation
- Patients with orbital and locoregional dissemination
- Patientsw ithm etastaticd isease.

8.2 Patients with High Risk Intraocular Disease

The International Retinoblastoma Staging System (IRSS) considers patients with completely resected retinoblastoma after enucleation of the affected eye to have Stage 1 disease (Table 8.2) Histopathological risk factors for extraocular relapse include invasion into the choroid, inside the sclera, the optic nerve and possibly, the anterior segment (National registry of retinoblastoma in Japan 1975). However, their impact as independent risk factors may not be homogeneous. The quality of the published evidence is hampered by the lack of prospective randomized studies, the rarity of the disease, and the diverse pathological criteria for defining the invasion of the ocular coats used by different groups. A thorough postenucleation histopathological staging is essential to define groups with different risks of relapse. This is a major limitation in developing countries where the enucleated eyes of patients with advanced disease are done in centers with no specialized pathological examination. Sometimes, pathological examination is never performed, and the risk of relapse cannot be estimated (Bowman et al. 2006). There are wide variations in the definitions of the degree of invasion to the ocular coats among many centers, which further complicates the interpretation of results from different groups. The International Retinoblastoma Staging Working Group found a great disparity in the processing of eyes, definition of pathology criteria, and treatment, in a survey that included large centers in developing and developed countries (Chantada et al. 2008). Therefore, a guideline for eye processing intended to be disseminated in developing countries, and providing consensus definitions for the different degrees of invasion to the ocular coats has been agreed upon and published (see chapter 3).

Table 8.2. International staging schema for patients with retinoblastoma (Chantada et al. 2006a)

Stage 0. Patients treated conservatively

Stage I. Eye enucleated, completely resected histologically

Stage II. Eye enucleated, microscopic residual tumor

Stage III. Regional extension
(a) Overt orbital disease
(b) Preauricular or cervical lymph node extension

Stage IV. Metastatic disease
(a) Hematogenous metastasis (without CNS involvement)
  1. Single lesion
  2. Multiple lesions
(b) CNS extension (with or without any other site of regional or metastatic disease)
  1. Prechiasmatic lesion
  2. CNS mass
  3. Leptomeningeal and CSF disease

Additionally, there is controversy about which patients with high risk pathology risk factors need adjuvant therapy. The treating physician has to decide whether to prescribe adjuvant chemotherapy to all patients with putative risk factors, or to avoid it in controversial cases and aggressively treat those who relapse. In situations where the pathological examination of enucleated eyes is not entirely reliable, the first option is reasonable, whereas in specialized centers, especially those under prospective studies, a more precise identification of patients at risk can be done. The availability of treatment for extraocular relapse with high dose chemotherapy and stem cell rescue needs to be considered in this decision, since patients who relapse with distant metastatic disease can be rescued only by this treatment (Chantada et al. 2004a). On the other hand, adjuvant chemotherapy does not eliminate the possibility of extraocular relapse, and in groups with low relapse rates, its benefit is not proven.

8.2.1 Choroidal Invasion

Choroidal invasion has been determined to be a pathological risk factor for extraocular relapse in many series (Chantada et al. 2004a; Shields et al. 1993; Khelfaoui et al. 1996; Finger et al. 2002). It has been suggested that once the tumor reaches the choroid, it may gain access to the systemic circulation giving rise to hematogenous metastasis. Some studies suggest that choroidal invasion may only be relevant when it is combined with postlaminar optic nerve invasion (Chantada et al. 2004a; Shields et al. 1993). In both retrospective and prospective studies, the relapse rate for patients with isolated choroidal invasion (without postlaminar optic nerve invasion) treated with enucleation alone and no adjuvant therapy has been lower than 5% (Chantada et al. 2004a, b; Schvartzman et al. 1996) and, therefore, the role of chemotherapy in isolated choroidal invasion is controversial.

Most centers discriminate between different degrees of invasion to the choroid (denominated major and minor, full and partial, massive and focal by different groups) and some recommend adjuvant chemotherapy for the cases with more advanced disease. However, comparison among published series has been complicated by the lack of a standardized definition for discriminating between the various degrees of choroidal invasion, and so, the International Retinoblastoma Staging Working Group recently reached a consensus about this issue (Table 8.3). In addition, since only a few sections

Table 8.3. Consensus definition for grading choroidal invasion. International Retinoblastoma Working Group

Massive choroidal invasion: The full thickness of the choroid should be invaded (at least one cell adherent to the sclera) *or* largest dimension greater than 3 mm or tumor noted grossly.

of the enucleated eye are routinely examined, choroidal invasion may be missed. The current treatment protocol from the Children's Oncology Group (COG ARET 0332) prescribes adjuvant chemotherapy with carboplatin, etoposide and vincristine for patients with either isolated massive choroidal invasion or any degree of choroidal invasion in an eye that also has any degree of optic nerve extension (including pre-laminar). Other groups (such as most Latin American centers) do not routinely use adjuvant therapy for isolated choroidal invasion or when it is combined with less than postlaminar optic nerve involvement.

8.2.2 Optic Nerve Invasion

The lamina cribrosa constitutes the anatomical landmark for the limits of the eye. Patients with prelaminar or intralaminar invasion of the optic nerve are not clearly at higher risk for extraocular disease (Chantada et al. 1999a; Shields et al. 1994; Magramm et al. 1989). However, when the tumor extends beyond the lamina cribrosa (microscopically outside the eye), most authors agree that the risk of extraocular relapse increases, even when the resection margin is free of tumor (Magramm et al. 1989). To our knowledge, the largest reported series included 66 patients in New York from 1922 to 1986, and only 42% survived (Magramm et al. 1989). Other smaller series identified postlaminar optic nerve invasion as a risk factor and adjuvant treatment was recommended (Khelfaoui et al. 1996; Shields et al. 1994; Honavar et al. 2002; Stannard et al. 1979).

Recently, there has been considerable debate about whether patients with postlaminar optic nerve invasion need adjuvant therapy to prevent extraocular relapse. Honavar et al found that patients with postlaminar optic nerve invasion who received adjuvant chemotherapy had a better outcome than those who only were observed after enucleation in their retrospective series of 29 patients treated over 25 years (Honavar et al. 2002). Other series failed to show any benefit of chemotherapy to prevent extraocular relapse (Stannard et al. 1979; Uusitalo et al. 2001). The Garrahan group performed a recent analysis of 61 patients with postlaminar optic nerve disease treated on three consecutive treatment protocols and reported a 94%

overall survival rate with tailored therapy (Chantada et al. 2007a). Patients who had postlaminar optic nerve involvement together with full choroidal invasion and/or scleral invasion and those with greater than 1 mm of invasion through the optic nerve or greater than 30% of extension through the optic nerve were at higher risk of relapse and adjuvant chemotherapy was recommended. Better results were found by using a more intensive regimen at higher doses providing a better CNS coverage. Patients without other high risk features (30% of the whole population) were managed without adjuvant therapy. However, it should be stressed that the subgroups were small and the results should be confirmed in a larger cohort, possibly in an international study.

The length of the optic nerve stump and the extent of invasion through the lamina may also be important. A retrospective study reported that patients with an optic nerve stump shorter than 5 mm were at higher risk of relapse, independent of the presence of optic nerve invasion (Rubin et al. 1985). The estimation of this parameter may be misleading since it may vary depending on when it is measured. Abramson et al. (2003a) showed that the optic nerve shrinks up to a 30% of its overall length after fixation, so this parameter should be standardized for adequate analysis. Uusitalo et al. (2001) also prescribed adjuvant chemotherapy for their 7/11 cases with disease extending at least 1 mm beyond the posterior extent to the lamina cribrosa and no further treatment for the remaining four cases with less than that. In that series, no patient had concomitant scleral invasion andn oner elapsed.

8.3 Patients with Microscopic Residual Disease after Enucleation

In most instances, these children present with advanced intraocular disease, often with glaucoma and, on occasions, buphthalmia, but no evidence of overt disease and the treating group recommends enucleation as primary treatment. Pathological examination of the enucleated eye then shows microscopical residual disease, designated as IRSS stage 2 (National registry of retinoblastoma in Japan 1975). This can be manifested in two ways: tumor invasion through the optic nerve extending beyond the resection margin and/or extension through the choroid, across the sclera into the orbit. In both instances, adjuvant treatment is mandatory since the microscopically seeded tumor cells will inevitably lead to disease relapse if not treated. In order to accurately assign a proper stage, a comprehensive pathological examination of the enucleated eye is essential. A short optic nerve stump may result in tumor invasion through the resection margin that could be avoided if a longer stump had been obtained. Consequently, enucleation should be done by an experienced ophthalmologist to obtain a long optic nerve stump (of at least 10 mm), thereby avoiding leaving a tumor residue (Abramson and Ellsworth 1980); however, massive buphthalmia may lead to a difficult procurement of an adequate optic nerve stump. Patients with a short optic nerve stump with tumor beyond the resection margin should be treated in the same way as those with an appropriate stump. The value of a second look operation to access to the remaining optic nerve stump and achieve a deeper resection is not known. The enucleated eye should be examined by an experienced ocular pathologist, and it is essential to obtain a transverse section of the distal end of the optic nerve prior to opening the globe in all patients. The pathologist should also measure the optic nerve length and report if the optic nerve appeared grossly enlarged. Cases where the optic nerve appears massively enlarged and seen at imaging studies done before enucleation are considered IRSS stage 3 and they should usually be treated with neoadjuvant chemotherapy and delayed enucleation (Fig. 8.1) (Chantada et al. 2006a). Microscopic optic nerve invasion usually goes undetected by imaging studies, even when MRI is used (de Graaf et al. 2006). The pathologist should also assess the occurrence of microscopic invasion of the subarachnoid space. This is an uncommon feature of retinoblastoma and these patients should receive the same treatment than those with tumor at the resection margin of the optic nerve. The pathologist should also assess the tumor extension to the sclera. Artifactual scleral invasion may be seen when tumor "floating" cells are seen on the sclera due to inadequate handling of the specimen. Scleral invasion occurs inevitably with concomitant invasion to the full width of the choroid.

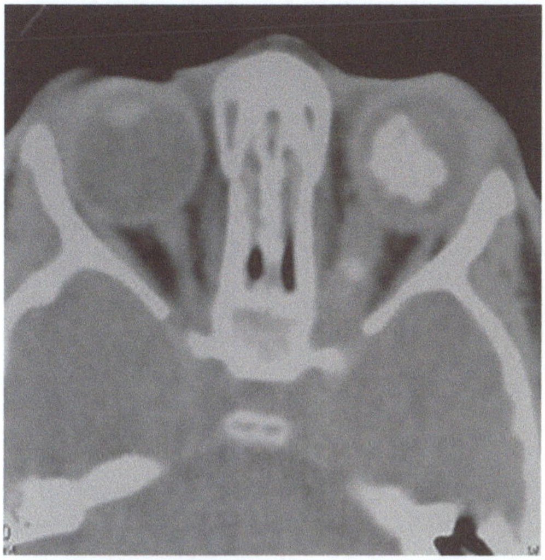

Figure 8.1

Computed tomography scan showing massively enlarged optic nerve in a patient with retinoblastoma

The optimal treatment of patients with a microscopic residual disease is under investigation. It should include multimodal therapy including enucleation, radiotherapy and chemotherapy. However, the best regimen has yet to be determined. Data regarding treatment of patients with tumor invasion to the cut end are very limited and no randomized trial has ever been reported. The traditional approach for the postenucleation treatment of these patients included adjuvant systemic and intrathecal chemotherapy along with radiotherapy (Chantada et al. 2004b; Magramm et al. 1989; Howarth et al. 1980; Zelter et al. 1991; Grabowski and Abramson 1987). The survival rate for these patients ranged from 40% to 70%. Intrathecal chemotherapy usually included methotrexate, cytarabine, and dexamethasone, which may not be active in retinoblastoma and is potentially neurotoxic. Therefore, current regimens omit intrathecal chemotherapy and use more intensive intravenous therapy including agents at higher doses and with better penetration to the CNS, such as carboplatin (Chantada et al. 2004b). Current chemotherapy regimens include moderately intensive systemic chemotherapy including: carboplatin, etoposide, and vincristine, as per the Central America AHOPCA (Asociacion de Hemato-oncologia Pediatrica de Centro America) protocol or more intensive regimens including these drugs (or cisplatin) in combination with cyclophosphamide, and anthracyclines, such as idarubicin or doxorubicin, in the COG, SFCE (French Society of Pediatric Oncology), and Hospital Garrahan studies. There has not been a comparative analysis between the two approaches and both could be considered standard.

Early reports supported the used of prophylactic cranial radiotherapy (Zelter et al. 1988). However, more recent series included orbital radiotherapy (including the chiasm in the radiation field) at a dose of 45 Gy (Schvartzman et al. 1996; Chantada et al. 2004b). However, even though this treatment is less toxic than cranial radiotherapy, severe orbital hypoplasia and endocrinological dysfunction, leading to growth hormone deficiency or hypopituitarism may occur. Therefore, South African investigators developed a localized radiotherapy technique using Iodine seeds with initial encouraging preliminary results (Stannard et al. 2002). Other groups investigated the role of intensive chemotherapy followed by autologous stem cell rescue to avoid radiotherapy in these patients; however, the long term toxicity of this treatment is also substantial (Gallie B, unpublished). The role of orbital radiotherapy has not been prospectively evaluated and only a cooperative multicentric study could provide an answer to that question. Current series report a 70–80% survival in this cohort and leptomeningeal relapse is the most common adverse event, but all reported results include few patients (Chantada et al. 2004b; Antoneli et al. 2003).

8.3.1 Trans-Scleral Invasion

The treatment of patients with microscopic extension through the sclera is even more controversial. To our knowledge, there are no series specifically reporting their outcome and no consensus treatment guidelines are available. The current COG and AHOPCA protocols for these patients give adjuvant chemotherapy with carboplatin, etoposide and vincristine. However, the current protocol at the Hospital Garrahan uses more intensive chemotherapy, since previous results with lower dose regimens were relatively discouraging (Chantada et al. 2004b). The use of orbital radiotherapy is controversial and most current protocols avoid it. According to our preliminary results, most extraocular relapses included the CNS, so they would not likely be avoided if orbital radiotherapy were given. Therefore, the current treatment of patients with microscopical transscleral disease (if the resection margin of the optic nerve is free of tumor) is adjuvant chemotherapy, and the use of orbital radiotherapy is under investigation.

8.3.2 Future Directions

Since up to one third of the patients with microscopic residual disease or high risk features relapse and eventually die, and many of those who survive suffer from cosmetic and functional sequelae, newer treatments should be developed. One approach would be to try to identify them preoperatively to give neoadjuvant chemotherapy in order to downstage the disease, thereby avoiding orbital irradiation (Bellaton et al. 2003). In a series of 184 initially enucleated patients with unilateral retinoblastoma at the Hospital Garrahan, glaucoma and buphthalmia were significantly associated by multivariate analysis with the occurrence of microscopically disseminated disease. Therefore, patients with these features may be considered for preoperative chemotherapy in the context of a controlled study. An adequate standardization of the histopathology features is essential, as described above. The investigation of minimally disseminated disease at diagnosis by PCR techniques could potentially be a way of identifying those cases requiring postoperative treatment (Yamane et al. 1999).

8.4 Orbital and Locoregional Disease

Disease that has massively spread outside the eye into the orbit and is evident by imaging studies is considered to be IRSS stage 3 because of regional dissemination (Chantada et al. 2006a). Dissemination to the preauricular or cervical lymph nodes may be encountered, but the eye lacks lymphatic drainage except for the conjunctiva, so dissemination through this route is seldom seen. Patients with malignant preauricular adenopathy are also categorized as Stage 3 in the IRSS (Fig. 8.2) (Chantada et al. 2006a). Since, occasionally, preauricular lymph node enlargement may be caused by inflammatory phenomena, confirmatory biopsy should be considered in unclear cases.

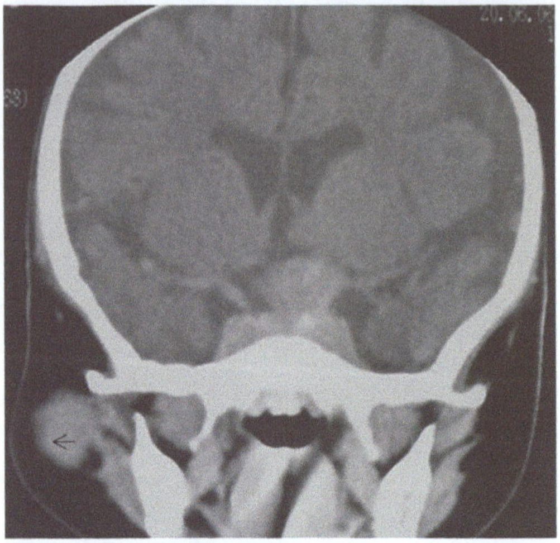

Figure 8.2

Preauricular adenopathy (*arrow*) in a patient with retinoblastoma

Patients who present with overt orbital retinoblastoma should be extensively screened for distant metastasis since 30–40% of them may harbor at least one metastatic site (Chantada et al. 2003). Patients with overt extraocular dissemination are seen more frequently in developing countries, probably because of delayed diagnosis (Antoneli et al. 2003; Chantada et al. 1999b). In series from developed countries, less than 10% of the patients present with extraocular tumor extension. However, in contemporary series from mid-income countries, such as Mexico, Turkey, Argentina, and Brazil, the occurrence of extraocular extension ranged from 10% to 40% (Chantada et al. 2004b; Antoneli et al. 2003; Leal-Leal et al. 2004; Ozkan et al. 2006). In lower income countries, such as Tanzania, survival rates are lower than 30% (Bowman et al. 2006).

A careful extent of disease evaluation is mandatory in cases with overt orbital extension, since the tumor may already have been disseminated to distant sites (Table 8.1), and detecting occult metastatic disease is critical, since IRSS stage 4 patients need to receive more intensive therapy to provide them the best chance of cure. A bone marrow examination (aspiration and biopsy of multiple sites) should be performed, and immunocytology, for example, with the ganglioside GD2, may increase the sensitivity of this examination in this patient cohort (Chantada et al. 2006b). Examination of the CSF by lumbar puncture followed by cell count and microscopical examination of the cytocentrifugate should be done in all patients. Retinoblastoma cells tend to adhere to the glass walls of the tubes used for the CSF collection leading to false negative results (Stannard et al. 1975). Fixing the cells in a 50% alcohol solution, immunophenotyping and a careful microscopical examination of the centrifugate (even when the cell count is 0) may help reducing the false negative rate of this procedure (Stannard et al. 1975). The whole neuraxis should be examined, preferentially with MRI in all patients with tumor extending to the resection margin of the optic nerve to detect occult dissemination. Even though tumor extension through the optic nerve into the CNS, including the chiasm, may be considered as a loco-regional extension, the current IRSS considers any form of CNS invasion to be stage 4b since the prognosis of these patients has been very poor (Chantada et al. 2006a).

Treatment of patients with overt extraocular dissemination should be multidisciplinary, including the pediatric oncologist, ophthalmologist and radiotherapist. In the past, initial orbital exenteration was considered in these patients in order to achieve a complete resection of the tumor. However, nowadays this mutilating surgical procedure is seldom necessary, since retinoblastoma is highly responsive to modern chemotherapy and the tumor usually responds dramatically to chemotherapy, allowing for a more conservative surgical approach. Therefore, the standard therapy for retinoblastoma with overt orbital or regional extension is preoperative chemotherapy followed by resection of any residual orbital mass and adjuvant chemotherapy and radiotherapy (Fig. 8.3). With this approach, 60–85% of patients can be cured (Antoneli et al. 2003; Chantada et al. 2003; Doz et al. 1994). The chemotherapy regimen should include drugs with good CNS penetration like the ones used for treating microscopically disseminated disease. Current protocols usually give two or three cycles preoperatively and 4–6 postoperatively. Local control should then be consolidated with orbital irradiation (40–45 Gy). In many cases, massive necrosis is seen after preoperative chemotherapy and it is not possible to assess the extension to the optic nerve. In these cases, including the chiasm in the radiation field is advisable. When the preauricular and/or cervical lymph nodes are involved, most authors include them in the radiation field, but there is no evidence that this has a prognostic impact, especially in those cases who achieve a complete response to neoadjuvantc hemotherapy.

8.4.1 Orbital Relapse

Orbital relapse may occur after enucleation (Hungerford et al. 1987). This event can be detected at follow up examinations by palpating the orbital socket during routine ophthalmological examinations or by the presence of an overt orbital mass (Fig. 8.4). Orbital relapses should be documented by biopsy, especially in heritable cases where secondary malignancies are possible. Occasionally, an orbital relapse occurs in a patient enucleated after an attempt for ocular preservation (Chantada et al. 2007b). Treatment of these patients depends on the treatment received before this event. As in cases with massive orbital disease detected at diagnosis, a comprehensive extent of disease evaluation is mandatory to rule out distant metastatic disease. When isolated orbital relapse occurs in patients who had been treated only with enucleation, the treatment is the same as that for patients with orbital disease at diagnosis, and the results are comparable (Chantada et al. 2003). When this event occurs in patients with a previous history of chemotherapy, given for chemoreduction or as adjuvant therapy in cases with pathology risk factors, especially in those who had already received orbital radiotherapy, treatment should be individualized using previously unused

a

b

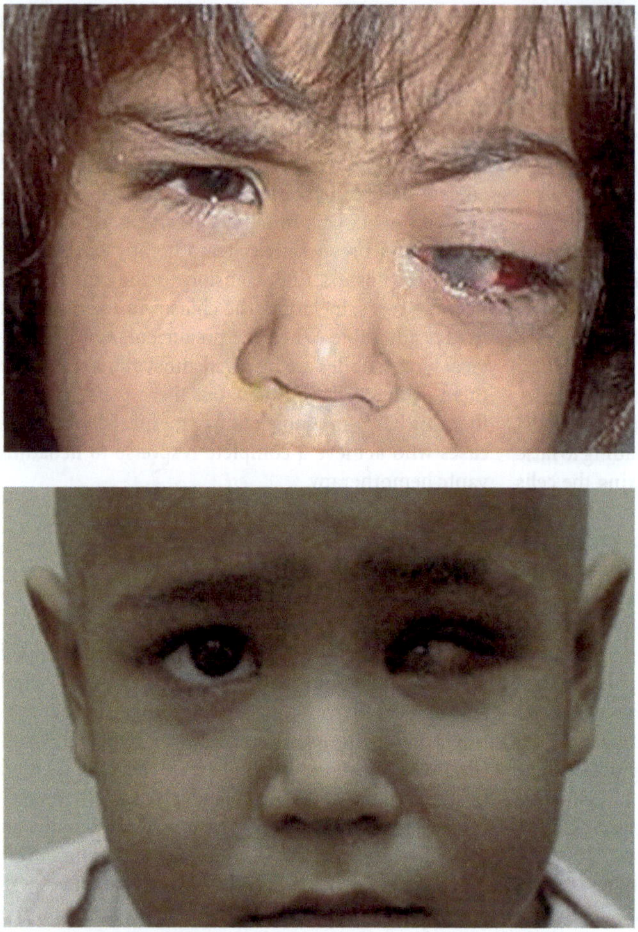

Figure 8.3

Shrinkage of orbital disease in a patient with overt orbital retinoblastoma at diagnosis and after two cycles of chemotherapy, including carboplatin, etoposide, cyclophosphamide, idarubicin and vincristine

agents. Some of these patients can be salvaged with current treatments (Chantada et al. 2007b). Consolidation with high dose chemotherapy with autologous stem cell rescue may be indicated in patients with chemosensitive disease and a history of previous orbital radiotherapy (Chantada et al. 2007b).

8.4.2 Special Situations

In very uncommon situations, orbital retinoblastoma can develop after an invasive surgical procedure involving, for example, vitrectomy or vitreous puncture, or any other intraocular surgery (Shields et al. 2000).

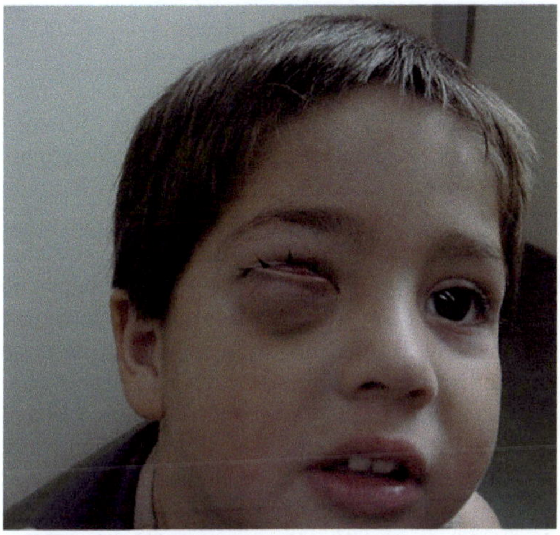

Figure 8.4

Orbital relapse in a patient enucleated for unilateral retinoblastoma. The family detected the orbital mass because the prosthesis was not fitting well

Most these cases have been reported where the surgeon was not aware of the presence of retinoblastoma. All children with unsuspected retinoblastoma who undergo intraocular surgery should be treated with adjuvant chemotherapy and radiotherapy to attempt to prevent an orbital relapse.

8.5 Metastatic Disease

8.5.1 Stage 4a: Metastatic Disease Without CNS Involvement

The IRSS designates patients with distant metastatic disease, but without CNS involvement to be stage 4a. These patients have had a poor prognosis when treated with conventional therapy, but may be cured when therapy is intensified to include high-dose chemotherapy with autologous stem cell rescue (ASCR).

A number of older publications described the results of treatment with conventional dose chemotherapy (usually vincristine, doxorubicin, cyclophosphamide, cisplatin, and etoposide) and radiation therapy. Despite occasional reports of long-term event-free survival (Abramson and Andracchi 1997), the bulk of the evidence suggested that the prognosis remained grim with such an approach (Abramson 2005). More recent publications using aggressive conventional chemotherapy confirmed the dismal prognosis. Argentine investigators noted that all 26 patients with distant metastases died (The Committee for the National Registry of Retinoblastoma 1992), and Brazilian investigators noted that only 1 of 14 patients (7%) with distant metastases survived (Abramson et al. 2003b).

Case reports had suggested that the use of high-dose chemotherapy with ASCR might be beneficial for patients with metastatic retinoblastoma (Abramson et al. 2003b; Abiose 1979), and subsequently, Institute Curie investigators reported the results of 25 patients with high-risk retinoblastoma treated with high-dose carboplatin, etoposide, and cyclophosphamide, followed by ASCR (Abramson 2005). Five of eight patients with metastases not involving the CNS were event-free survivors 11–70 months after high-dose chemotherapy. Three had central nervous system relapses and died of disease 10–20 months after high-dose chemotherapy. Three other patients had disease that progressed during induction with conventional induction chemotherapy and never received high-dose chemotherapy. In total, then, 5 of 11 patients (45%) with metastatic disease, not initially involving the central nervous system, were event-free survivors.

Memorial Sloan-Kettering Cancer Center investigators initially reported the results of 4 patients with stage 4a disease treated with intensive chemotherapy and high-dose chemotherapy with ASCR, and subsequently reported an expanded series in abstract form (Leal-Leal et al. 2006; Gunduz et al. 2006). All had bone marrow and/or bone metastases, and some also had liver and orbit disease. Induction chemotherapy consisted of vincristine, a platinum agent, cyclophosphamide, and etoposide (+/− doxorubicin), and the high-dose regimen was carboplatin and thiotepa-based. Seven of 10 patients were event-free survivors at a median of 84 months (Abiose 1979). Two relapsed in the CNS at 7 and 10 months after the diagnosis of metastatic disease (prior to high-dose chemotherapy).

These two failures were associated with treatment delays due to fungal infection ($n=1$) and insurance denial ($n=1$), and the patients later died of progressive tumor. One patient relapsed in the CNS 16 months after the diagnosis of metastatic disease and later died of progressive tumor. The remaining 7 patients were failure-free and alive at 16–130 months after the diagnosis of metastatic disease.

Other groups have also published small series and the overall results appear promising. German investigators treated 5 patients, 3 of whom had stage 4a disease, with a regimen very similar to that used in New York (Abramson et al. 2004). None of those 3 patients received radiation therapy and they were event-free survivors at 24, 69, and 124 months from diagnosis of metastatic disease. St. Jude investigators reported 4 patients treated with intensive therapy, including high-dose chemotherapy with stem cell rescue, but their regimens (carboplatin-etoposide, busulfan-cyclophosphamide-melphalan, cyclophosphamide-etoposide, cyclophosphamide-topotecan) did not include thiotepa (Rodriguez-Galindo et al. 2004). Radiation therapy was used for bone metastases. Two of the 4 patients were long-term survivors. CHLA investigators included 2 patients with stage 4a disease in their report (The Committee for the National Registry of Retinoblastoma 1992). One patient with orbit, bone and bone marrow disease received high-dose cyclophosphamide, thiotepa, and etoposide, with stem cell rescue, but died of disease at 10 months. Another patient had an isolated bone metastasis and received high-dose carboplatin, etoposide, and melphalan, with stem cell rescue, but died at 23 months due to a secondary Ewing sarcoma. Most recently, a Japanese report included 3 patients with stage 4a disease treated with intensive therapy, including high-dose melphalan-based chemotherapy with ASCR (Abramson et al. 2004). One of the 3 patients received radiation therapy. All 3 patients were event-free survivors at 38, 107, and 113 months.

The overall experiences suggest that addition of high-dose chemotherapy with ASCR is associated with improved survival for patients with stage 4a retinoblastoma. The inclusion of thiotepa in the regimen may be associated with a lower risk of CNS recurrence (the most likely site of failure) due to the excellent CNS penetration of that agent.

8.5.2 Stage 4b: Distant Metastatic Disease with CNS Involvement

The results of treatment of these patients with conventional therapy are very poor, and affected patients seldom survive (Schvartzman et al. 1996; Chantada et al. 2004b; Ozkan et al. 2006; Leal-Leal et al. 2006; Gunduz et al. 2006). Only limited data are available regarding the prognosis of patients with metastatic retinoblastoma involving the central nervous system disease (IRSS stage 4b) treated with high-dose chemotherapy and ASCR. The French Society of Paediatric Oncology (SFOP) experience included 4 stage 4b patients who received high-dose carboplatin, etoposide and cyclophosphamide with stem cell rescue. Three died of CNS disease, and one was free of disease at 63 months (Abramson 2005). The CHLA report included 4 patients with stage 4b disease, none of whom survived (The Committee for the National Registry of Retinoblastoma 1992). None received high-dose chemotherapy, but is unclear whether any had been treated with the intention to include high-dose chemotherapy in the regimen, even though none ultimately received such therapy. The Japanese report included 2 patients with stage 4b disease and both died of disease (Abramson et al. 2004).

8.5.3 Future Research

The Children's Oncology Group has proposed a study of multimodality therapy for extraocular retinoblastoma (COG ARET 0321) and hopes that other cooperative groups or major centers around the world will participate. In this study, patients with stage 2 & 3 extraocular retinoblastoma (orbital disease, regional nodal disease, and/or optic nerve margin positivity) will receive aggressive conventional chemotherapy and involved-field external beam radiation therapy. Those with stage 4a and 4b metastatic disease (as well as those with trilateral retinoblastoma) will receive aggressive conventional induction chemotherapy, have autologous stem cells harvested, receive high-dose carboplatin, thiotepa and etoposide with ASCR, and then (depending on response) will be considered for external beam radiation therapy.

References

Abiose A (1979) Pattern of retinal diseases in Lagos. Ann Ophthalmol1 1(7):1067–1072

Abramson DH (2005) Retinoblastoma in the 20th century: past success and future challenges the Weisenfeld lecture. Invest Ophthalmol Vis Sci 46(8):2683–2691

Abramson DH, Andracchi S (1997) Orbital avitene granuloma formation after enucleation for intraocular retinoblastoma. Am J Ophthalmol 123(4):567–569

Abramson DH, Ellsworth RM (1980) The surgical management of retinoblastoma. Ophthalmic Surg 11(9):596–598

Abramson DH, Schefler AC, Almeida D et al (2003a) Optic nerve tissue shrinkage during pathologic processing after enucleation for retinoblastoma. Arch Ophthalmol 121(1):73–75

Abramson DH, Beaverson K, Sangani P et al (2003b) Screening for retinoblastoma: presenting signs as prognosticators of patient and ocular survival. Pediatrics 112(6 Pt 1): 1248–1255

Abramson DH, Beaverson KL, Chang ST et al (2004) Outcome following initial external beam radiotherapy in patients with Reese-Ellsworth group Vb retinoblastoma. Arch Ophthalmol 122(9):1316–1323

Antoneli CB, Steinhorst F, de Cassia Braga Ribeiro K et al (2003) Extraocular retinoblastoma: a 13-year experience. Cancer 98(6):1292–1298

Bellaton E, Bertozzi AI, Behar C et al (2003) Neoadjuvant chemotherapy for extensive unilateral retinoblastoma. Br J Ophthalmol 87(3):327–329

Bowman RJ, Mafwiri M, Luthert P et al (2006) Outcome of retinoblastoma in east Africa. Pediatr Blood Cancer 50(1):160–162

Chantada GL, de Davila MT, Fandino A et al (1999a) Retinoblastoma with low risk for extraocular relapse. Ophthalmic Genet 20(3):133–140

Chantada G, Fandino A, Manzitti J et al (1999b) Late diagnosis of retinoblastoma in a developing country. Arch Dis Child 80(2):171–174

Chantada G, Fandino A, Casak S et al (2003) Treatment of overt extraocular retinoblastoma. Med Pediatr Oncol 40(3):158–161

Chantada GL, Dunkel IJ, de Davila MT et al (2004a) Retinoblastoma patients with high risk ocular pathological features: who needs adjuvant therapy? Br J Ophthalmol 88(8):1069–1073

Chantada G, Fandino A, Davila MT et al (2004b) Results of a prospective study for the treatment of retinoblastoma. Cancer1 00(4):834–842

Chantada G, Doz F, Antoneli CB et al (2006a) A proposal for an international retinoblastoma staging system. Pediatr Blood Cancer 47(6):801–805

Chantada GL, Rossi J, Casco F et al (2006b) An aggressive bone marrow evaluation including immunocytology with GD2 for advanced retinoblastoma. J Pediatr Hematol Oncol 28(6):369–373

Chantada GL, Casco F, Fandino AC et al (2007a) Outcome of patients with retinoblastoma and postlaminar optic nerve invasion. Ophthalmology 114(11):2083–2089

Chantada GL, Dunkel IJ, Antoneli CB et al (2007b) Risk factors for extraocular relapse following enucleation after failure of chemoreduction in retinoblastoma. Pediatr Blood Cancer 49(3):256–260

Chantada GL, Doz F, Orjuela M, Qaddoumi I, Sitorus R, Kepak T, Furmanchuk A, Castellanos M, Sharma T, Chevez-Barrios P, Rodriguez-Galindo C, on behalf of the International Retinoblastoma Staging Working Group (2008) World disparities in risk definition and management of retinoblastoma. A report from the International Retinoblastoma Staging Working Group. Pediatr Blood Cancer 50(3):692–694

de Graaf P, Moll AC, Imhof SM et al (2006) Retinoblastoma and optic nerve enhancement on MRI: not always extraocular tumour extension. Br J Ophthalmol 90(6):800–801

Doz F, Khelfaoui F, Mosseri V et al (1994) The role of chemotherapy in orbital involvement of retinoblastoma. The experience of a single institution with 33 patients. Cancer 74(2):722–732

Finger PT, Harbour JW, Karcioglu ZA (2002) Risk factors for metastasis in retinoblastoma. Surv Ophthalmol 47(1):1–16

Grabowski EF, Abramson DH (1987) Intraocular and extraocular retinoblastoma. Hematol Oncol Clin North Am 1(4):721–735

Gunduz K, Muftuoglu O, Gunalp I et al (2006) Metastatic retinoblastoma clinical features, treatment, and prognosis. Ophthalmology 113(9):1558–1566

Honavar SG, Singh AD, Shields CL et al (2002) Postenucleation adjuvant therapy in high-risk retinoblastoma. Arch Ophthalmol 120(7):923–931

Howarth C, Meyer D, Hustu HO et al (1980) Stage-related combined modality treatment of retinoblastoma. Results of a prospective study. Cancer 45(5):851–858

Hungerford J, Kingston J, Plowman N (1987) Orbital recurrence of retinoblastoma. Ophthalmic Paediatr Genet 8(1):63–68

Khelfaoui F, Validire P, Auperin A et al (1996) Histopathologic risk factors in retinoblastoma: a retrospective study of 172 patients treated in a single institution. Cancer 77(6):1206–1213

Leal-Leal C, Flores-Rojo M, Medina-Sanson A et al (2004) A multicentre report from the Mexican Retinoblastoma Group. Br J Ophthalmol 88(8):1074–1077

Leal-Leal CA, Rivera-Luna R, Flores-Rojo M et al (2006) Survival in extra-orbital metastatic retinoblastoma: treatment results. Clin Transl Oncol 8(1):39–44

MacKay CJ, Abramson DH, Ellsworth RM (1984) Metastatic patterns of retinoblastoma. Arch Ophthalmol 102(3):391–396

Magramm I, Abramson DH, Ellsworth RM (1989) Optic nerve involvement in retinoblastoma. Ophthalmology 96(2):217–222
(1992) National registry of retinoblastoma in Japan (1975–1982). The Committee for the National Registry of Retinoblastoma. Nippon Ganka Gakkai Zasshi 96(11):1433–1442
Ozkan A, Pazarli H, Celkan T et al (2006) Retinoblastoma in Turkey: survival and clinical characteristics 1981–2004. Pediatr Int 48(4):369–373
Rodriguez-Galindo C, Wilson MW, Haik BG et al (2003) Treatment of metastatic retinoblastoma. Ophthalmology1 10:1237–1240
Rubin CM, Robison LL, Cameron JD et al (1985) Intraocular retinoblastoma group V: an analysis of prognostic factors. J Clin Oncol 3(5):680–685
Schvartzman E, Chantada G, Fandino A et al (1996) Results of a stage-based protocol for the treatment of retinoblastoma. J Clin Oncol 14(5):1532–1536
Shields CL, Shields JA, Baez KA et al (1993) Choroidal invasion of retinoblastoma: metastatic potential and clinical risk factors. Br J Ophthalmol 77(9):544–548
Shields CL, Shields JA, Baez K et al (1994) Optic nerve invasion of retinoblastoma. Metastatic potential and clinical risk factors. Cancer 73(3):692–698
Shields CL, Honavar S, Shields JA et al (2000) Vitrectomy in eyes with unsuspected retinoblastoma. Ophthalmology 107(12):2250–2255
Stannard CE, Sealy R, Sevel D et al (1975) Treatment of malignant meningitis in retinoblastoma. Br J Ophthalmol 59(7):362–365
Stannard C, Lipper S, Sealy R et al (1979) Retinoblastoma: correlation of invasion of the optic nerve and choroid with prognosis and metastases. Br J Ophthalmol 63(8):560–570
Stannard C, Sealy R, Hering E et al (2002) Postenucleation orbits in retinoblastoma: treatment with 125I brachytherapy. Int J Radiat Oncol Biol Phys 54(5):1446–1454
(1992) Survival rate and risk factors for patients with retinoblastoma in Japan. The Committee for the National Registry of Retinoblastoma. Jpn J Ophthalmol 36(2):121–131
Uusitalo MS, Van Quill KR, Scott IU et al (2001) Evaluation of chemoprophylaxis in patients with unilateral retinoblastoma with high-risk features on histopathologic examination. Arch Ophthalmol 119(1):41–48
Yamane S, Shirai C, Arimoto A et al (1999) Disseminated retinoblastoma successfully treated with myeloablative chemotherapy – implication for molecular detection of minimal residual disease. Bone Marrow Transplant 23(9):971–974
Zelter M, Gonzalez G, Schwartz L et al (1988) Treatment of retinoblastoma. Results obtained from a prospective study of 51 patients. Cancer 61(1):153–160
Zelter M, Damel A, Gonzalez G et al (1991) A prospective study on the treatment of retinoblastoma in 72 patients. Cancer 68(8):1685–1690

Second Malignancies and Other Long Term Effects in Retinoblastoma Survivors

C. Rodriguez-Galindo

Contents

9.1 Introduction 115
9.2 Second Malignancies. 115
9.2.1 Osteosarcoma 117
9.2.2 Soft Tissue Sarcomas 119
9.2.3 Skin Cancers 120
9.2.4 Lung Cancer and Other Common Cancers of Adulthood 120
9.2.5 Hematologic Malignancies 121
9.2.6 Trilateral Retinoblastoma 121
9.3 Other Long Term effects. 123
9.3.1 Orbital Growth and Facial Asymmetry 123
9.3.2 Visual Outcome 123
9.3.3 Cognitive and Functional Development of Patients with Retinoblastoma 123
9.3.4 Other Late Effects 124
References. 124

9.1 Introduction

Retinoblastoma is a cancer in the very young, and patients are very susceptible to the long term effects that the disease and the treatments administered may have in organ development and function. More importantly, patients with bilateral retinoblastoma are born with a germ-line mutation of the *RB1* gene, probably the most potent tumor suppressor gene, and are at risk of developing cancers throughout their lives; in this regard, retinoblastoma may be *just the beginning*.

9.2 Second Malignancies

The cumulative incidence of second cancers in patients with germ-line mutations of the *RB1* gene increases steadily with age, up to 30–60% at 40–50 years of age, although a more recent study estimates a considerably lower risk (Mohney et al. 1998; Kleinerman et al. 2005; Wong et al. 1997; Eng et al. 1993). Patients with nonhereditary retinoblastoma are not at an increased risk (Kleinerman et al. 2005; Wong et al. 1997; Eng et al. 1993). Most information on second malignancies in retinoblastoma survivors has derived from the prospective follow-up of a cohort of 1,601 survivors of retinoblastoma who were diagnosed between 1914 and 1984 at institutions in Boston and New York. The sequential updated analyses of this cohort have provided (and continue to provide) the most reliable description of cancer risk in this population (Kleinerman et al. 2005, 2000, 2007; Wong et al. 1997; Eng et al. 1993; Yu et al. 2009).

C. Rodriguez-Galindo and M.W. Wilson (eds.), *Retinoblastoma*, Pediatric Oncology,
DOI 10.1007/978-0-387-89072-2_9, © Springer Science+Business Media, LLC 2010

In the most recent analysis, the median follow-up for patients with hereditary and non-hereditary retinoblastoma was 25.2 years and 29.5 years, respectively (Kleinerman et al. 2005). The standardized incidence ratio (SIR) in these studies was calculated as the ratio of the observed number of cancers to the expected number from the Connecticut Tumor Registry. The incidence of second cancers was significantly elevated in survivors of hereditary retinoblastoma (SIR 19 vs. 1.2 in nonhereditary retinoblastoma patients), and almost any neoplasm has been described in this population (Wong et al. 1997) (Kleinerman et al. 2005). For hereditary retinoblastoma, the greatest risk (SIR > 100) was for neoplasms of bone, connective and soft tissue, eye and orbit, and nasal cavities. An increased risk (SIR > 10) was also noted for pineoblastoma, melanoma, CNS malignancies, and neoplasms of the buccal cavity and corpus utery. The lowest risk (SIR < 10) was seen for neoplasms of the lung, breast, and colon (Kleinerman et al. 2005) (Table 9.1).

The cumulative incidence of a second neoplasm after 30 years from diagnosis of retinoblastoma is greater than 30% (Mohney et al. 1998; Kleinerman et al. 2005; Wong et al. 1997; Fletcher et al. 2004). Reports differ on the risk, and cumulative incidences in excess of 50% have been reported (Wong et al. 1997; Fletcher et al. 2004). The more accurate data probably derives from the Boston-New York cohort, which illustrates the changes in cancer risk estimates with longer follow-up. The cumulative incidence of second cancers at 50 years in survivors of hereditary retinoblastoma was estimated to be 51% in the analysis reported by Wong et al. in 1997 (Wong et al. 1997). This figure decreased to 36% in the analysis of the same cohort reported by Kleinerman et al. in 2005, (Kleinerman et al. 2005) probably reflecting the lower doses of scatter radiation received by patients treated in the more recent eras. Although patients have a lifetime risk of developing additional malignancies, the second malignancy usually occurs in the first decade after the diagnosis of retinoblastoma. Median age at diagnosis of a second neoplasm is 15–17 years (Wong et al. 1997; Abramson and Frank 1998). However, there continues to be an increased risk of developing second malignancy-associated death throughout the retinoblastoma survivor's life (Yu et al. 2009).

Table 9.1. Risk and type of new cancers in 963 survivors of hereditary retinoblastoma (adapted from Kleinerman et al. 2005)

Cancer site	Observed	SIR (95% CI)
All sites	260 (100%)	19 (16–21)
Bone	75 (28.8%)	360 (283–451)
Soft tissue	34 (13%)	122 (84–170)
Nasal cavities	32 (12.3%)	1,111 (760–1,569)
Melanoma	29 (11.1%	28 (18–40)
Eye and orbit	17 (6.5%)	266 (155–426)
Brain	10 (3.8%)	13.6 (6.5–25)
Breast	10 (3.8%)	3.96 (1.9–7.3)
Corpus uteri	7 (2.7%)	20 (8.0–41)
Buccal cavity	7 (2.7%)	20 (8.2–42)
Lung	5 (1.9%)	5.94 (1.9–14)
Pineoblastoma	5 (1.9%)	90.8 (29–212)
Colon	3 (1.1%)	6.28 (1.3–18)
Hodgkin lymphoma	3 (1.1%)	3.4 (0.7–10)
Bladder	2 (0.7%)	6.15 (0.7–22)
Thyroid	2 (0.7%)	3.34 (0.4–12)
Leukemia	2 (0.7%)	2.25 (0.3–8.1)

SIR Standardized incidence ratio

Furthermore, survivors of a second neoplasm appear to have an increased risk of developing a third and a fourth malignancy, which occur at shorter intervals. The cumulative incidence of a third neoplasm is 22% at 10 years from the second cancer, and it occurs at a median of 5.8 years (Abramson et al. 2001).

Radiation therapy plays a major role in the risk of second neoplasms in patients with hereditary retinoblastoma. The second tumorigenic event (*second hit*) is usually chromosomal in nature, often as a result of mitotic recombination errors (Zhu et al. 1992; Harbour 2001). This second hit is very sensitive to environmental factors, such as ionizing radiation, thus explaining the increased risk of radiation-induced malignancies in survivors of retinoblastoma (Weinberg 1991). Radiation results in a significant increase in the incidence of second cancers in patients with hereditary disease; the cumulative probability of developing a second malignancy is 38% in irradiated vs. 21% in non-irradiated patients (Kleinerman et al. 2005). The greatest risk (SIR > 100) is for neoplasms of bone, soft tissues, nasal cavities and orbits, and for pineoblastoma. The risk of developing a second cancer appears to correlate with the timing of radiation as well ; children receiving radiation therapy during their first year may have a higher risk of developing a second cancer (Yu et al. 2009; Abramson and Frank 1998). However, the need for earlier radiation may also be an indication of a biologically and clinically more aggressive disease. Changes in radiation techniques over the years are having an impact on cancer risk. As shown in the cohort reported by Kleinerman et al., the use of orthovoltage prior to 1960 was associated with a higher risk of second malignancies than radiation techniques used in subsequent decades; the cumulative incidence of second cancers at 40 years was 32.9% and 26.3%, respectively (Kleinerman et al. 2005). With the evolving treatment approaches for intraocular retinoblastoma, which may decrease the overall need for external beam radiation, and the development of newer radiation techniques, such as conformal, intensity-modulated and proton-beam radiation, it is likely that further decrease in cancer risk will be observed. In a cohort of British retinoblastoma survivors born before 1950, prior to the routine use of radiation therapy, less than 15% of second tumors were sarcomas, highlighting the important role of radiation therapy in the development of those malignancies (Fletcher et al. 2004).

Traditionally, an excess risk has been attributed solely to the use of radiation therapy. In survivors of childhood cancer, there is a documented increased risk of developing second malignancies, particularly osteosarcoma, associated with the combined use of chemotherapy and radiation therapy (Tucker et al. 1987). A similar phenomenon may occur in retinoblastoma survivors, and the most recent analyses suggest a synergistic effect in carcinogenic risk with the use of chemotherapy. The overall risk of developing cancer in hereditary retinoblastoma patients who received radiation and chemotherapy was 25, compared with 19 for those who received only radiation. Most of this difference was accounted for by the higher risk noted for osteosarcomas; the SIR was 539 for combined treatment and 302 for radiation only (Kleinerman et al. 2005).

Sarcomas of bone and soft tissues account for more than 40% of all second neoplasms, followed by neoplasms of the nasal cavities and melanoma (Kleinerman et al. 2005; Wong et al. 1997) (Table 9.1). Sarcomas in general and osteosarcoma in particular, are cancers of the young retinoblastoma survivor; 76% of all cancers in the irradiated patients occurring <25 years are sarcomas vs. 33% in non-irradiated patients. Conversely, 76% of cancers diagnosed at <25 years of age are sarcomas, whereas sarcomas represent less than 50% of cancers in older patients; in non-irradiated patients, the proportion was 33% in <25 years and 8% in >25 years (Kleinerman et al. 2005;Fl etcher et al. 2004).

9.2.1 Osteosarcoma

Osteosarcoma, as a second malignancy, is often associated with retinoblastoma (Fig. 9.1). In the general population, only 7% of osteosarcomas follow other malignancies, and almost half of these cases occur in retinoblastoma survivors (Hauben et al. 2003). Likewise, although multifocal OS accounts for only 4% of all osteosarcomas, 25% of those occur in retinoblastoma survivors (Jaffe et al. 2003). Osteosarcoma is the most common malignancy in survivors of retinoblastoma, both in the irradiated and the non-irradiated areas, and account for 25–40% of all second malignancies (Kleinerman et al. 2005; Yu et al. 2009; Abramson and Frank 1998; Aerts et al. 2004; Acquaviva et al. 2006; Moll et al. 2001). Half to two-thirds of osteosarcomas occur in the irradiated fields of the skull and face (Kleinerman et al. 2005; Abramson and Frank 1998; Aerts et al. 2004; Acquaviva et al. 2006; Moll et al. 2001); one-third of tumors develop in the extremities, and less than 10% in the trunk (Kleinerman et al. 2005). The SIR is 360; it is higher in irradiated fields (SIR 406), but it is still significantly increased in non-irradiated fields (SIR 69). Osteosarcoma occurring in the irradiated retinoblastoma patient accounts for 30% of all osteosarcomas of the head and neck (Daw et al. 2000).

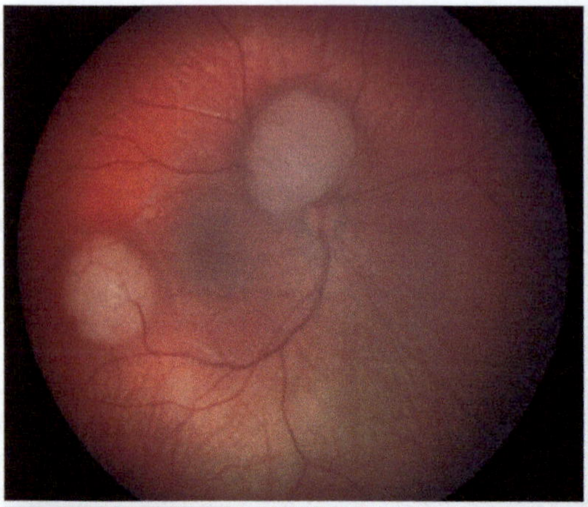

a

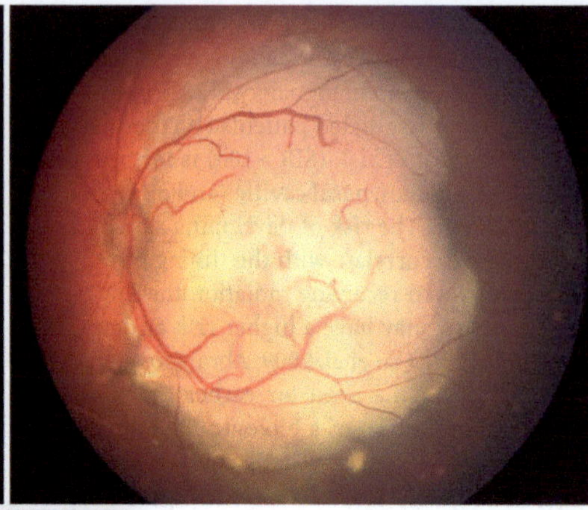

b

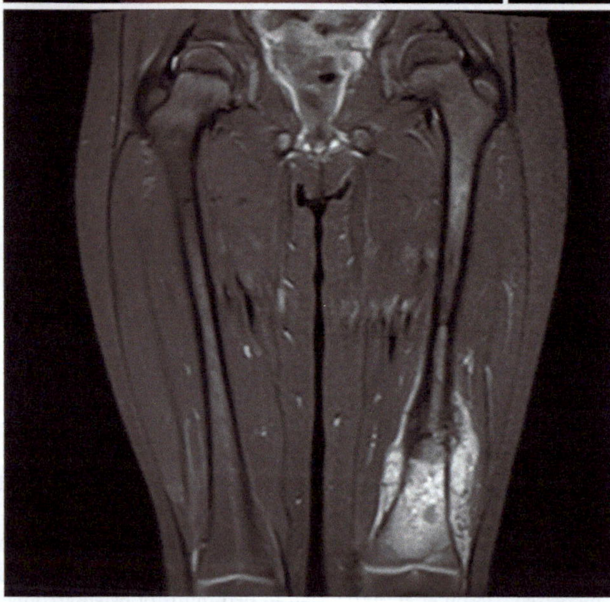

c

Figure 9.1 a c

Funduscopic images of the right a and left b eyes of a 2 month-old infant with bilateral retinoblastoma, successfully treated with chemoreduction and focal treatments, without external beam radiation therapy. At 6 years of age, the patient presented with left leg pain, and MRI showed a destructive lesion in the L distal femur c pathology showed osteosarcoma

Clinical presentation is similar to conventional osteosarcoma, and clinical behavior does not seem to be different; less than 20% of the cases are metastatic (Abramson et al. 2005). Osteosarcomas occur in the young ages, both in irradiated and non-irradiated fields, usually peaking during the adolescent years (Abramson and Frank 1998; Aerts et al. 2004; Chauveinc et al. 2001). However, osteosarcomas occurring during the first decade of life are usually in the irradiated fields (Chauveinc et al. 2001). With appropriate multidisciplinary treatment, secondary osteosarcoma occurring in retinoblastoma survivors is curable (Stine et al. 2003; Dunkel et al. 1998); however, a major limitation is the common occurrence in the head and neck, sites where local control is challenging (Acquaviva et al. 2006; Moll et al. 2001; Daw et al. 2000).

Ewing sarcoma, although rare, has also been described in retinoblastoma survivors. It accounts for 15–25% of all bone tumors, almost always occurring outside the radiation field (Mohney et al. 1998; Moll et al. 2001). Ewing sarcoma in retinoblastoma survivors accounts for approximately 16% of cases of Ewing sarcoma occurring as a second malignancy (Spunt et al. 2006).

9.2.2 Soft Tissue Sarcomas

Soft tissue sarcomas are the second most common malignancy in retinoblastoma survivors, with a SIR of 122, and account for approximately 10–15% of all second malignancies (Kleinerman et al. 2005; Yu et al. 2009; Bisogno et al. 2004). Soft tissue sarcomas are closely associated with the use of radiation; SIR is much higher in irradiated fields (140) than in non-irradiated fields (23). In the Boston–New York cohort, the cumulative risk for soft tissue sarcomas at 50 years after radiation therapy was 13.1% (Kleinerman et al. 2005, 2007). Approximately, 10% of all secondary sarcomas in children surviving cancer occur in retinoblastoma survivors (Bisogno et al. 2004).

As it occurs for osteosarcoma, most soft tissue sarcomas occur in the irradiated fields; sarcomas of the head and face account for 70% of the cases, with the remaining being in the trunk (20%) and limbs (<5%) (Kleinerman et al. 2005, 2007; Abramson and Frank 1998; Aerts et al. 2004; Acquaviva et al. 2006; Moll et al. 2001). A very characteristic spectrum of histologies has been described (Table 9.2). Leiomyosarcoma is the most common subtype, accounting for approximately one-third of the cases, followed by fibrosarcoma, malignant fibrous histiocytoma, rhabdomyosarcoma, non-specified sarcomas, and liposarcoma. When compared with the normal population, SIR is significantly elevated for leiomyosarcoma (390), fibrosarcoma (398), and rhabdomyosarcoma (279), but also higher for malignant fibrous histiocytoma (100) and liposarcoma (99) (Kleinerman et al. 2007). There is a correlation between radiation

Table 9.2. Risk and type of soft tissue sarcomas in 963 survivors of hereditary retinoblastoma (adapted from Kleinerman et al. 2007)

	Treatment					
	All treatments		Radiation		No radiation	
Histology	Observed	SIR (95% CI)	Observed	SIR	Observed	SIR
Total	69 (100%)	184 (143–233)	66	212 (164–270)	3	47 (9.4–137)
Soft tissue sarcoma NOS	10 (14.5%)	96 (46–177)	10	115 (55–211)	0	0.0 (0.0–218)
Fibrosarcoma	13 (18.8%)	398 (211–681)	13	475 (253–813)	0	0.0 (0.0–691)
Malignant fibrous histiocytoma	12 (17.4%)	100 (52–175)	11	110 (55–197)	1	51 (0.66–284)
Liposarcoma	3 (4.3%)	99 (20–286)	3	120 (24–351)	0	0.0 (0.0–329)
Leiomyosarcoma	23 (33.3%)	390 (247–585)	22	476 (298–720)	1	78 (1.0–436)
Rhabdomyosarcoma	8 (11.6%)	279 (120–551)	7	281 (112–578)	1	271 (3.5–1,510)

SIR standard incidence ratio, *NOS* no otherwise specified

exposure and histologic subtype; fibrosarcoma, rhabdomyosarcoma, malignant fibrous histiocytoma, and non-specified subtypes almost always occur in the irradiated fields. Conversely, leiomyosarcoma and liposarcoma commonly arise in the non-irradiated fields (Kleinerman et al. 2007). Although secondary sarcomas in childhood cancer survivors are associated with increasing doses of anthracyclines or alkylators, (Henderson et al. 2007) the use of chemotherapy does not appear to increase the risk of developing soft tissue sarcomas in retinoblastoma survivors; however, the combined use of radiation and chemotherapy appears to increase the risk of developing leiomyosarcoma when compared with radiation alone (Kleinerman et al. 2007).

Soft tissue sarcomas are malignancies of the young survivor, and more than half the tumors are diagnosed in the first 30 years from retinoblastoma (Kleinerman et al. 2007; Abramson and Frank 1998; Aerts et al. 2004). Fibrosarcoma, rhabdomyosarcoma, and malignant fibrous histiocytoma predominantly occur 10–20 years from retinoblastoma diagnosis, whereas non-specified sarcomas occur across all time intervals. An exception to the rule is leiomyosarcoma, which more commonly (78%) occurs after 30 years from retinoblastoma diagnosis, and typically outside the irradiated fields; SIR for this subtype after 30 years is 435 (Kleinerman et al. 2007). Very common locations for leiomyosarcoma are the uterus and bladder (Mohney et al. 1998; Kleinerman et al. 2005; Kleinerman et al. 2007; Yu et al. 2009; Venkatraman et al. 2003), and may also occur as a radiation induced malignancy in the paranasal sinuses (Dunkel eta l. 1998).

The liposarcoma risk also increases with increasing age (Kleinerman et al. 2007). Alteration of *RB1* gene has been demonstrated in both lipomas and liposarcomas. An interesting observation is the increased incidence of lipomas in survivors of hereditary retinoblastoma. Lipomas were present in 3.6% of patients with hereditary retinoblastoma, compared with only 0.6% in patients with sporadic disease (Li et al. 1997). The incidence of a second neoplasm appears to be higher in those patients with lipomas; 30% of patients with lipoma developed a second malignant neoplasm, compared with 12% of patients without lipoma. These data suggest that the presence of lipomas could be a clinical marker of susceptibility to second neoplasms (Li et al. 1997).

Sarcoma risk and location do not seem to differ by sex, except for leiomyosarcomas. In males, 64% of primaries were in the face, whereas for females, 58% of tumors were in the pelvic area, highlighting the relevance of uterine primaries (Kleinerman et al. 2007).

9.2.3 Skin Cancers

Skin cancers account for 16–19% of all second cancers in survivors of hereditary retinoblastoma, and occur both inside and outside the irradiated fields, usually within the first three decades of life (Mohney et al. 1998; Kleinerman et al. 2005; Yu et al. 2009; Abramson and Frank 1998). The highest risk is for melanoma, but basal cell and squamous cell carcinomas are also common. The SIR for melanoma is 28 in the radiation field and 15 outside the irradiated areas. Skin cancer also accounts for approximately one-third of all third tumors (Abramson and Frank 1998).

9.2.4 Lung Cancer and Other Common Cancers of Adulthood

In recent years, with improvements in treatment that have resulted in longer survival rates, it has become apparent that patients with hereditary retinoblastoma are also at risk of developing epithelial cancers late in adulthood (Yu et al. 2009; Fletcher et al. 2004). The SIR is elevated for lung, breast, colon, buccal cavity, bladder, and corpus uteri neoplasms (Kleinerman et al. 2005) (Table 9.1). Lung cancer appears to be one of the most common (Kleinerman et al. 2000; Fletcher et al. 2004). This is not surprising since somatic mutations of the *RB1* gene are known to contribute to the development of lung cancer (Kleinerman et al. 2000; Harbour et al. 1988). Compared with the general population, hereditary retinoblastoma survivors have a higher mortality from lung cancer and all other epithelial cancers combined (standard mortality ratio 7.01 and 3.29, respectively) (Fletcher et al. 2004). Rather than epithelial, most bladder and uterine cancers (and a large proportion of colon neoplasms) are probably leiomyosarcomas (Kleinerman et al. 2005, 2007). There is an increased incidence of breast cancer in irradiated patients, but this increased risk is similar for patients with hereditary and nonhereditary retinoblastoma; the breast dose from scatter radiation is approximately 0.4 Gy (Kleinerman et al. 2005). New reported excess risks include carcinomas of the salivary glands and tongue; low doses of radiation (<5 Gy) have been associated with secondary salivary cancers (Kleinerman et al. 2005). It is possible that most of the excess cancer risks might be preventable by limiting exposure to DNA damaging agents, such as tobacco and UV light.

9.2.5 Hematologic Malignancies

Patients with hereditary retinoblastoma have a slightly increased risk of developing hematologic malignancies with a SIR of 2.25 (SIR 1.27 in non-hereditary cases) (Kleinerman et al. 2005). The use of etoposide may add an additional risk to this patient population (Smith et al. 1994). Etoposide-related leukemia shows a dose-response relation with the highest risk associated with cumulative doses greater than 4,000 mg/m^2 (Smith et al. 1994; Pui et al. 1991). Also associated with dosage schedule, there is a higher leukemogenic potential when the medication is administered weekly than when administered every 3 or 4 weeks (Pui et al. 1991). The cumulative doses of etoposide and other topoisomerase-II inhibitors, such as anthracyclines used in patients with retinoblastoma, are significantly lower, and it is therefore assumed that the risk of treatment-related leukemia is minimal. Therapy-related acute myeloid leukemia after the treatment of retinoblastoma has been reported, although its occurrence appears to be very low (Nishimura et al. 2001; Gombos et al. 2007).

9.2.6 Trilateral Retinoblastoma

Trilateral retinoblastoma refers to the association of bilateral retinoblastoma with an asynchronous

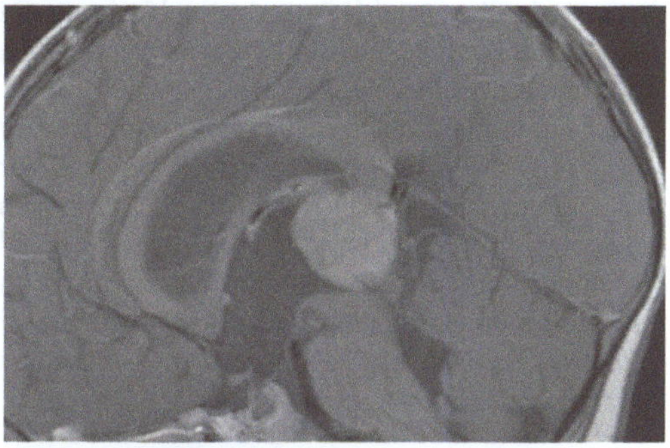

Figure 9.2

MRI showing a 2×2×2 cm pineal gland mass in a 3-year-old survivor of bilateral retinoblastoma. Resection of the mass was performed, and pathology showed pineoblastoma

intracranial tumor (Fig. 9.2) (Kivelä 1999; Amoaku et al. 1996; Blach et al. 1994). The SIR for trilateral retinoblastoma is 90.8, and it seems to be associated with the use of radiation therapy (SIR is 0 in non-irradiated patients) (Kleinerman et al. 2005). Tumors comprising trilateral retinoblastoma are primitive neuroectodermal tumors exhibiting varying degrees of neuronal or photoreceptor differentiation, suggesting an origin from the germinal layer of primitive cells (Marcus et al. 1998). This association can occur in 3–9% of patients with the genetic form, and appears to be more common in familial cases. The prognosis is almost uniformly fatal. Trilateral retinoblastoma was the principal cause of death from retinoblastoma during the first decade of life in the United States (Blach et al. 1994). The majority of these tumors are pineoblastomas, but in 20–25% of the cases, the tumors are suprasellar or parasellar. The association of bilateral retinoblastoma with a tumor in the pineal gland and a fourth primary of suprasellar location is called quadrilateral retinoblastoma.

In most cases, trilateral retinoblastoma resembles undifferentiated retinoblastomas with the more frequent formation of Homer–Wright rosettes. The median age at diagnosis of trilateral retinoblastoma is 23–48 months, (Kivelä 1999; Amoaku et al. 1996; Blach et al. 1994; Holladay et al. 1991) and the interval between the diagnosis of bilateral retinoblastoma and the diagnosis of the brain tumor is usually more than 20 months (Kivelä 1999; Paulino 1999). Suprasellar tumors are usually diagnosed earlier, (Paulino 1999) and in 15–20% of the cases, the intracranial tumor antecedes the diagnosis of retinoblastoma, (Amoaku et al. 1996) In recent years, with the more widespread use of chemoreduction treatments for patients with bilateral retinoblastoma and decrease in the use of radiation, the incidence of trilateral retinoblastoma has decreased dramatically, almost to the point that patients with the genetic form of retinoblastoma are now considered to be almost protected against this fatal complication (Shields et al. 2001). However, approximately 5% of patients with bilateral disease develop pineal cysts; which appear to be a *forme fustre* of trilateral retinoblastoma (Fig. 9.3) (Rodriguez-Galindo et al. 2003; Beck-Popovic et al. 2006).

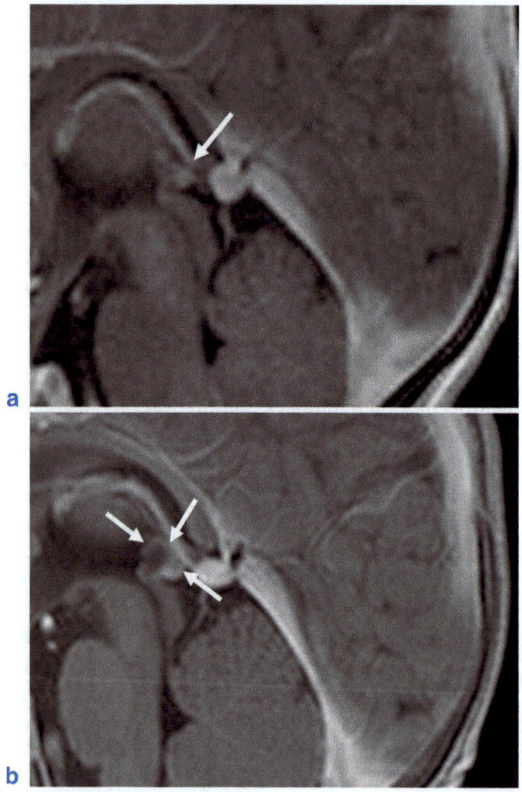

Figure 9.3 a,b

a MRI performed at diagnosis of retinoblastoma in a 6-month-old infant, showing a solid pineal gland (*arrow*) measuring 3 × 4 mm. b MRI performed in the same patient, 7 months later, showing a solid and cystic pineal gland (*arrows*) measuring 8 × 6 mm

The prognosis for patients with trilateral retinoblastoma is dismal; patients die of disseminated neuroaxis disease in less than 9 months (Kivelä 1999; Holladay et al. 1991; Paulino 1999). The rare survivors are usually those diagnosed with screening imaging, and treated with intensive chemotherapy with or without craniospinal radiation (Kivelä 1999). Pineoblastoma occurring in non-retinoblastoma patients is also associated with a poor prognosis. However, with an appropriate aggressive multimodal approach, these patients can be cured. Pineoblastoma is a chemosensitive neoplasm, and it appears to have a steep dose-response curve for alkylating agents. Studies in older patients with primary pineoblastoma have recently shown that a treatment with complete resection and intensive alkylator- and cisplatin-based therapy, followed by craniospinal irradiation (36 Gy with boost to pineal gland to 59 Gy), and consolidation with high-dose chemotherapy and autologous stem cell rescue, may produce survival rates in more than two thirds of the patients (Gururangan et al. 2003). It is therefore possible that similar treatment guidelines could be used for trilateral retinoblastoma. One must, however, consider the serious long term toxicities of such doses of radiation in the very young child. Therefore, current strategies are directed towards avoiding irradiation using intensive chemotherapy followed by consolidation with autologous stem cell rescue, an approach similar to those being used in the treatment of brain tumors in infants.

Because of the poor prognosis of trilateral retinoblastoma, screening neuroimaging is a common practice. One fourth of the cases in the literature correspond to cases found during screening (Kivelä 1999). Given the short interval between the diagnosis of retinoblastoma and the occurrence of trilateral retinoblastoma, routine screening might detect the majority of cases within two years (Kivelä 1999). While it is not clear whether early diagnosis can impact survival, (Moll et al. 2000) it is usually recommended to perform neuroimaging every 6 months until 5 years of age (Kivelä 1999; Paulino 1999; Singh et al. 1999).

9.3 Other Long Term effects

9.3.1 Orbital Growth and Facial Asymmetry

Because their orbital growth is still in progress, children treated for retinoblastoma are at risk of developing functionally and cosmetically significant bony orbital abnormalities. These sequelae become evident by early adolescence, when orbital growth is largely complete, and the result is the "hourglass facial deformity" (Yue and Benson 1996). Enucleation and evisceration, which cause orbital contraction, as well as radiotherapy, which induces arrest of bone growth, adversely affect orbital growth. In children treated for bilateral retinoblastoma, the impact of enucleation in orbital development is not different from that of irradiation. Final orbital volumes after enucleation correlate with the size of the prosthetic implant, but there are no differences in final orbital volumes based on the type of implant (Kaste et al. 1997; Lyle et al. 2007).

Delay of radiation therapy should therefore be a goal when designing treatment for children with bilateral retinoblastoma. Studies show that the therapeutic strategy of chemoreduction and aggressive focal treatments can successfully delay the use of radiation therapy for at least 6 to 7 months, (median age 21 months) (Rodriguez-Galindo et al. 2003; Shields et al. 2002). In addition to theoretically decreasing the risk of second cancers, delaying radiation therapy may also allow more complete facial and orbital growth, thus reducing the degree of midfacial deformities (Yue and Benson 1996; Kaste et al. 1997). However, with the use of a multidisciplinary approach, the dose of radiation needed for disease control may also be reduced (Merchant et al. 2002).

9.3.2 Visual Outcome

Visual outcome is frequently good in children treated for retinoblastoma, (Ek et al. 2002) however, maculopathy (Rougier et al. 1997) and deficits in acuity, (Ek et al. 2002) visual fields and dark adaptation, (Ek et al. 2002) and in visuomotor integration (Ross et al. 2001) have been reported for many patients. Visual outcome correlates with the intraocular stage and, more importantly, tumor location. Visual acuity 20/40 or better can be achieved in 90% of eyes with extramacular tumors, and in 24% of eyes with macular tumors. Overall, half the eyes may achieve a final visual acuity of 20/40 or better, and two-thirds have visual acuity of 20/200 or better (Demirci et al. 2005). However, visual outcome is not always easily predicted on the basis of the initial presentation (Hall et al. 1999). These findings suggest that visual function in survivors of retinoblastoma is influenced by more distal elements of the visual system, including the primary visual cortex. Because retinoblastoma affects the visual system at an age in which the central nervous system is still developing, (Huttenlocher et al. 1982) differences in visual outcome among retinoblastoma patients may be due, at least in part, to disease- or treatment-induced differences in visual field development in the primary visual cortex. New imaging technology, such as functional MRI and diffusion tensor imaging, may be used to evaluate changes in the visual pathways and the primary visual cortex (Morita et al. 2000). Visual rehabilitation and follow-up is discussed in chapter 10.

9.3.3 Cognitive and Functional Development of Patients with Retinoblastoma

Patients with retinoblastoma suffer a potential restriction in their development due to their visual limitations. However, few studies have addressed the development of these young children. Interestingly, the earliest papers describing cognitive development in this population suggested that children with retinoblastoma might have above average or superior intelligence (Thurrell and Josephson 1966; Williams 1968; Levitt et al. 1972; Eldridge et al. 1972). These findings were based on a small number of patients and were never confirmed or unconfirmed, but the idea of superior intelligence became part of the "lore" among clinicians working with the retinoblastoma population. In the report of Ek et al, a population-based study from Sweden, 22 children with retinoblastoma were assessed at 4 and 6 years of age (Ek et al. 2002). Both bilateral and unilateral patients showed above average developmental quotients, with the bilateral group showing higher scores in the superior range. Only two children in the cohort demonstrated below average development, and both of them were bilateral patients who received radiation therapy in the first month of life. The authors concluded that bilateral retinoblastoma is associated with superior cognitive capacities. The other recent series involved 54 patients who were assessed prior to the age of 42 months with the Bayley Scales of Infant Development (Ross et al. 2001). There was no indication of superior intelligence in this cohort, but neither was there an indication of increased difficulties. The average mental and motor development scores were in the normal range and did not differ from population norms. Thus, although children with retinoblastoma do not appear to be at-risk developmentally, questions regarding the developmental trajectory for this population remain.

9.3.4 Other Late Effects

Platinum compounds are commonly used to treat retinoblastoma. While the effects on hearing of cisplatin are well documented, there is conflicting evidence concerning the potential ototoxic effects of carboplatin. While it is usually assumed that carboplatin ototoxicity is extremely rare, there are very few studies investigating cumulative incidence of and prognostic factor for ototoxicity secondary to this platinum agent. In the two studies reported, no cases of carboplatin-induced hearing loss were documented (Smits 2006; Lambert et al. 2008). However, very careful age-appropriate evaluations of hearing function, including tympanometry, otoacoustic emission measurement, and visual reinforced audiometry, must be performed (Smits 2006).

References

Abramson DH, Frank C (1998) Second nonocular tumors in survivors of bilateral retinoblastoma. A possible age effect on radiation-related risk. Ophthalmology 105:573–580

Abramson DH, Melson MR, Dunkel IJ, Frank CM (2001) Third (fourth and fifth) nonocular tumors in survivors of retinoblastoma. Ophthalmology 108:1868–1876

Abramson DH, Lawrence SD, Beaverson KL, Lee TC, Rollins IS, Dunkel IJ (2005) Systemic carboplatin for retinoblastoma: change in tumour size over time. Br J Ophthalmol 89:1616–1619

Acquaviva A, Ciccolallo L, Rondelli R et al (2006) Mortality from second tumour among long-term survivors of retinoblastoma: a retrospective analysis of the Italian retinoblastoma registry. Oncogene 25:5350–5357

Aerts I, Pacquement H, Doz F et al (2004) Outcome of second malignancies after retinoblastoma: a retrospective analysis of 25 patients treated at the Institut Curie. Eur J Cancer 40:1522–1529

Amoaku WMK, Willshaw HE, Parkes SE, Shah KJ, Mann JR (1996) Trilateral retinoblastoma: a report of five patients. Cancer 78:858–863

Beck-Popovic M, Balmer A, Maeder P, Braganca T, Munier FL (2006) Benign pineal cysts in children with bilateral retinoblastoma: a new variant of trilateral retinoblastoma? Pediatr Blood Cancer 46:755–761

Bisogno G, Sotti G, Nowicki Y et al (2004) Soft tissue sarcoma as a second malignant neoplasm in the pediatric age group. Cancer 100:1758–1765

Blach LE, McCormick B, Abramson DH, Ellsworth RM (1994) Trilateral retinoblastoma – incidence and outcome: decade of experience. Int J Radiat Oncol Biol Phys 29:729–733

Chauveinc L, Mosseri V, Quintana E et al (2001) Osteosarcoma following retinoblastoma: age at onset and latency period. Ophthalmic Genet 22:77–88

Daw NC, Mahmoud HH, Meyer WH et al (2000) Bone sarcomas of the head and neck in children: the St. Jude Children's Research Hospital experience. Cancer 88:2172–2180

Demirci H, Shields CL, Meadows AT, Shields JA (2005) Long-term visual outcome following chemoreduction for retinoblastoma. Arch Ophthalmol 123:1525–1530

Dunkel IJ, Gerald WL, Rosenfield N, Strong E, Abramson DH, Ghavimi F (1998) Outcome of patients with a history of bilateral retinoblastoma treated for a second malignancy: the Memorial Sloan-Kettering experience. Med Pediatr Oncol 30:59–62

Ek U, Seregard S, Jacobson L, Oskar K, TRampe E, Kock E (2002) A prospective study of children treated for retinoblastoma: cognitive and visual outcomes in relation to treatment. Acta Ophthalmol Scand 80:294–299

Eldridge R, O'Meara K, Kitchen D (1972) Superior intelligence in sighted retinoblastoma patients and their families. J Med Genet 9:331–335
Eng G, Li FP, Abramson DH et al (1993) Mortality from second tumors among long-term survivors of retinoblastoma. J Natl Cancer Inst 85:1121–1128
Fletcher O, Easton D, Anderson K, Gilham C, Jay M, Peto J (2004) Lifetime risks of common cancers among retinoblastoma survivors. J Natl Cancer Inst 96:357–363
Gombos DS, Hungerford J, Abramson DH et al (2007) Secondary acute myelogenous leukemia in patients with retinoblastoma. Ophthalmology 114:1378–1383
Gururangan S, McLaughlin C, Quinn J et al (2003) High-dose chemotherapy with autologous stem-cell rescue in children and adults with newly diagnosed pineoblastomas. J Clin Oncol 21:2187–2191
Hall LS, Ceisler E, Abramson DH (1999) Visual outcomes in children with bilateral retinoblastoma. J AAPOS 3:138–142
Harbour J (2001) Molecular basis of low-penetrance retinoblastoma. Arch Ophthalmol 119:1699–1704
Harbour JW, Lai SL, Whang-Peng J, Gazdar AF, Minna JD, Kaye FJ (1988) Abnormalities in structure and expression of the human retinoblastoma gene in SCLC. Science2 41:353–357
Hauben EI, Arends J, Vandenbrouke JP, van Asperen CJ, Van Marck E, Hogendoorn PCW (2003) Multiple primary malignancies in osteosarcoma patients. Incidence and predictive value of osteosarcoma subtype for cancer syndromes related with osteosarcoma. Eur J Human Genet1 1:611–618
Henderson TO, Whitton J, Mertens AC et al (2007) Secondary sarcomas in childhood cancer survivors: a report from the Childhood Cancer Survivor Study. J Natl Cancer Inst 99:300–308
Holladay DA, Holladay A, Montebello JF, Redmond KP (1991) Clinical presentation, treatment, and outcome of trilateral retinoblastoma. Cancer 67:710–715
Huttenlocher PR, de Courten C, Garey LJ, Van der Loos H (1982) Synaptogenesis in human visual cortex – evidence for synapse elimination during normal development. Neurosci Lett 13:247–252
Jaffe N, Pearson P, Yasko AW, Lin P, Herzog C, Raymond K (2003) Single and multiple metachronous osteosarcoma tumors after therapy. Cancer 98:2457–2466
Kaste S, Chen G, Fontanesi J, Crom D, Pratt CB (1997) Orbital development in long-term survivors of retinoblastoma. J Clin Oncol 15:1183–1189
Kivelä T (1999) Trilateral retinoblastoma: a meta-analysis of hereditary retinoblastoma associated with primary ectopic intracranial retinoblastoma. J Clin Oncol 17:1829–1837
Kleinerman RA, Tarone RE, Abramson DH, Seddon JM, Li FP, Tucker MA (2000) Hereditary retinoblastoma and risk of lung cancer. J Natl Cancer Inst 92:2037–2039
Kleinerman RA, Tucker MA, Tarone RE et al (2005) Risk of new cancers after radiotherapy in long-term survivors of retinoblastoma: an extended follow-up. J Clin Oncol 23:2272–2279
Kleinerman RA, Tucker MA, Abramson DH, Seddon JM, Tarone RE, Fraumeni JF (2007) Risk of soft tissue sarcomas by individual subtype in survivors of hereditary retinoblastoma. J Natl Cancer Inst 99:24–31
Lambert MP, Shields C, Meadows AT (2008) A retrospective review of hearing in children with retinoblastoma treated with carboplatin-based chemotherapy. Pediatr Blood Cancer 50:223–226
Levitt EA, Rosenbaum AL, Willerman L, Levitt M (1972) Intelligence of retinoblastoma patients and their siblings. Child Dev 43:939–948
Li FP, Abramson DH, Tarone RE, Kleinerman RA, Fraumeni JFJ, Boice JD (1997) Hereditary retinoblastoma, lipoma, and second primary cancers. J Natl Cancer Inst 89:83–84
Lyle CE, Wilson MW, Li CS, Kaste SC (2007) Comparison of orbital volumes in enucleated patients with unilateral retinoblastoma: hydroxyapatite implants versus silicone implants. Ophthal Plast Reconstr Surg 23:393–396
Marcus DM, Brooks SE, Leff G et al (1998) Trilateral retinoblastoma: insights into histogenesis and management. Surv Ophthalmol 43:59–70
Merchant TE, Gould C, Hilton N et al (2002) Ocular preservation after 36 Gy external beam radiation therapy for retinoblastoma. J Pediatr Hematol Oncol 24:246–249
Mohney B, Robertson D, Schomberg P, Hodge D (1998) Second nonocular tumors in survivors of heritable retinoblastoma and prior radiation therapy. Am J Ophthalmol 126:269–277
Moll A, Imhof S, Schouten-van Meeteren AYN, Boers M (2000) Trilateral retinoblastoma: is the location of the intracranial tumor important. Cancer 88:965–966
Moll AC, Imhof SM, Schouten-van Meeteren AYN, Kuik DJ, Hofman P, Boers M (2001) Second primary tumors in hereditary retinoblastoma: a register-based study, 1945–1997. Ophthalmology 108:1109–1114
Morita T, Kochiyama T, Yamada H et al (2000) Difference in the metabolic response to photic stimulation of the lateral geniculate nucleus and the primary visual cortex of infants: a fMRI study. Neurosci Res 38:63–70
Nishimura S, Sato T, Ueda H, Ueda K (2001) Acute myeloblastic leukemia as a second malignancy in a patient with hereditary retinoblastoma. J Clin Oncol 19:4182–4183
Paulino AC (1999) Trilateral retinoblastoma: is the location of the intracranial tumor important? Cancer 86:135–141
Pui C-H, Ribeiro RC, Hanckok M (1991) Acute myeloid leukemia in children treated with epipodophyllotoxins for acute lymphoblastic leukemia. N Engl J Med 325:1682–1687
Rodriguez-Galindo C, Wilson MW, Haik BG et al (2003) Treatment of intraocular retinoblastoma with vincristine and carboplatin. J Clin Oncol 21:2019–2025
Ross G, Lipper EG, Abramson D, Preiser L (2001) The development of young children with retinoblastoma. Arch Pediatr Adolesc Med 155:80–83

Rougier P, Bugat R, Douillard JY et al (1997) Phase II study of irinotecan in the treatment of advanced colorectal cancer in chemotherapy-naive patients and patients pretreated with fluorouracil-based chemotherapy. J Clin Oncol1 5:251–260

Shields CL, Meadows AT, Shields JA, Carvalho C, Smith A (2001) Chemoreduction for retinoblastoma may prevent intracranial neuroblastic malignancy (trilateral retinoblastoma). Arch Ophthalmol 119:1269–1272

Shields CL, Honavar SG, Meadows AT et al (2002) Chemoreduction plus focal therapy for retinoblastoma: factors predictive of need for treatment with external beam radiotherapy or enucleation. Am J Ophthalmol 133:657–664

Singh AD, Shields CL, Shields JA (1999) New insights into trilateral retinoblastoma. Cancer 86:3–5

Smith MA, Rubinstein L, Ungerleider RS (1994) Therapy-related acute myeloid leukemia following treatment with epipodophyllotoxins: estimating the risks. Med Pediatr Oncol 23:86–98

Smits A, Swen SJ, Goverts T, Moll AC, Imhof SM, Schouten-van Meeteren AY (2006) Assessment of hearing in very young children receiving carboplatin for retinoblastoma. Eur J Cancer 42:492–500

Spunt SL, Rodriguez-Galindo C, Fuller CE et al (2006) Ewing sarcoma-family of tumors that arise after treatment of primary childhood cancer. Cancer 107:201–206

Stine KC, Saylors RL, Saccente S, Becton DL (2003) Long-term survival in osteosarcoma patients following retinoblastoma using doxorubicin, cisplatin and methotrexate. Med Pediatr Oncol 41:77–78

Thurrell RJ, Josephson TS (1966) Retinoblastoma and intelligence. Psychosomatics 7:368–370

Tucker MA, D'Angio GJ, Boice JD et al (1987) Bone sarcomas linked to radiotherapy and chemotherapy in children. N Engl J Med 317:588–593

Venkatraman L, Goepel JR, Steele K, Dobbs SP, Lyness RW, McCluggage WG (2003) Soft tissue, pelvic, and urinary bladder leiomyosarcoma as second neoplasm following hereditary retinoblastoma. J Clin Pathol 56:233–236

Weinberg R (1991) The tumor suppressor genes. Science 254:1138–1146

Williams M (1968) Superior intelligence of children blinded from retinoblastoma. Arch Dis Child 43:204–210

Wong FL, Boice JD, Abramson DH et al (1997) Cancer incidence after retinoblastoma. Radiation dose and sarcoma risk. JAMA 278:1262–1267

Yu CL, Tucker MA, Abramson DH et al (2009) Cause-specific mortality in long-term survivors of retinoblastoma. J Natl Cancer Inst 101:581–591

Yue N, Benson M (1996) The hourglass deformity as a consequence of orbital irradiation for bilateral retinoblastoma. Pediatr Radiol 26:421–423

Zhu X, Dunn J, Goddard A et al (1992) Mechanisms of loss of heterozygosity in retinoblastoma. Cytogenet Cell Genet 59:248–252

Visual Rehabilitation

M.E. Hoehn

Contents

10.1 Introduction 127
10.2 Spectacles 127
10.3 Patching or Pharmacologic Penalization 129
10.4 Cataract Surgery 129
10.5 Strabismus Surgery 131
10.6 Low Vision 131
10.7 Conclusion 132
References 132

10.1 Introduction

Visual rehabilitation for children with retinoblastoma can be challenging. These children have unique problems that are uncommon in most pediatric ophthalmology patients. It is important to remember that these patients are either undergoing active treatment, which can be arduous for both the child and the family or they are cancer survivors, having already dealt with a long period of treatment-related issues. When proposing therapeutic options, one must consider the child as a whole. For example, is the child so sick from chemotherapy that nausea and vomiting make patching unrealistic? Is the retinal pathology, from both the tumor and the treatment, so extensive that the visual potential is questionable, and therefore patching may or may not be of any benefit? Is the child complaining that the glasses prescribed make everything smaller, and therefore does not want to wear them? These and other questions should be considered and discussed with the family. Care should be individualized, and every attempt should be made to maximize the patient's vision, as well as to facilitate his or her access to low vision aids and services.

10.2 Spectacles

Spectacles are something that the ophthalmologist prescribes every day. Yet, the patient with retinoblastoma can make this seemingly simple task very challenging. This is especially true when trying to convince the parent and the child that spectacles are necessary in the setting of a monocular patient.

C. Rodriguez-Galindo and M.W. Wilson (eds.), *Retinoblastoma*, Pediatric Oncology,
DOI 10.1007/978-0-387-89072-2_10, © Springer Science+Business Media, LLC 2010

It is absolutely essential that monocular patients wear polycarbonate lenses at all times in order to protect the good eye (Drack et al. 1993). They also need appropriate sports goggles for any significant sporting endeavor. A list of these can be found on the web site of the American Academy of Ophthalmology (http://www.aao.org/eyesmart/injuries/eyewear.cfm). The task of convincing patients to wear protective eyewear is even more challenging when the patient has good vision in the remaining eye. In such cases, it is sometimes possible to perform a manifest refraction and find a small degree of refractive error (even a quarter of a diopter). The child may find this small correction subjectively better, and therefore be more inclined to wear the spectacles. If no refractive error is found, then, proper counseling and coaxing must be used to convince the child to use spectacles in order to protect the good eye.

It is important to keep in mind that the goal of prescribing glasses for the patient with retinoblastoma – or any patient with visual impairment – is to help the patient, not to be insistent that the patient must wear the "correct" refraction. Even with the use of the trial frame, prescribing glasses for patients with low vision often involves trial and error. This should be discussed with the patient and family, so that they are prepared for the possibility of multiple changes in glasses over a short period of time.

Just because the cycloplegic refraction is prescribed does not mean that it is the best pair of spectacles for the patient. Some patients with low vision may be myopic, but may not like to wear the correction because of minification. Such patients will complain that the glasses make everything look smaller. Using the trial frames, it may be possible to determine if a lower amount of myopic correction makes an improvement. Actually, some myopic patients prefer no correction for distance vision and a reading add for near vision due to the magnifying properties of the reading aid. Hence, the reading aid provides an easy and inexpensive magnifier. As before, a non-cycloplegic refraction in a pair of trial frames can assist in determining if a reading aid should be used and how much power should be put into the reading aid.

Another major problem with patients with retinoblastoma is retinoscopy. Often, one retinoscopes the elevated tumor mass giving an artificially high hyperopic correction. In such cases, it is important to consider where the child is in his or her treatment. If the child is undergoing active chemotherapy, the tumor mass may shrink and it may be best to defer glasses until the tumor is smaller, allowing a more accurate refraction. If the child has been out of therapy for some time, and the tumor has been stable, then a trial of the glasses is prudent.

If a child is not wearing his or her spectacles, and complaining, "I don't like them," ask why. Does the child not see well with them? Do they not make a difference in the child's vision? Do they hurt his or her face/ears/nose? Do they not like the way they look? Is the child teased about them? Once you have the answer, try to solve the problem. If the child does not see well with the spectacles or if they do not really help, try a dry, subjective refraction. Letting the child walk around in a pair of trial frames to see how he or she likes them may also be helpful. If the child complains of discomfort, inspect the glasses. Do they need adjustment? Are they broken or too small for the child's face? If they are repairable, suggest an adjustment at an optical store. Many parents do not realize that this must be done frequently with children's glasses because of wear and tear. They also do not realize that it is a free service at most optical stores. If the glasses are broken or too small, recheck the prescription, and arrange for a new pair. If the child does not like the way the spectacles look, ask if another frame might help. If the child is being teased, review with him or her the importance of the glasses. Be encouraging and positive about the spectacles, and how they improve the child's vision and life.

An additional consideration when prescribing spectacles is the facial features of the child. Due to radiation or early enucleation, the child may have one or both eyes that are significantly enophthalmic in appearance. If this is the case, consider prescribing a +6.00 or +7.00 sphere for an already poorly seeing eye or an anophthalmic socket with a prosthesis. This will give the optical illusion of a larger and therefore more symmetric appearing eye.

10.3 Patching or Pharmacologic Penalization

When proposing patching or atropine penalization to the patient with retinoblastoma, once again consider the overall clinical picture. Is the diagnosis so new that the family is overwhelmed, and the thought of doing anything else is impossible? Is the child undergoing chemotherapy and experiencing so much nausea and vomiting that patching the good eye is not a practical option? Is the retina of the "bad" eye so distorted from residual tumor and treatment scars that vision may not improve? Has the parent been diligently trying to patch, but the child consistently runs into things or shuts down altogether while wearing the patch? Remember that these are not "normal" amblyopic eyes. They often have extensive pathology that precludes improvement in vision even with the most rigorous patching regimen. However, visual improvement can occur, even in eyes with extensive macular pathology. Some of these eyes develop an ectopic fovea and good vision. Even if an ectopic fovea does not develop, visual improvement can be seen.

Often, there is no way to tell which eye will improve with occlusion therapy. Therefore, when deciding to prescribe penalization therapy, one must again consider the child as a whole.

Sometimes, especially in eyes that have received external beam radiation in very young children, sensitivity to the patch adhesive can occur. Consider an eye pad with Hypafix (registered trademark) as an adhesive, either as a sheet that completely covers the eye pad or in strips as if patching an eye after surgery. Atropine can also be helpful in this situation, although the use of atropine in very dense amblyopia is somewhat controversial and poorly studied (Pediatric Eye Disease Investigator Group 2003; Pediatric Eye Disease Investigator Group 2005). Another option is the use of an over-the-spectacle "soft" patch. This can be effective if properly positioned, so that the nasal aspect is securely tucked under the nosepiece of the glasses and the temporal side is completely smoothed out under the temple earpiece of the glasses. As with all other amblyopia treatments, the "soft" patch can be effective if it is actually used on a regular and sufficient basis. Atropine and soft patches over the glasses are not the best first choice, but can be helpful if adhesive patches fail.

Whatever method is chosen, a discussion with the family regarding realistic outcomes is necessary. As stated previously, the retinal pathology may be so extensive that there may not be an improvement in the vision. The possibility that the child will not be able to function while patched should be discussed with the family. In such cases, the patching will need to be stopped. This risk must be weighed against the fact that a significant number of eyes do improve, and the family should be encouraged to try amblyopia treatment. However, if the parents have tried and failed with amblyopia treatment, they need permission to stop. The parents need the reassurance that their child's poor vision is due to the disease and not due to their lack of diligence.

10.4 Cataract Surgery

Once an eye that has retinoblastoma develops a cataract, the physician and family are faced with a difficult situation. Pediatric cataract surgery is not like adult cataract surgery. Pediatric cataract surgery presents a greater technical challenge. That plus the inherent risk of cataract surgery, namely infection and hemorrhage (both suprachoroidal (Ling et al. 2004) and intraocular), make eyes with both retinoblastoma and a cataract a unique challenge. Furthermore, there is the added worry of tumor dissemination and reactivation (Honavar et al. 2001).

While rare, reactivation has been well-documented in the literature and should be included in a proper informed consent. Because of this concern, the minimum time of tumor quiescence before proceeding with cataract extraction should be 12 months (Moshfeghi et al. 2005).

Once a cataract develops, a decision whether or not to proceed with cataract surgery must be made on the basis of both declining visual function and inability to monitor tumor progression (Honavar et al. 2001). Early, small cataracts that do not interfere with visual function or tumor visualization (classically less than 3 mm in size) (Wright and Spiegel 2003) can be watched. The visual impact of larger cataracts can be difficult to assess due to patient age, inability to adequately test vision, and impact of retinal pathology.

Even in the verbal child, exactly when to proceed with cataract surgery can be a difficult decision. In general, a preschool child with 20/70 or 20/80 vision (Wright and Spiegel 2003), and an older child with 20/60 vision will need cataract surgery. However, the baseline acuity of the eye should be remembered. If the eye had poor vision prior to cataract development then a significant decline from baseline is more important than the actual acuity. For example, an eye may have an initial best-corrected acuity of 20/60 based on retinal pathology. When the vision declines significantly enough to affect the visual function of the child, then cataract surgery is indicated. When a "significant enough" decline in acuity occurs, it is patient dependent. A discussion with the family of when the benefits outweigh the risks is best. However, if at any time the ocular oncologist is having difficulty in visualizing the tumor, proceeding with cataract surgery is prudent. Otherwise, the eye will require enucleation, in order to prevent occult tumor activity (Honavar et al. 2001).

Before proceeding with cataract surgery, it is always wise to discuss the surgery with the child's ocular oncologist, so that coordination of care can be arranged. The oncologist can assure the cataract surgeon of tumor quiescence and be involved in the post-operative care as needed.

Because of the risk of retinoblastoma reactivation, we advocate the following surgical approach. After an appropriate incision or incisions have been created and a viscoelastic substance has been used to reform the anterior chamber, a continuous curvilinear capsulorrhexis is created. Irrigation and aspiration of the lens material is then performed. An appropriate intraocular lens (IOL) is placed in the capsular bag. The viscoelastic substance is removed, acetylcholine chloride (Miochol) or carbachol (Miostat) is used to constrict the pupil, and the eye is closed. The posterior capsule is left intact if at all possible, and a YAG capsulotomy is performed in 6–8 weeks or as needed. This can be done under general anesthesia in co-ordination with the ocular oncologist during an evaluation under anesthesia (EUA). This method is preferred so as to maintain the capsular barrier between the vitreous cavity and the anterior chamber, in order to decrease the risk of spread of the retinoblastoma from the back to the front of the eye.

The calculation of the IOL for a child is a subject of much debate. Since the growth of the eye cannot be predicted, at best, an "educated guess" must be made as to what lens power the eye will require for the majority of the patient's life. The age of the child and the status of the fellow eye must be taken into account. In general, the younger the child, the shorter the eye, and the higher the IOL required. However, this will not be the case for the duration of the child's life, and so a lower-power IOL should be implanted (Wright and Spiegel 2003). As stated previously, how much the eye will grow and how much the refraction will change is unknown, so a "best guess" must be made as to how much lower the power of the IOL should be. Different surgeons use different formulas, and these are available in various books on the topic. Whatever formula is used, my colleagues and I prefer a monofocal IOL with post-operative bifocal spectacles or reading glasses, depending on the final refraction.

For post-operative care, antibiotic and steroid drops or ointment should be used. A similar follow-up schedule should be employed with the exception of possible coordination of an examination under anesthesia with the child's ocular oncologist with the YAG capsulotomy.

As mentioned previously, the YAG capsulotomy can be performed under general anesthesia. A YAG mounted on a rolling table is utilized. After the child has been induced and the airway secured (either with laryngeal mask airway or with endotracheal tube, depending on the anesthetist's preference), the child is rolled onto the shoulder opposite the eye to receive the laser. The child's head is then positioned into the laser. Placement of a pillow or "donut" under the child's cheek opposite the eye to be lasered is helpful (Kerr 2000). A lid speculum is also helpful with an assistant using balanced salt solution to keep the eye lubricated. The capsulotomy is then performed keeping in mind that a child's posterior capsular opacification is usually much thicker than that of an adult's, and therefore, more energy must be used. Because children have a more solidified vitreous than adults, the capsular opacity should be completely obliterated after it has been removed from the posterior aspect of the IOL; otherwise, the opacity will adhere once again to the posterior aspect of the IOL. This is unlike adults, in whom the capsular opacity tends to fall posteriorly into the vitreous cavity.

10.5 Strabismus Surgery

Many times, eyes that have been treated for retinoblastoma develop strabismus. As with all other cases of an ocular deviation, the first principles of strabismus management must be followed. Maximize the vision with spectacles if needed, treat any amblyopia, and then proceed with surgery (Elkington and Khay 1988). Sometimes, a non-sensory strabismus can coexist with retinoblastoma. For example, if it is an accommodative esotropia, obtain a good refraction and employ a trial of spectacles. As previously noted, retinoscopy in these patients can be challenging. However, one's best attempt should be made, and the prescription given. Occasionally, the spectacles, especially in the cases of hyperopia with esotropia, will reduce or eliminate the strabismus. Even in a sensory deviation, consider spectacles if they have never been tried before, since they may reduce the deviation and improve the vision (Rosenbaum and Santiago 1999). However, most strabismus seen in patients with retinoblastoma is sensory and not amenable to spectacle correction. Therefore, strabismus surgery will be needed. In the case of a sensory deviation, the choice to have a surgery must remain with the patient and/or the patient's family. Sometimes, the patient or family feel that the eye turn is the "least of their problems" and do not wish to undergo further surgery. Other times, the patient or family is anxious to have the deviation corrected for psychosocial reasons. In general, my colleagues and I recommend waiting until the child is 3–5 years old before correcting the strabismus with surgery. Doing so allows the tumor to become quiescent (as most cases of retinoblastoma have been treated and have remained stable for one or more years at this point). It also allows the patient and family to recover from the diagnosis of "cancer," which is an extremely stressful event; this will also give time for stabilization of the deviation as well as growth of the child, which decreases anesthesia risks.

My colleagues and I recommend that the strabismus surgeon consults the ocular oncologist before operating to make sure that there are no contraindications to surgery. Also, a discussion with the ocular oncologist about what treatments were given previously can help with surgical planning. Radioactive plaques and cryotherapy can cause significant scarring leading to a more challenging strabismus operation.

The informed consent is the same as for other strabismus procedures. As with all sensory deviations, a proper informed consent should include the possibility of a return of the deviation, as eyes with poor vision tend to drift. The same surgical technique as with all other strabismus operations should be employed. Consideration should be given to overcorrecting the deviation, since eyes with poor vision do tend to deviate again over time. If this route is chosen, discussion with the patient should include this topic, as patients can sometimes be unhappy when one type of strabismus turns into another, unless they know beforehand that such an outcome is intended.

10.6 Low Vision

As alluded to earlier, many patients treated for retinoblastoma have poor vision and require low vision aids and services. It is imperative that these patients receive assistance in obtaining these. Questioning the family about the services they are receiving is recommended. Many children in these circumstances cannot function in school without assistance with visual tasks. A range of aids is available, and the choice of aids must be age and patient appropriate. Prescribing low vision aids is often a process of trial and error: What works for one person does not necessarily work for another. Encourage parents and patients to keep trying, until they find the low vision aids that work best for them. Also, there is great variability in the availability of low vision services depending on location. Some states and schools offer a great deal of help; others do not. It is helpful to know the resources available in one's area of practice so as to guide patients for services. Encourage the patient and family to keep trying to find the best low vision aids and resources to increase the patient's function as much as possible. Remember that the low vision aids needed, will change as the child grows and matures. Sometimes, young children can use the same reading material as their peers, but cannot continue to do so as they advance in school because the print becomes smaller. Also, as the child grows, he or she will be able to utilize more sophisticated aids and devices. Therefore, periodic re-assessment is needed.

10.7 Conclusion

Visual rehabilitation for the patient with retinoblastoma must be approached differently than for other children. However, with consideration of the underlying pathology and the child's overall needs, the endeavor can make a huge difference in the lives of these children.

References

Drack A, Kutschke PJ, Stair S, Scott WE (1993) Compliance with safety glasses wear in monocular children. J Pediatr Ophthalmol Strabismus 30(4):249–252

Elkington AR, Khay PT (1988) Squint, the ABCs of eyes. BMJ 297(6648):608–611

Honavar SG, Shields CL, Shields JA, Demirci H, Naduvilath TJ (2001) Intraocular surgery after treatment of retinoblastoma. Arch Ophthalmol 119(11):1613–1621

Kerr NC (2000) Yag Laser capsulotomy with a standard upright laser for children under general anesthesia. Poster present at: 26th annual meeting of the American Association for Pediatric Ophthalmology and Strabismus; Apr 12–16, San Diego, CA

Ling R, Cole M, James C, Kamalarajah S, Foot B, Shaw S (2004) Suprachoroidal haemorrhage complicating cataract surgery in the UK: epidemiology, clinical features, management, and outcomes. Br J Ophthalmol 88(4):478–480

Moshfeghi D, Wilson M, Grizzard S et al (2005) Intraocular surgery after treatment of germline retinoblastoma. Arch Ophthalmol 123:1008–1012

Pediatric Eye Disease Investigator Group (2003) A comparison of atropine and patching treatments for moderate amblyopia by patient age, cause of amblyopia, depth of amblyopia, and other factors. Ophthalmology 110(8):1632–1637; discussion 1637–1638

Pediatric Eye Disease Investigator Group (2005) Randomized trial of treatment of amblyopia in children aged 7 to 17 years. Arch Ophthalmol 123(4):437–447

Rosenbaum A, Santiago A (1999) Clinical strabismus management principles and surgical techniques. W.B. Saunders, Philadelphia, p 18

Wright K, Spiegel P (eds) (2003) Pediatric ophthalmolgy and strabimus, 2nd ed. Springer, New York, p 466

Retinoblastoma in Developing Countries

G.L. Chantada · S. Luna-Fineman · I. Qaddoumi · A. Furmanchuk · J. Wilimas

Contents

11.1 Introduction 133
11.2 Delayed Diagnosis 134
11.2.1 Causes of Delayed Diagnosis 135
11.2.2 Preventing Late Diagnosis 135
11.3 Special Problems in the Treatment of Retinoblastoma in Less Developed Countries 137
11.4 Resources to Address this Global Problem . . . 138
References 140

11.1 Introduction

The term developing countries refers to nations with relatively low per capita income, usually poorly industrialized societies lacking basic services for health and sanitation with widespread poverty and low literacy rates. Access to health care is limited in these societies. This term has been criticized and alternatives like, "less developed country," have been proposed, but developing country is the most widely used term and will be used throughout this article. There is some variability in opinion as to which countries are developing countries based only on the gross domestic per capita product. Therefore, the Human Development Index (HDI) was developed as a reliable indicator. This index is a comparative measure of life expectancy, education, literacy, and general standard of living. Most countries can be included into one of three groups (low, intermediate, and high). They can also be classified as developed, developing, and under-developed countries. Some countries with an acceptable HDI may have wide inequities in the care they provide to different segments of their societies and this will have an impact on the results of treatment of children with cancer (Scopinaro and Casak 2002).

Childhood cancer often receives little attention in the less developed societies because other problems, such as infection, poor hygiene, and malnutrition are given higher priority. As these problems are gradually controlled, pediatric cancer becomes an important cause of mortality, and many less developed countries have started programs to address this problem (Howard et al. 2007). Pediatric cancer in developing countries has unique problems that influence the care of children with the disease. Late diagnosis and refusal

C. Rodriguez-Galindo and M.W. Wilson (eds.), *Retinoblastoma*, Pediatric Oncology,
DOI 10.1007/978-0-387-89072-2_11, © Springer Science+Business Media, LLC 2010

of treatment, abandonment of therapy are the most common problems faced in this setting and need to be addressed appropriately (Spinetta et al. 2002).

Retinoblastoma is unique among pediatric malignancies in that survival rates in industrialized countries have improved over the last decades to reach the current figure of over 95% without the introduction of any form of therapy other than enucleation. The most likely explanation for these excellent results is that good access to health care and adequate education of parents promote early consultation of a specialist, who makes the diagnosis and provides appropriate treatment. In this setting, current efforts are directed toward increasing the eye preservation rate while decreasing the risk of secondary malignancies. In less affluent societies, retinoblastoma is still a life threatening disease and survival rates as low as 30% have been reported from East African countries (Bowman et al. 2006). Up to one third of patients with retinoblastoma died of metastatic disease, according to a report from Uzbekistan (Mouratova 2003). However, there is limited published information about the situation of retinoblastoma in developing countries. In less developed countries, patients present with advanced disease, often extending outside the eye giving rise to distant metastasis (Kaimbo et al. 2002). Leukocoria and strabismus, the most common presenting signs of retinoblastoma in affluent societies are relatively less frequent in developing countries and the patients present often with buphthalmia, proptosis, or neurologic signs (Kaimbo et al. 2002; Chang et al. 2006). There is little chance of cure for these children who are diagnosed with a curable disease that delay has made incurable. The situation in countries with mid-level HDI is gradually improving with current survival figures higher than 80% in countries like Argentina, Brazil, Mexico, and Turkey (Leal-Leal et al. 2004; Ozkan et al. 2006; Ribeiro Kde and Antoneli 2007; Chantada et al. 2004). However, in this setting, patients often present with locally advanced disease that is curable, but only in the context of a highly specialized medical facility. There is also inequity in the care that children with cancer receive in these countries, and so only a few patients receive adequate therapy (Scopinaro and Casak 2002).

It has been hypothesized that the incidence of retinoblastoma may be higher in some developing areas as discussed in chapter 2 and some maternal diet habits, such as low vegetable and fruit intake have been implicated (Orjuela et al. 2005). It is estimated that over 80% of children under 15 years worldwide live in less developed countries and so, it can be assumed that worldwide, more children are dying of retinoblastoma than surviving it.

11.2 Delayed Diagnosis

Delayed diagnosis of retinoblastoma is a major problem in developing countries. Patients present with advanced intraocular disease, often followed by extraocular dissemination. Although there is controversy as to whether delayed diagnosis is associated with advanced disease in other pediatric malignancies, the natural history of retinoblastoma in documented familial cases states that the disease advances from an intraocular limited stage to a metastatic stage in a time period measured by months (Pollock et al. 1991; Abramson et al. 1998). There is no controversy that children with advanced disease do worse than those with localized disease. Although multiple factors are implicated in late diagnosis of retinoblastoma in developing countries, specific events have been involved. The time from first symptom to diagnosis of retinoblastoma (lag time), measured in weeks or months, has been linked to a higher risk of advanced disease and loss of vision (Erwenne and Franco 1989; Chantada et al. 1999a). Delay in referral to an ophthalmologist correlates with advanced disease and inability to save vision (Erwenne and Franco 1989; Butros et al. 2002). Many groups found that delays greater than 6 months from initial symptoms to contact with a physician correlate with locoregional disease and greater than 12 months with metastatic disease (central nervous system and distant) (Leal-Leal et al. 2004; Chantada et al. 1999a; Ozdemir et al. 2007; Rodrigues et al. 2004). Industrialized countries also report advanced intraocular disease leading to decreased eye-survival. Older patients (>5 years of age) are usually not thought to be at risk for retinoblastoma by most physicians and might be diagnosed late (Aguirre Neto et al. 2007). Although leukocoria is the most common symptom at diagnosis, other signs such as strabismus, squinting, or decrease in visual acuity are ignored by parents and primary care providers, delaying diagnosis.

11.2.1 Causes of Delayed Diagnosis

Causes of delay in diagnosis in developing countries can be divided into:

1. Poorh ealths ervices
2. Lacko fa warenessi nh ealthc arep roviders
3. Generals ocietalp roblems.

(1) *Poor health services*: Developing countries may lack primary care facilities and enough secondary and tertiary referral centers for prompt therapy. Moreover, rural areas and long distances from major hospitals make it difficult for families to travel and access care. In countries without insurance services, the lack of insurance and worry over cost of care delays parents from consulting a physician.

(2) *Lack of awareness in health care providers*: Cancer continues to be taboo in developing counties. Health care providers and ophthalmologists do not think of retinoblastoma as a curable disease. Ignorance about the early symptoms (leukocoria, strabismus, pain, irritability in the young) and curability is frequent. Occasionally, early symptoms are misdiagnosed as toxoplasmosis, Coat's disease, amblyopia, or even conjunctivitis. Developing countries use Public Heath Assistants for Primary Care Providers, who have limited education about childhood cancer. These providers were found to refer patients later in the course of disease. Education has been shown to increase awareness as well as early referrals (see below).

(3) *General societal problems*: In developing countries, parents and family members are usually the first to notice an abnormality in the eye. However, only a fraction seek medical attention and often not until late in the course of the disease, when vision is impaired or the eye is completely destroyed. Parental level of education correlates with late diagnosis (Chantada et al. 1999a). Parents having only elementary school education seek care later than parents with high school or higher education (Chantada et al. 1999a). The lack of trust in the medical establishment hampers early enucleation allowing for progression of disease. Distance to the specialized ophthalmologist prolongs referral time. Although level of poverty has not been studied, lack of health insurance and fear of costs are always a concern among parents, even in developed countries. Infectious disease and malnutrition continue to be the most common causes of death in children of the developing world. The most common causes of blindness in these children are vitamin A deficiency and trachoma. Childhood cancer has not yet impacted them as it has in industrialized countries. So, governmental agencies do not include retinoblastoma as a priority.

11.2.2 Preventing Late Diagnosis

Programs in early detection must include education about symptoms (leucocoria, strabismus, squinting, poor vision, heterochromia, irritability, pain, glaucoma, and proptosis), immediate referral (to ophthalmologists and oncologists), patient education regarding the different treatment modalities and their appropriate allocation (chemotherapy, local control, and enucleation) and genetic counseling. However, early detection programs or general population/physician education are rare. A pioneering program was developed in Brazil with country-wide programs through the media, hospitals, and health care centers. Antoneli et al. reported a reduction in lag time from 8 to 5.8 months from first symptom. They were able to measure significant decrease in referral to tertiary care centers within 3 years (C. Antoneli, personal communication). Honduras implemented a retinoblastoma awareness program in conjunction with nation-wide vaccination programs. A decrease from 73% to 35% incidence of extra ocular disease was documented only 2 years after the national campaign (Leander et al. 2006). Their patients sought care earlier and abandoned therapy less frequently. Similar public awareness campaigns have been implemented in Mexico and other countries with limited resources, under the sponsorship of the International Network for Cancer Treatment and Research (material available at www.inctr.org) (Fig. 11.1).

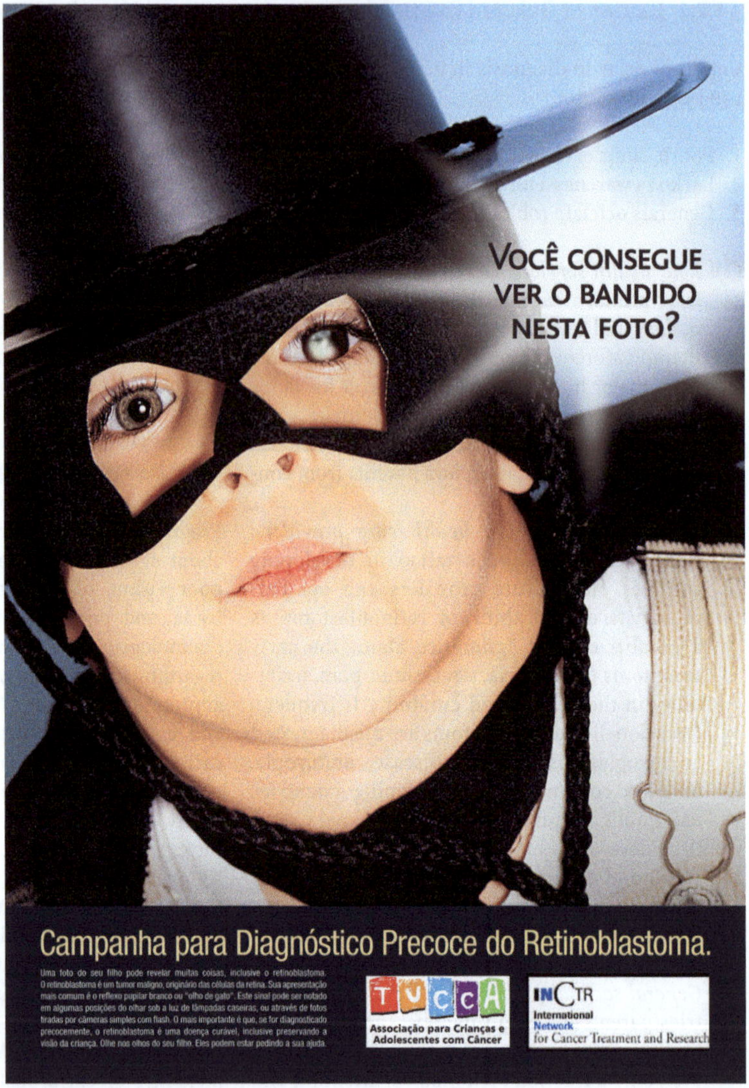

Você consegue ver o bandido nesta foto?
Campanha para Diagnóstico Precoce do Retinoblastoma.
Uma foto do seu filho pode revelar muitas coisas, inclusive o retinoblastoma. O retinoblastoma é um tumor maligno, originário das células da retina. Sua apresentação mais comum é o reflexo pupilar branco ou "olho de gato". Este sinal pode ser notado em algumas posições do olhar sob a luz de lâmpadas caseiras, ou através de fotos tiradas por câmeras simples com flash. O mais importante é que, se for diagnosticado precocemente, o retinoblastoma é uma doença curável, inclusive preservando a visão da criança. Olhe nos olhos do seu filho. Eles podem estar pedindo a sua ajuda.
TUCCA
Associação para Crianças e Adolescentes com Câncer
INCTR
International Network for Cancer Treatment and Research

Figure 11.1

Public Awareness Campaign Sponsored by INCTR
Can You See the Bandit in This Picture?
Campaign for Retinoblastoma Early Diagnosis
A photo of your child can tell many things. Including when he has retinoblastoma. Retinoblastoma is a malignant eye tumor in children, derived from retinal cells. The most common early sign observed is a white pupil reflex (cat's eye). It is usually visible in some artificial light or in photographs where a flash has been used. Early diagnosis is crucial, as if it is detected early, retinoblastoma is curable and the eyes may be saved. Look into your child's eyes. They might need your help

Campaigns for promoting early diagnosis are the first step in improving public awareness of retinoblastoma. However, there is no question that it will take general societal changes, eliminating poverty, giving education to health care professionals and the general population, and prioritizing children's health care through governmental agencies to improve the overall care and outcomes of retinoblastoma and all childhood cancers.

Treatment abandonment is also frequent (Arora et al. 2007). It has a major impact in the care of retinoblastoma since timely enucleation could save a child's life when conservative treatments have failed. Patients may become lost to follow up, usually because of migration or other socioeconomic problems (Menon et al. 2007). Patients with intraocular retinoblastoma treated conservatively need prolonged follow up, usually lasting for years, so every effort to prevent follow up drop outs should be undertaken. Units treating retinoblastoma should develop a specialized social work network to detect and prevent treatment abandonment.

11.3 Special Problems in the Treatment of Retinoblastoma in Less Developed Countries

Publications describing treatment in mid-income countries are abundant in retinoblastoma. They use modern chemoreduction, associated with local control (transpupillary thermotherapy, photocoagulation, and cryotherapy) for early disease and radiation therapy in case of failure or advanced disease (Chantada et al. 2005; Antoneli et al. 2006; Gunduz et al. 2004). Therapies and outcomes in less developed countries are under-reported. Little is known from some parts of Africa, vast areas of Asia including China and some Latin American countries (Bowman et al. 2006; Li et al. 2004). Results come from highly specialized centers in large cities in countries such as Brazil, Mexico, Turkey, India, or Argentina, and the situation in smaller centers may be different. Nevertheless, in these countries, organized treatment groups have used prospective protocols and published significant information for the treatment of retinoblastoma.

In recent years, there has been a trend towards moving to chemotherapy to increase the eye salvage rate in intraocular retinoblastoma in developed countries. This treatment, called chemoreduction, proved to be valuable for reducing the number of enucleated eyes, but its major value was to reduce the use of external beam radiotherapy that is associated with a higher risk for second malignancies. There have been some reports of this treatment modality in mid income countries that have highlighted specific regional particularities (Menon et al. 2007; Chantada et al. 2005; Antoneli et al. 2006; Sohajda et al. 2006). Chemoreduction poses significant challenges to treating physicians in this setting, as it can only be considered in the setting of a multidisciplinary approach that is often unavailable. In under-developed countries, enucleation will cure almost 100% of the patients with intraocular disease that could be candidates for chemoreduction. In this setting, chemoreduction should seldom be offered to patients with unilateral retinoblastoma or patients in whom close follow-up is not possible. Treating physicians should also consider that relapses may occur up to 4–5 years later, needing further local treatment and even enucleation, so close and extended follow-up is mandatory (Shields et al. 2004). Chemoreduction and focal therapy are available only in large specialized tertiary centers in most developing countries and patients must travel long distances for treatment and follow-up. Establishing the remission status of a tumor and providing local therapy requires experience and the availability of technology, so it is recommended that patients that have been treated conservatively should be followed up at the same institution. Moreover, abandonment of therapy is very common in many developing countries and prolonged therapies might hasten abandonment and poor outcomes (Howard et al. 2006). Patients in developing countries usually present with advanced disease, usually with vitreous seeding and it is difficult to avoid external beam radiotherapy in these situations (Chantada et al. 2005). Trying to preserve eyes with advanced disease may put the patient at risk for extraocular relapse if close follow - up and judicious criteria for timely enucleation are not available. A study from Brazil and Argentina showed that chemoreduction is not associated with an increased risk for extraocular relapse (Chantada et al. 2006). Establishing a chemoreduction program in developing countries is expensive and time consuming.

Human and technological resources are intensively required for these programs (Wilson et al. 2006). Patients should be monitored with ocular examinations under anesthesia on a monthly basis for the first year and less frequently thereafter. Expensive lasers and brachytherapy plaques should be available for local treatment. After considering all these constraints, however, we believe that chemoreduction is justified in mid income countries where poor services for rehabilitation of handicapped children are available. According to published evidence from mid-income countries, chemoreduction was able to reduce significantly the number of bilaterally enucleated patients as well as to decrease the overall number of enucleated eyes (Chantada et al. 2005). The choice of the chemotherapy regimen is also important. Myelosuppressive regimens should be avoided in situations where the patient is unlikely to receive proper supportive therapy. There is no solid evidence of the superiority of more intensive regimens for chemoreduction. Regimens with carboplatin alone or in combination with vincristine are well tolerated and permit affected children to return home between chemotherapy cycles (Rodriguez-Galindo et al. 2003; Dunkel et al. 2007). A chemotherapy protocol tailored to disease extension, trying to avoid etoposide and limiting the number of chemotherapy cycles in patients with less advanced disease is advisable (Chantada et al. 2005). The lack of availability of some sophisticated local treatments may be responsible for some treatment failures, and the early use of radiation therapy is often required. The equipment for radiotherapy is obsolete in many developing countries and few centers can deliver adequate radiotherapy for these children. Vitreous extension is one consequence of advanced disease and therefore of poorer preservation rates in retinoblastoma. Since this event is more common in developing countries, innovative, less toxic treatments are justified for this population. Periocular administration of chemotherapy may be a way of delivering higher levels of chemotherapy to the vitreous while reducing systemic toxicity (Abramson 2005). This modality may be cost-effective in less economically developed countries. However, few drugs other than carboplatin have beens tudied.

11.4 Resources to Address this Global Problem

Experience gained in the development of pediatric ophthalmology and oncology programs throughout the world should be applied to create programs to effectively diagnose and treat retinoblastoma. Retinoblastoma is rare but treatable and curable. The relatively small numbers of patients worldwide means that neither ophthalmologists nor oncologists in developing countries are likely to have the expertise to treat without expert advice. The fact that it is curable, often with enucleation alone, makes efforts for early diagnosis and treatment worthwhile and cost effective. The small numbers of experts in retinoblastoma centers have shown themselves willing to provide support to retinoblastoma centers in countries with limited resources. Fortunately, technology is available to facilitate provision of such advice and support. This section will cover the concept of twinning, use of technology including telemedicine and internet, development of protocols in developing countries, certain organizations which provide help and support, and cooperative endeavors.

Twinning, an organized cooperation or partnership between programs and people in resource rich and resource poor countries, has been remarkably successful in improving survival of children with cancer throughout the developing world (Howard et al. 2006; Veerman and Sutaryo 2005; Howard et al. 2004). These programs generally provide some degree of financial support and significant amounts of training, education, and organizational help provided by means of a great deal of personal involvement and cooperation. Successful twinning programs in retinoblastoma have been developed through twinning between ophthalmologists and oncologists at St. Jude Children's Research Hospital and those in Central America and Jordan. These efforts have included donation of equipment including RetCams, ultrasound, laser and cryotherapy units, training in the use of this equipment, visits to countries to promote the programs and problem solve and frequent consults and patient discussions. Meetings via internet or telemedicine have occurred at least monthly.

Concepts such as multidisciplinary teamwork and data collection and analysis have been emphasized.

Technology in the form of communication via telemedicine and the internet is central to the success of these programs. Real time conferences scheduled to discuss cases serve as an educational tool and problem "brain storming." The RetCam has facilitated educational efforts, international conferences, and meetings to discuss protocol development and individual patients and consults. A telemedicine program for retinoblastoma similar to an existing neuro-oncology program has been developed in Jordan and has improved treatment and survival of children with retinoblastoma in that country (Qaddoumi et al. 2007). The educational internet site, www.Cure4kids.org has several lectures and seminars about retinoblastoma. It also has the presentations from the 2007 international conference, Retinoblastoma: One world, one vision, which were also presented live via internet and teleconferencing. The ORBIS cybersite e-consultation site is a remarkable resource, which allows ophthalmologists anywhere in the world who have access to a computer and the internet to post case histories, drawings, photographs, and questions about specific patients and get rapid, free, expert consultation. The RetCam allows ophthalmologists to photograph retinal images and document presence of disease and response to therapy. This also facilitates expert consultation, particularly in complicated patients. RetCams are expensive and generally not available in countries with limited resources but might be provided in selected regional Centers of Excellence developed to provide more sophisticated care, particularly for patients with bilateral disease to avoid blindness. The partnership between the Fund for Ophthalmic Knowledge (New York, USA) and the Hospital Garrahan (Buenos Aires, Argentina) started in 1995 and became one pioneering twinning effort in retinoblastoma. It provided training, technology supply, expert advise and more recently support of research programs (Carcaboso et al. 2007). Since retinoblastoma presents specific challenges in developing countries, research studies should be done in that setting to cover their specific needs. An important function of twinning programs is to teach clinicians in resource-poor areas how to develop and use the tools for clinical investigation while providing the best possible care. So, evidence-based diagnosis, treatment, and outcome improvement is strengthened by twinning programs.

Improvements in patient care and survival are dependent upon the development of disease specific protocols and supportive care guidelines. These need not be complicated but should be designed to clearly outline treatment and address specific important local problems through carefully outlined questions and treatment, data collection, and analysis. Treatment protocols must be developed or modified by taking into account local conditions and available resources (Howard et al. 2006). However, they should also be based on specific information from the medical literature. For example, a treatment protocol in sub-Saharan Africa might concentrate on earlier diagnosis and enucleation while in Guatemala, with an organized retinoblastoma program, development of a protocol for radioactive implants might be a consideration. Much of the current published evidence for the treatment of extraocular retinoblastoma comes from developing countries such as Brazil, Argentina, Mexico, and Turkey (Leal-Leal et al. 2004; Ozkan et al. 2006; Chantada et al. 2004; Chantada et al. 1999b; Leal-Leal et al. 2006; Antoneli et al. 2003; Gunduz et al. 2006).

There are many organizations throughout the world that provide help to patients with retinoblastoma and the programs that treat these patients. This section is not intended to be comprehensive and will mention only some of the many dedicated groups. Already mentioned have been ORBIS international, a nonprofit humanitarian organization dedicated to blindness prevention (www.orbis.org) and the retinoblastoma program and educational web site (www.Cure4kids.org) at St. Jude Children's Research Hospital. The Childhood Eye Cancer Trust (www.chect.org.uk) is a United Kingdom charity for families and individuals affected by retinoblastoma which offers support and information, funds, research, and raises public awareness. Daisy's Eye Cancer Fund (www.daisyseyecancerfund.org), also in the United Kingdom, has a global approach, focusing on developing countries, particularly in Africa. Retinoblastoma Solutions (www.retinoblastomasolutions.org) in Canada, provides information on genetics and testing.

Retinoblastoma International (www.retinoblastoma.net) supports research, education, clinical care, early diagnosis, and awareness programs and has an outreach program with Mexico. The International Network for Cancer Treatment and Research (www.inctr.org) has developed educational programs and organized international treatment programs.

There are many organized programs and cooperative endeavors which have made an impact on the treatment of retinoblastoma in countries with limited resources and serve as examples of successful approaches. Once again, space allows only a few programs to be mentioned. In collaboration with INCTR, the Mexican Retinoblastoma Group was created in January 2003 and has developed a national registry, early diagnosis and education programs and a treatment protocol. The group has annual meetings and is working to improve the treatment of retinoblastoma nationally (Leal-Leal et al. 2004). The Association of Central American Pediatric Hematologists/Oncologists (AHOPCA) has developed a common protocol for Central America and has monthly meetings with the members of the retinoblastoma programs at St. Jude Children's Research Hospital and the Hospital Garrahan Program in Argentina. The Children's Oncology Group has been working with physicians in India to strengthen programs there. Since retinoblastoma is a rare disease and patients are not cared for in a vacuum, it is important to also consider collaborations with organizations with a broader scope. Two such organizations are ORBIS, which has done a tremendous amount to improve treatment of retinoblastoma through support of programs, donation of equipment, education and the cybersite consultation site, and the International Agency for the Prevention of Blindness (www.iapb.org) which has more extensive programs dealing with eye diseases.

In summary, retinoblastoma is a rare but treatable and curable disease which can and should be addressed at some level in most areas throughout the world. Delay in diagnosis and abandonment of therapy are common in developing countries. Programs to educate medical personnel and the general population, and essentially human development might lead to early diagnosis and better outcome. There are many existing programs and organizations which provide examples of successful approaches and support. Even very simple approaches, such as early diagnosis with enucleation will save lives and can progress to improved therapy as conditions improve. Sophisticated therapy with chemoreduction and local therapy should be attempted only in specialized institutions with adequate patient follow-up.

References

Abramson DH (2005) Periocular chemotherapy for retinoblastoma: success with problems? Arch Ophthalmol 123(1):128–129; author reply 129

Abramson DH, Mendelsohn ME, Servodidio CA et al (1998) Familial retinoblastoma: where and when? Acta Ophthalmol Scand 76(3):334–338

Aguirre Neto JC, Antoneli CB, Ribeiro KB et al (2007) Retinoblastoma in children older than 5 years of age. Pediatr Blood Cancer 48(3):292–295

Antoneli CB, Steinhorst F, de Cassia Braga Ribeiro K et al (2003) Extraocular retinoblastoma: a 13-year experience. Cancer 98(6):1292–1298

Antoneli CB, Ribeiro KC, Steinhorst F et al (2006) Treatment of retinoblastoma patients with chemoreduction plus local therapy: experience of the AC Camargo Hospital, Brazil. J Pediatr Hematol Oncol 28(6):342–345

Arora RS, Eden T, Pizer B (2007) The problem of treatment abandonment in children from developing countries with cancer. Pediatr Blood Cancer

Bowman RJ, Mafwiri M, Luthert P, et al (2008) Outcome of retinoblastoma in east Africa. Pediatr Blood Cancer 50(1):160–162

Butros LJ, Abramson DH, Dunkel IJ (2002) Delayed diagnosis of retinoblastoma: analysis of degree, cause, and potential consequences. Pediatrics 109(3):E45

Carcaboso AM, Bramuglia GF, Chantada GL et al (2007) Topotecan vitreous levels after periocular or intravenous delivery in rabbits: an alternative for retinoblastoma chemotherapy. Invest Ophthalmol Vis Sci 48(8):3761–3767

Chang CY, Chiou TJ, Hwang B et al (2006) Retinoblastoma in Taiwan: survival rate and prognostic factors. Jpn J Ophthalmol 50(3):242–249

Chantada G, Fandino A, Manzitti J et al (1999a) Late diagnosis of retinoblastoma in a developing country. Arch Dis Child 80(2):171–174

Chantada GL, Fandino A, Mato G et al (1999b) Phase II window of idarubicin in children with extraocular retinoblastoma. J Clin Oncol 17(6):1847–1850

Chantada G, Fandino A, Davila MT et al (2004) Results of a prospective study for the treatment of retinoblastoma. Cancer 100(4):834–842

Chantada GL, Fandino AC, Raslawski EC et al (2005) Experience with chemoreduction and focal therapy for intraocular retinoblastoma in a developing country. Pediatr Blood Cancer 44(5):455–460

Chantada GL, Dunkel IJ, Antoneli CB, et al (2007) Risk factors for extraocular relapse following enucleation after failure of chemoreduction in retinoblastoma. Pediatr Blood Cancer 49(3):256–260

Dunkel IJ, Lee TC, Shi W, et al (2007) A phase II trial of carboplatin for intraocular retinoblastoma. Pediatr Blood Cancer 49(5):643–648

Erwenne CM, Franco EL (1989) Age and lateness of referral as determinants of extra-ocular retinoblastoma. Ophthalmic Paediatr Genet 10(3):179–184

Gunduz K, Gunalp I, Yalcindag N et al (2004) Causes of chemoreduction failure in retinoblastoma and analysis of associated factors leading to eventual treatment with external beam radiotherapy and enucleation. Ophthalmology111(10):1917– 1924

Gunduz K, Muftuoglu O, Gunalp I et al (2006) Metastatic retinoblastoma clinical features, treatment, and prognosis. Ophthalmology 113(9):1558–1566

Howard SC, Pedrosa M, Lins M et al (2004) Establishment of a pediatric oncology program and outcomes of childhood acute lymphoblastic leukemia in a resource-poor area. JAMA 291(20):2471–2475

Howard SC, Ortiz R, Baez, LF et al (2007) Protocol-based treatment for children with cancer in low income countries in Latin America: a report on the recent meetings of the Monza International School of Pediatric Hematology/Oncology (MISPHO)--Part II. Pediatr Blood Cancer 48(4):486–490

Howard SC, Marinoni M, Castillo L et al (2007) Improving outcomes for children with cancer in low-income countries in Latin America: a report on the recent meetings of the Monza International School of Pediatric Hematology/Oncology (MISPHO)-Part I. Pediatr Blood Cancer 48(3):364–369

Kaimbo WK, Mvitu MM, Missotten L. (2002) Presenting signs of retinoblastoma in Congolese patients. Bull Soc Belge Ophtalmol (283):37–41

Leal-Leal C, Flores-Rojo M, Medina-Sanson A et al (2004) A multicentre report from the Mexican Retinoblastoma Group. Br J Ophthalmol 88(8):1074–1077

Leal-Leal CA, Rivera-Luna R, Flores-Rojo M et al (2006) Survival in extra-orbital metastatic retinoblastoma: treatment results. Clin Transl Oncol 8(1):39–44

Leander C, Fu LC, Pena A, et al (2007) Impact of an education program on late diagnosis of retinoblastoma in Honduras. Pediatr Blood Cancer 49(6):817–819

Li YP, Feng GG, Yi YZ (2004) Present status and developmental trend of retinoblastoma research in China. [Zhonghua yan ke za zhi] Chin J Ophthalmol 40(4): 217–219

Menon BS, Juraida E, Alagaratnam J et al (2007) Chemoreduction for intraocular retinoblastoma in Malaysia. J Pediatr Hematol Oncol 29(1):2–4

Mouratova T. (2003) Retinoblastoma in Uzbekistan. Bull Soc Belge Ophtalmol (289):63–69

Orjuela MA, Titievsky L, Liu X et al (2005) Fruit and vegetable intake during pregnancy and risk for development of sporadic retinoblastoma. Cancer Epidemiol Biomarkers Prev 14(6):1433–1440

Ozdemir H, Tacyildiz N, Unal E et al (2007) Clinical and epidemiological characteristics of retinoblastoma: correlation with prognosis in a Turkish pediatric oncology center. Pediatr Hematol Oncol 24(3):221–231

Ozkan A, Pazarli H, Celkan T et al (2006) Retinoblastoma in Turkey: survival and clinical characteristics 1981–2004. Pediatr Int 48(4):369–373

Pollock BH, Krischer JP, Vietti TJ (1991) Interval between symptom onset and diagnosis of pediatric solid tumors. J Pediatr 119(5):725–732

Qaddoumi I, Mansour A, Musharbash A et al (2007) Impact of telemedicine on pediatric neuro-oncology in a developing country: the Jordanian–Canadian experience. Pediatr Blood Cancer 48(1):39–43

Ribeiro Kde C, Antoneli CB (2007) Trends in eye cancer mortality among children in Brazil, 1980–2002. Pediatr Blood Cancer 48(3):296–305

Rodrigues KE, Latorre Mdo R, de Camargo B (2004) Delayed diagnosis in retinoblastoma. J Pediatr 80(6):511–516

Rodriguez-Galindo C, Wilson MW, Haik BG et al (2003) Treatment of intraocular retinoblastoma with vincristine and carboplatin. J Clin Oncol 21(10):2019–2025

Scopinaro MJ, Casak SJ (2002) Paediatric oncology in Argentina: medical and ethical issues. Lancet Oncol 3(2):111–117

Shields CL, Mashayekhi A, Cater J et al (2004) Chemoreduction for retinoblastoma: analysis of tumor control and risks for recurrence in 457 tumors. Trans Am Ophthalmol Soc 102:35–44, discussion 44–35

Sohajda Z, Damjanovich J, Bardi E et al (2006) Combined local treatment and chemotherapy in the management of bilateral retinoblastomas in Hungary. J Pediatr Hematol Oncol 28(6):399–401

Spinetta JJ, Masera G, Eden T et al (2002) Refusal, noncompliance, and abandonment of treatment in children and adolescents with cancer: a report of the SIOP Working Committee on Phychosocial Issues in Pediatric Oncology. Med Pediatr Oncol 38(2):114–117

Veerman AJ, Sutaryo, Sumadiono (2005) Twinning: a rewarding scenario for development of oncology services in transitional countries. Pediatr Blood Cancer 45(2):103–106

Wilson MW, Haik BG, Rodriguez-Galindo C (2006) Socioeconomic impact of modern multidisciplinary management of retinoblastoma. Pediatrics 118(2): e331–e336

Appendix

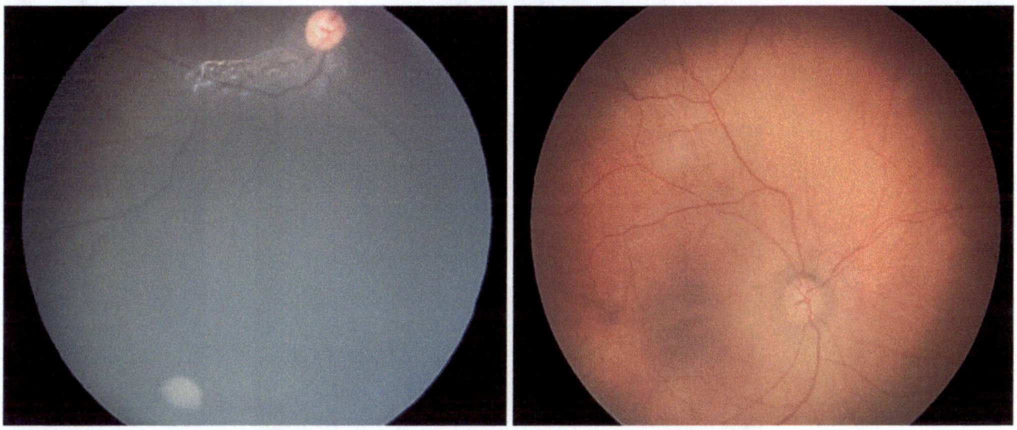

a b

Figures 1a and 1b

Group A retinoblastoma – Tumor ≤ 3 mm in greatest dimension confined to the retina and located > 3 mm from the foveola and > 1.5 mm from the optic disc

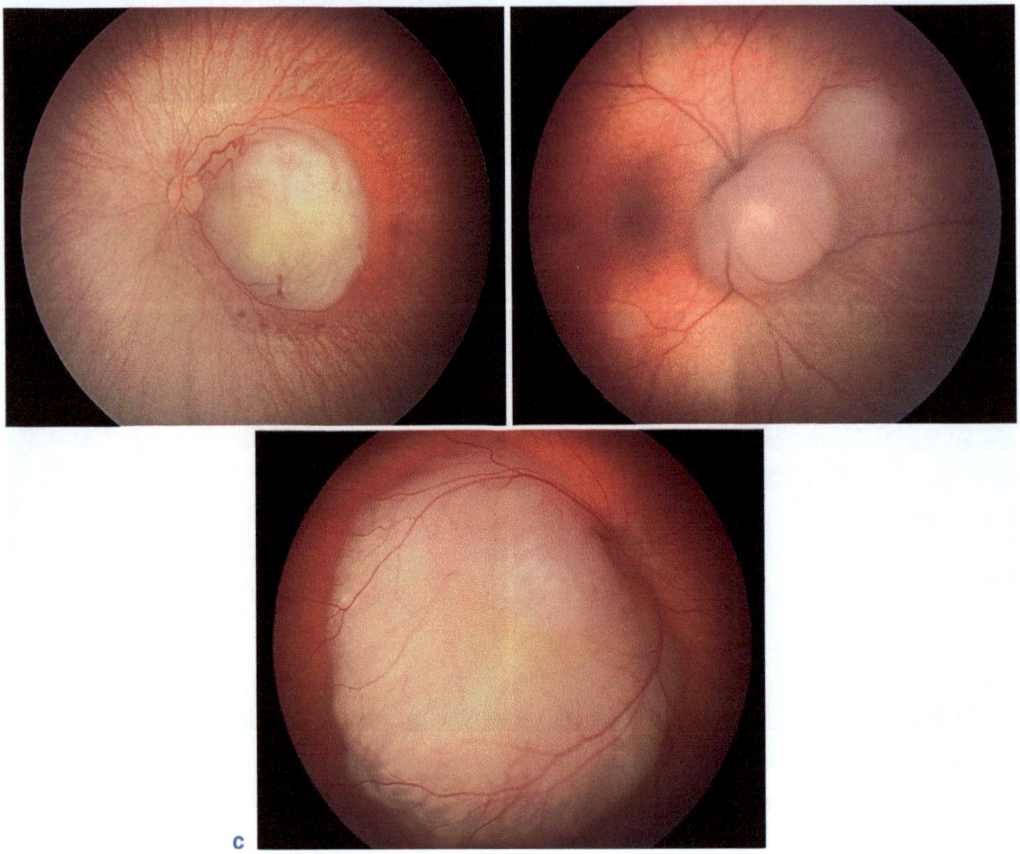

a b c

Figures 2a, 2b, and 2c

Group B retinoblastoma – Tumors confined to the retina not in group A and with subretinal fluid ≤ 3mm from the base of the tumor

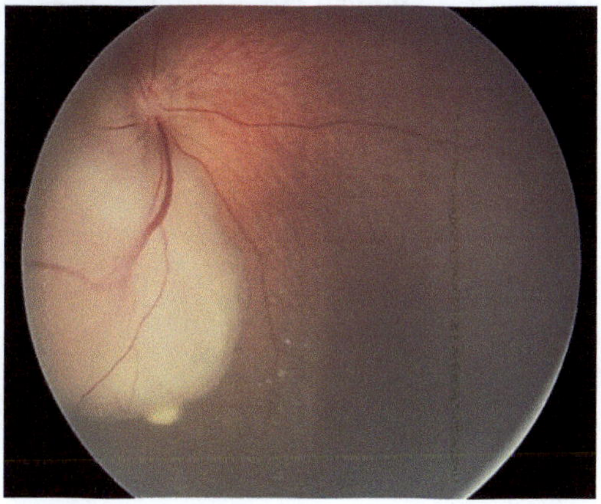

Figure 3

Group C Retinoblastoma – Tumor with vitreous or subretinal seeding ≤ 3mm from the tumor

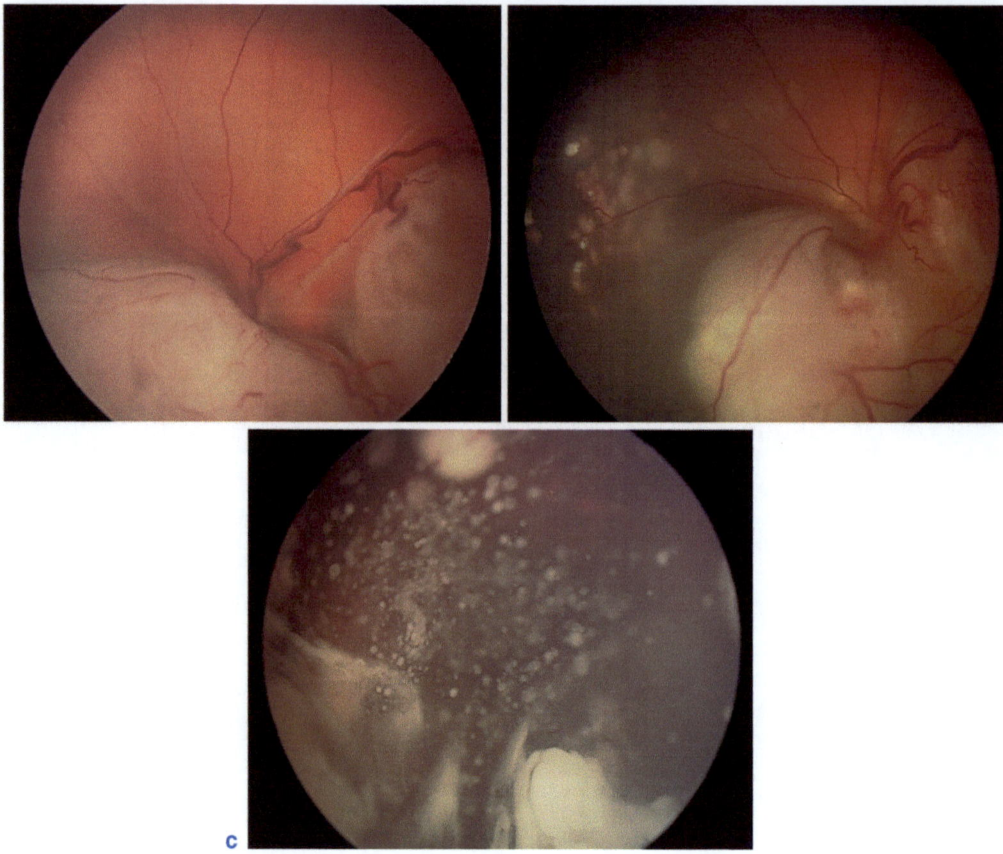

a b c

Figures 4a, 4b, and 4c

Group D retinoblastoma – Presence of subretinal fluid alone > 6 mm from the tumor, or vitreous or subretinal seeding > 3 mm from tumor

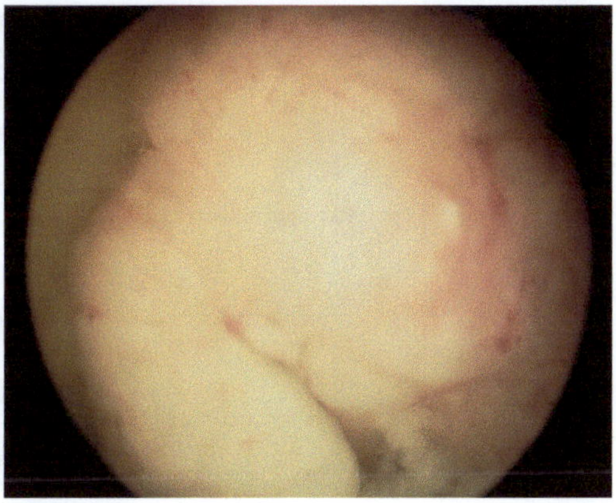

Figure 5

Group E retinoblastoma – Advanced intraocular retinoblastoma, with more than 2/3 of the globe filled with tumor

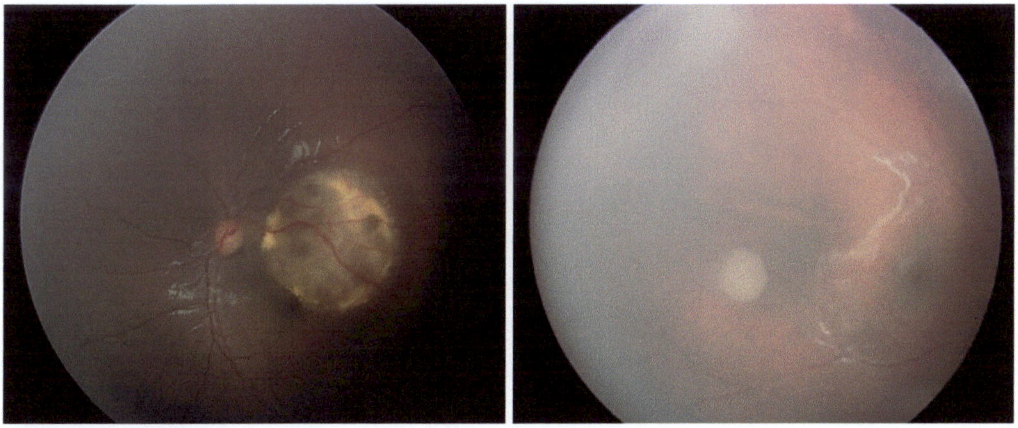

a b

Figure 6a and 6b

Retinal astrocytomas in a 5 yo girl with neurofibromatosis type 1 (a) and in a 10 mo infant with tuberous sclerosis (b)

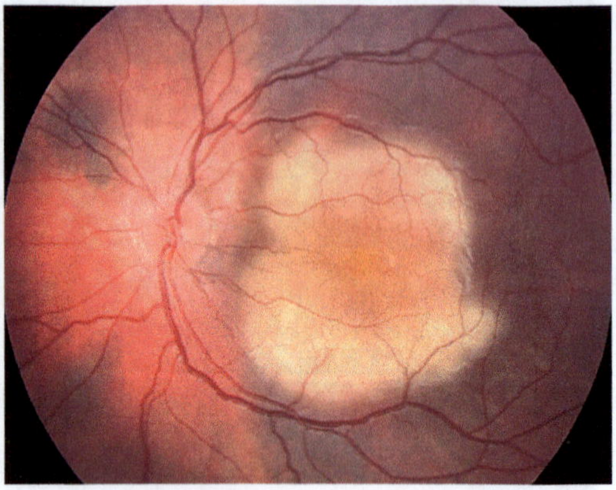

Figure 7

Choroidal osteoma – Low line calcific choroidal lesion within the macula

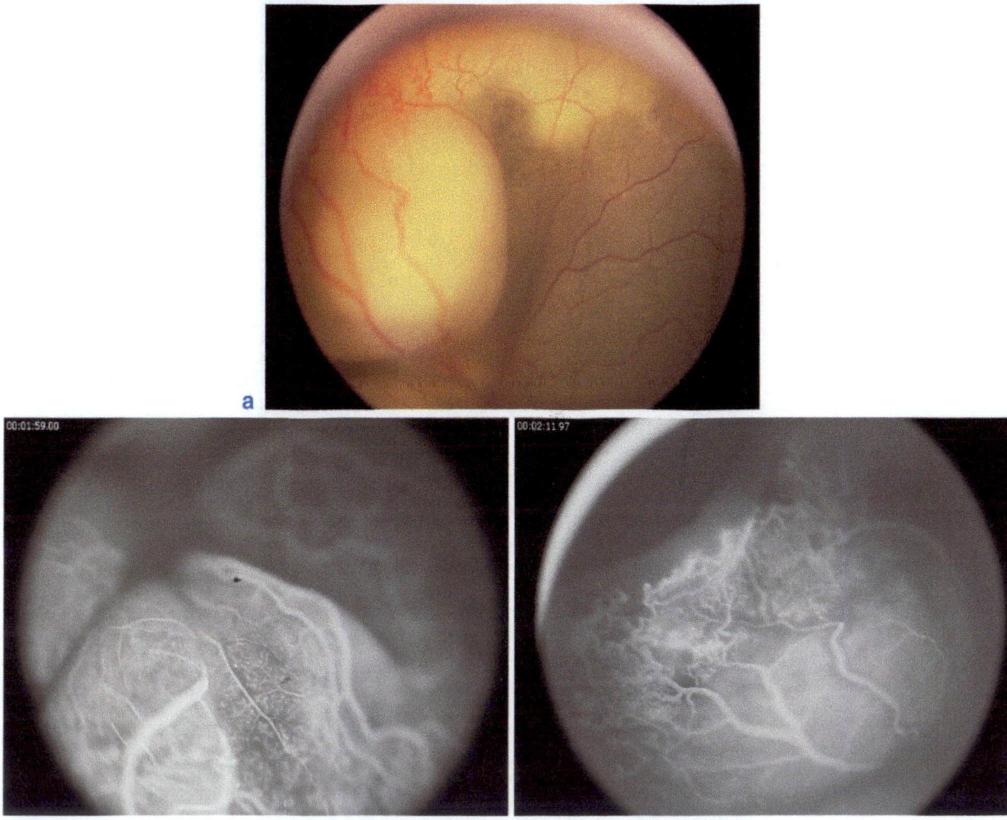

Figures 8a, 8b, and 8c

Coats disease a: Exudative retinal detachment with mustard colored subretinal fluid. b,c: Fluorescein angiograms highlight the telangiectatic vessels characteristic of Coats disease

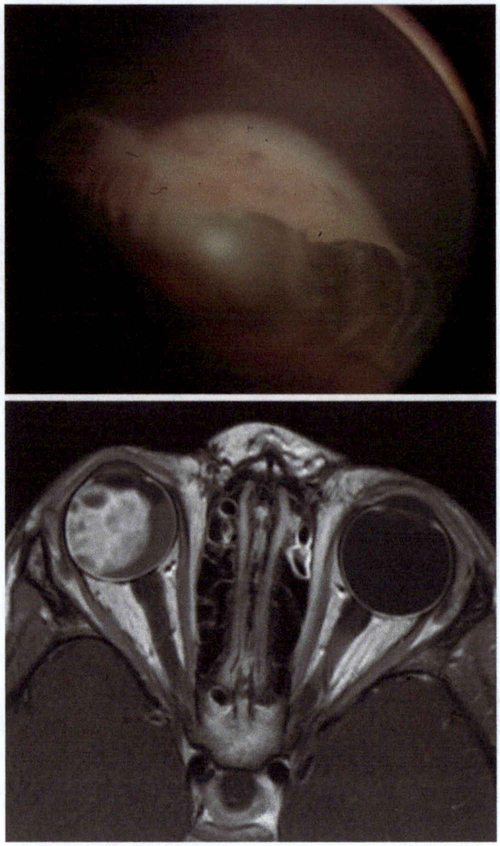

a

b

Figures 9a and 9b

Medulloepithelioma –Variably pigmented cilliary body mass. MRI highlights characteristic intralesional cysts

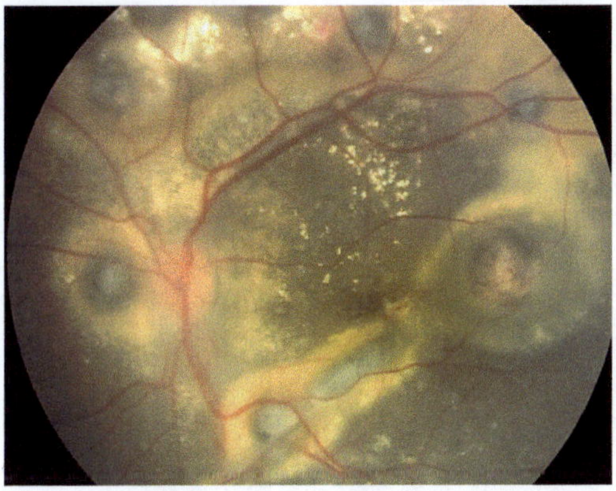

Figure 10

Toxocara chorioretinitis – multiple subretinal foci of choroidal inflammation with associated exudates

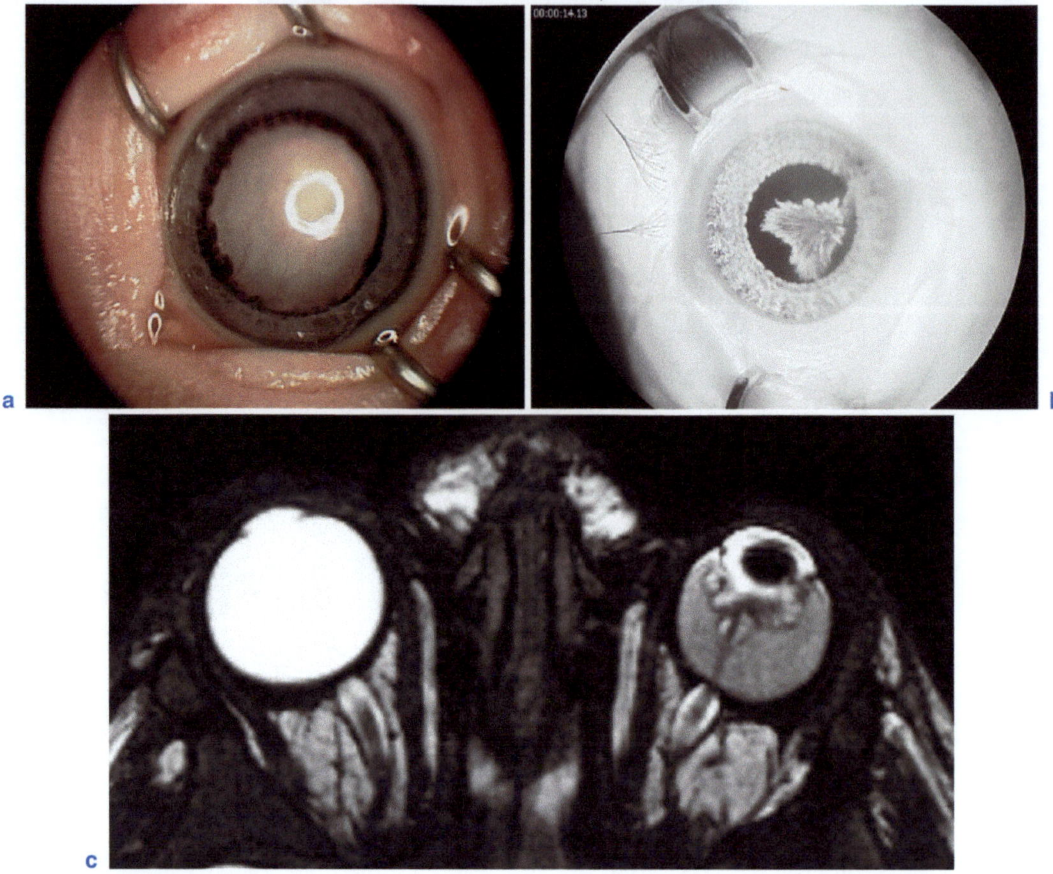

Figures 11a, 11b, 11c

Persistent Fetal Vasculature (previously known as Persistent Hyperplastic Primary Vitreous) Examination shows small eye with hypoplastic iris and retrolental membrane. Fluorescein angiogram and MRI highlight the fibrovascular stalk extending to the optic nerve

Subject Index

A

Aberrants plicing 50
Adjuvantc hemotherapy 69–70
Argong reenl asert herapy 95
ASCR. *See* Autologous stem cell rescue
Autologous stem cell rescue (ASCR) 78–79,1 11–112

B

Brachytherapy 97–98. *See also* Episcleral plaque brachytherapy
Braggp eak 57

C

Cancerg enetics 1–2
Capsulotomy. *See* YAGc apsulotomy
Carboplatin 81–82
– CCI 75
– human-derived fibrin protein sealant 76–77
– intravenous and subconjunctival administration 75
Carboplatino totoxicity 124
Cataracts urgery 129–131
CGH. *See* Comparative genomic hybridization
Chemotherapy
– adjuvant 69–70
– agents
– – carboplatin 71,8 1–82
– – cisplatin 84–85
– – cyclophosphamide 83–84
– – doxorubicin 82–83
– – etoposide 82
– – thiotepa 85–86
– – topotecan 71,8 5
– – vincristine 71,8 1
– extraocularr etinoblastoma
– – metastatic 78–79
– – orbital and locoregional 77–78
– intraocularr etinoblastoma
– – bilateral 70–72
– – intravitreal and intrarterial delivery 77
– – therapy-related leukemia 73
– – tumor formation 72–73
– – unilateral 69–70
– ocularp harmacokinetics 68–69
– periocülara dministration
– – carboplatin 75–77
– – transscleral drug delivery mechanisms 68, 73–75
– research and emergent therapies
– – suicide gene therapy 80–81
– – topotecan 80
– – transgenic mouse models 79–80
Choroidalo steoma 148
Cisplatin 84–85
Clinical and histopathologic features
– clinical history 26–27
– differential diagnosis 27–28
– endophytic growth pattern 31
– examination under anesthesia 28–29
– exophytic growth pattern 31–32
– eyes,p rocessing 37–39
– fine needle aspiration biopsy 30
– fleurettes 33, 35
– Flexner-Wintersteiner rosettes 33, 35
– grouping and staging 30
– Homer Wright rosettes 33, 35
– initial clinical assessment 27
– initialp resentation 25–26
– metastasis 36
– mixed endophytic and exophytic tumor growth 32
– multifocal calcifications and necrosis 32, 34
– necrotic growth pattern 32, 33
– optic nerve invasion 33–34, 36
– prognostic factors 37
– pseudorosettes 32, 34
– trilateral retinoblastoma 37
– uveal invasion 34–36
Coats disease 149
Comparative genomic hybridization (CGH) 43–44
Coulomb-controlled iontophoresis (CCI) 75
Cryotherapy 96–97
Cyclophosphamide 83–84

D

Delayed diagnosis
– chemoreduction and focal therapy 137–138
– early detection programs 135
– human development index (HDI) 133
– lack of awareness 135
– lasers and brachytherapy plaques 138
– poor health services 135
– public awareness campaign 136, 137
– resources
– – ORBIS cybersite e-consultation site 139
– – organizations and programs 139–140
– – twinning concept 138
– societal problems 135
– strabismus and leukocoria 134
Differential diagnosis 27–28
Doxorubicin 82–83

E

Epidemiology
- biologicu nderpinnings 15–16
- factors 11
- genderd ifferences 15
- populationd ifferences
- - global incidence data 12
- - highest incidence registries 12–13
- - IARC 14
- potentialh ypotheses
- - diagnosticin terval 19–20
- - diet 18–19
- - *in vitro* fertilization (IVF) 17
- - nonoccupationalp arental exposures 18
- - parentala ge 16–17
- - parentalo ccupations 16
- - screening and media campaigns 20
- - UVe xposure 17–18
- - virala gents 19
- subpopulations 14–15
Epigeneticm utation 50
Episcleralp laqueb rachytherapy 58–59
Etoposide 82
Ewing'ss arcoma 119
External beamr adiotherapy 92, 99
Extraoculara ndm etastatic retinoblastoma treatment
- high risk intraocular disease
- - choroidali nvasion 105
- - histopathological risk factors 104
- - optic nerve invasion 105–106
- metastaticd isease
- - high-dosec hemotherapy and ASCR 78–79
- - withC NS 112
- - withoutC NS 111–112
- microscopic residual disease
- - artifactual scleral invasion 106
- - multivariatea nalysis 108
- - optic nerve stump 106
- - therapies 107
- - trans-sclerali nvasion 107–108
- orbital and locoregional disease 77–78
- - chemotherapy 109
- - dissemination 108
- - examination 109
- - orbitalr elapse 109–110
- signsa nds ymptoms 103

F

Finen eedlea spiration biopsy 30
FISH. *See* Fluorescence *In Situ* hybridization
Flexner-Wintersteiner rosettes 33,3 5
Fluorescence *In Situ* hybridization (FISH) 44, 49
Frameshift mutation 50

G

Geneticc ounseling
- environmentmental factors 48
- heritability 46–47
- molecular genetic testing 48
- *RB1* test strategies
- - aberrant splicing and epigenetic mutation 50
- - missense mutation 49
- - molecular genetic techniques 49–50
- - mosaicism 51
- - mutation identification 49–50
- - nonsense and frameshift mutation 50
- - parent of origin effect 51
- - penetrance mutation 51
- - prenatal testing 49
- - sporadic bilateral or familial 48–49
- - sporadic unilateral 49
- - translocations and gross deletions 50–51
Germline *RB1*m utation 48,7 2
Grossd eletions 50–51
Group Ar etinoblastoma 143
GroupB r etinoblastoma 144
GroupC r etinoblastoma 145
GroupD r etinoblastoma 146
GroupE r etinoblastoma 147

H

Hematogenous metastasis 105
Homer Wright rosettes 33,3 5
Human-derived fibrin protein sealant 76–77

I

In vitro fertilization (IVF) 17
Intensity-modulated radiation therapy 56–57
International Agency for Research in Cancer (IARC) 12, 14
International Retinoblastoma Staging System (IRSS) 104
Intraocular pressure (IOP) 7
Intraocular retinoblastoma
- bilateral 70–72
- choroidal invasion 105
- emerging treatments 99
- focal therapies
- - argon green laser 95
- - brachytherapy 97–98
- - cryotherapy 96–97
- - diode laser 95–96
- - external beam radiotherapy 92, 99
- - periocular chemotherapy 98
- - tumour responses 94
- histopathological risk factors 104
- intravitreal and intrarterial delivery 77
- optic nerve invasion 105–106
- primary treatments
- - enucleation 91–92
- - external beam radiotherapy 92
- - medial rectus muscle 91–92, 94
- - Reese–Ellsworth and International Classification Groups 93
- therapy-related leukemia 73
- tumor formation 72–73
- unilateral 69–70
IRSS. *See* International Retinoblastoma Staging System

L

Leiomyosarcoma 119

M

MDM2 and *MDMX* genes 3–4
Medulloepithelioma 150
Metastatic disease
- high-dose chemotherapy with ASCR 78–79
- with CNS 112
- without CNS 111–112

Microscopicr esiduald isease
- artifactual scleral invasion 106
- multivariatea nalysis 108
- optic nerve stump 106
- therapies 107
- trans-scleral invasion 107–108
Missensem utation 49
MLPA. *See*M ultiplex ligation-dependent probe amplification
Moleculararg eneticp rogression
- cell of origin 42–43
- genomic gain, post-*RB1* progressive events
- - 1q: *KIF14* 43–44
- - 2p: *NMYC* 44
- - 6p: *DEK* & *E2F3* 44
- genomic loss, post-*RB1*p rogressive events
- - 16q: *CDH11* 44–45
- - $p75^{NTR}$ 45
- M1 and M2 mutational events 42
- murinem odels
- - Cre-loxs ystem 46
- - limitations 46
- - *RB1* knockout mouse 45
- - viralo ncoprotein-induced 45–46
- *RB1* gene, protein and function 42
- senescence,t ransienta rrest 43
Mosaicism, *RB1*m utation 51
Multiplex ligation-dependent probea mplification 49

N

Nonsensem utation 50

O

Oculard rugt ransporters 69
ORBISc ybersitee -consultation site 139–140
Orbital and locoregional disease 77–78
- chemotherapy 109
- dissemination 108
- examination 109
- orbitalr elapse 109–110
Orthotopicx enograftm odel 6–7
Osteosarcoma 117–119

P

Periocularc hemotherapy 98
- carboplatin administration
- - CCI 75
- - human-derived fibrin protein sealant 76–77
- - intravenous and subconjunctival 75
- transscleral drug delivery
- - direct penetration pathway 73–74
- - factorsa ffecting 74
- - scleralp ermeability 74–75
Persistentf etal vasculature 152
Photocoagulation 95–96
Pineoblastoma 121, 122
Potential hypotheses, epidemiology
- diagnostic interval 19–20
- diet 18–19
- *in vitro* fertilization (IVF) 17
- nonoccupational parental exposures 18
- parentala ge 16–17
- parentalo ccupations 16
- screening and media campaigns 20
- UVe xposure 17–18
- virala gents 19
Preclinicalm odels
- limitations 6
- orthotopic xenograft model 6–7
- *RB1*g ene 5–6
Primary primitive neuroectodermal tumor (PNET) 15, 16, 36
Primarys ystemic chemotherapy 91–93
Protonb eam radiation therapy 57
Pseudorosettes 32, 34

R

Radiation therapy
- advantages 55–56
- extraocular and high-risk retinoblastoma 60–61
- management controversies 63–64
- nonmalignant side effects 63
- secondarym alignant tumors 61–62
- treatmentm ethods
- - coronal digital reconstruction 57
- - D-shaped fields 56
- - dose–volume curves 58
- - episcleral plaque brachytherapy 58–59
- - immobilization 59–60
- - intensity-modulated radiation therapy 56–57
- - proton beam radiation therapy 57–58
Radioactive isotopes, brachytherapy 97
RB1 gene
- inactivation 2–3
- mutation 70, 72, 92
- protein and function 42
Reese–Ellsworth Groups 56, 93
RetCam 139
Retinal astrocytomas 147
Retinal pigment epithelium (RPE) 68–69, 74
Retinal progenitor cells 7–8
RPE. *See* Retinal pigment epithelium

S

Second malignancy
- carboplatin ototoxicity 124
- cognitive and functional development 123–124
- cumulative incidence 115–116
- hematologic malignancies 121
- lung and epithelial cancers 120–121
- orbital growth and facial asymmetry 123
- osteosarcoma 117–119
- radiation therapy 116–117
- SIR 116–117
- skin cancers 120
- soft tissue sarcomas 119–120
- trilateral retinoblastoma 121–123
- visual outcome 123
Secondary genetic lesions
- conditional inactivation 4–5
- Rb and p53 pathways 3–4
Senescence, transient arrest 43
Simian virus 40 large T-antigen (TAg) 42, 45
SIR. *See* Standardized incidence ratio
Soft tissue sarcomas 119–120
Standardized incidence ratio (SIR)
- hematologic malignancies 121
- leiomyosarcoma 119
- radiation therapy 116–117
- risk and type, soft tissue sarcomas 119

Stereotacticr adiation therapy 57
Strabismuss urgery 131
Suicideg enet herapy 80–81

T

Thiotepa 85–86
Three-dimensionalr adiation therapy 56,6 1
Topotecan 71,8 5
Toxocarac horioretinitis 151
Translocations 50–51
Transpupillaryt hermotherapy (TTT) 95–96
Treatment. *See also*C hemotherapy
- extraocularr etinoblastoma
- – metastatic 78–79
- – orbital and locoregional 77–78
- high risk intraocular disease
- – choroidali nvasion 105
- – histopathological risk factors 104
- – optic nerve invasion 105–106
- metastaticd isease
- – high-dose chemotherapy and ASCR 78–79
- – withC NS 112
- – withoutC NS 111–112
- microscopic residual disease
- – artifactual scleral invasion 106
- – multivariate analysis 108
- – optic nerve stump 106
- – therapies 107
- – trans-scleral invasion 107–108
- orbital and locoregional disease 77–78
- – chemotherapy 109
- – dissemination 108
- – examination 109
- – orbitalr elapse 109–110
- signsa nds ymptoms 103
Trilateralr etinoblastoma 121–123
TTT. *See* Transpupillary thermotherapy

V

Vincristine 71, 81
Visual rehabilitation
- cataract surgery 129–131
- cycloplegic refraction 128
- low vision aids 131–132
- patching or atropine penalization 129
- polycarbonate lenses, spectacles 127–128
- retinoscopy 128
- strabismus surgery 131

Y

YAG capsulotomy 130

MIX
Papier aus verantwortungsvollen Quellen
Paper from responsible sources
FSC® C105338

If you have any concerns about our products,
you can contact us on
ProductSafety@springernature.com

In case Publisher is established outside the EU,
the EU authorized representative is:
Springer Nature Customer Service Center GmbH
Europaplatz 3, 69115 Heidelberg, Germany

Printed by Libri Plureos GmbH
in Hamburg, Germany